T0177531

The Right Price

The Right Price

A Value-Based Prescription for Drug Costs

Peter J. Neumann, Joshua T. Cohen, and
Daniel A. Ollendorf

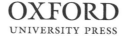

OXFORD
UNIVERSITY PRESS

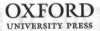

OXFORD
UNIVERSITY PRESS

Oxford University Press is a department of the University of Oxford. It furthers
the University's objective of excellence in research, scholarship, and education
by publishing worldwide. Oxford is a registered trade mark of Oxford University
Press in the UK and certain other countries.

Published in the United States of America by Oxford University Press
198 Madison Avenue, New York, NY 10016, United States of America.

CIP data is on file at the Library of Congress
ISBN 978-0-19-751287-6 (pbk.)
ISBN 978-0-19-751288-3 (hbk.)

DOI: 10.1093/oso/9780197512883.001.0001

Hardback printed by Bridgeport National Bindery, Inc., United States of America

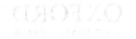

Contents

Contents

Acknowledgments

Writing a book is a marathon with its setbacks, doubts, and exhilarations. It also means a supporting cast who aid in the journey or cheer from the sidelines. We are grateful to many people who helped us reach the finish line.

Madison Silver provided excellent research assistance every step of the way and was instrumental in tracking down details and helping to shape the manuscript. Kristen Blanchard, Marlena Keisler, and Meghan Podolsky assisted skillfully in these efforts. Melissa Butchard worked tirelessly over two summers to ensure that supporting documentation was accurate.

David Kim read an early version of the manuscript and provided many helpful comments. Hildy Neumann also read and edited early versions of all of the emerging chapters and gave insights and editorial improvements. Chad Zimmerman, then at Oxford University Press, helped launch the project and supplied important early feedback. Sarah Humphreville, who in midcourse took over as our editor at Oxford University Press, shepherded the book in superb fashion, aided by Emma Hodgdon and Sujitha Logaganesan.

We have profited from countless discussions with colleagues at far-flung universities, research institutions, and private organizations. Although too numerous to list here, their research and insights are reflected in these pages and many of their papers referenced. We are especially grateful to colleagues at our Center for the Evaluation of Value and Risk in Health (CEVR) and at the Institute for Clinical Research and Health Policy Studies (ICRHPS) at Tufts Medical Center, including James Chambers, Julie Crowe, David Kim, Tara Lavelle, Anna Legassie, Paige Lin, and Natalia Olchanski, for their long-standing guidance and camaraderie. Thanks also to ICRHPS director, Harry Selker, and colleagues Karen Freund, Cathy Ide, David Kent, Debra Lerner, Susan Parsons, Robert Sege, Carol Seidel, and John Wong for creating such a stimulating environment in which to work and share ideas.

We emphasize that this book reflects the views of the authors and does not necessarily reflect those of members of ICRHPS, Tufts Medical Center, or other organizations. CEVR has been funded by government agencies, non-profit foundations, life science companies, industry trade groups, and others. None of these parties has supported this project or reviewed in advance what we have written.

We thank Steve Pearson for providing his recollections about the founding of the Institute for Clinical and Economic Review (ICER) and its evolution, controversies, and achievements. Steve also generously read and commented on an early version of the chapter on the history and influence of ICER to offer feedback and check for accuracy.

Finally, writing a book can be a joy, but it is also a commitment. We are thankful to have supporting spouses and families who continue to put up with us (most of the time). Collectively, the three of us have seven children and have been married for about 85 years. We are forever indebted to Carolyn Conte, Tobi Henzer, Keith Henzer, Hildy Neumann, Ariel Neumann, Anna Neumann, Alex Ollendorf, Matt Ollendorf, Jonathan Ollendorf, and Robin Ruthazer.

Preface

The pharmaceutical industry and its pricing methods provide an inviting target, easy to disparage and caricature. Even after accounting for discounts and rebates, average prices of leading brand-name drugs in the United States are two to four times higher than they are in Canada, Japan, and many European countries.[1] US per capita spending on prescription drugs is more than twice the level in the United Kingdom.[2,3] Prices for most new cancer drugs now exceed $100,000 per patient per year of treatment, despite the fact that many of these treatments seem to offer modest gains in life expectancy or lack such evidence at all.[4,5] With the advent of ever more targeted and powerful treatments, including cell- and gene-based therapies with multimillion dollar price tags, the need for sensible drug pricing and coverage policies will intensify.

Despite the controversies, there are few if any books dedicated to the question of what is a "fair" or "reasonable" drug price and how to think about the question. To be sure, the bookshelves fairly groan with works critical of pharmaceutical company practices, asserting or implying that drugs often deliver poor value for the money. Notable examples in the past decade or so include *Protecting America's Health*[6]; *Overdosed America: The Broken Promise of American Medicine*[7]; *Powerful Medicines: The Benefits, Risks, and Costs of Prescription Drugs*[8]; *The Truth About Drug Companies: How They Deceive Us and What to Do About It*[9]; *Selling Sickness: How the World's Biggest Pharmaceutical Companies Are Turning Us All Into Patients*[10]; *Bad Pharma: How Drug Companies Mislead Doctors and Harm Patients*[11]; *Ending Medical Reversal: Improving Outcomes, Saving Lives*[12]; *An American Sickness: How Healthcare Became Big Business and How You Can Take it Back*[13]; and *PhRMA: Greed, Lies and the Poisoning of America*.[14] Such accounts tend to highlight examples of disreputable behaviors and devote considerable attention to industry-wide reforms, rather than how to consider the costs and benefits of individual drug therapies.

There are also books that celebrate the scientific advances and breakthroughs that the drug industry has produced. A recent one is Peter Kolchinsky's *The Great American Drug Deal*, which argues that the temporarily high prices society pays for pharmaceuticals are well worth the cost when one consider the resulting abundance of inexpensive generics that benefit future generations in perpetuity. Kolchinsky calls for certain reforms to drug and health insurance industry practices to address problems in the marketplace but devotes little attention to how to measure the value that brand-name drugs deliver to patients and broader society.[15]

Health economists have certainly thought a lot about the value health interventions, whether drugs, devices, surgeries, lifestyle changes, or public health programs. There are many volumes on methods of *cost-effectiveness analysis*—a well-established approach for assessing the value of health technologies and services, including well-known how-to manuals,[16] popular reference guides,[17,18] and numerous works addressing theoretical and methodological issues and advances.[19-21] However, these references focus on the analytic tools researchers use and are aimed broadly at healthcare interventions, not at pharmaceuticals, per se. Textbooks on pharmacoeconomics—the branch of health economics "that identifies, measures, and compares the value and affordability of pharmaceutical" products[22]—generally offer guidance on measuring costs and therapeutic benefits but do not provide a broader perspectives on drug pricing policies.[23] Even the encyclopedic *Handbook of the Economics of the Biopharmaceutical Industry* reviews economic issues related to prescription drugs but provides a panoramic view of the industry, covering economic aspects of legal, regulatory, pricing, and health insurance topics, and industry dynamics pertaining to mergers, acquisitions, and alliances. The *Handbook* devotes only one of its 18 chapters to the valuation of pharmaceuticals.[24]

Most policy prescriptions for the pharmaceutical industry focus unsurprisingly on how to reduce drug prices. While lower prices are, of course, attractive to consumers, a single-minded focus on reducing drug prices ignores the fact that to a large degree, high drug prices are the consequence of deliberate policies stemming from the government's well-accepted and long-standing intention to grant drug firms temporary monopolies through patent protection to encourage companies to undertake risky investments in the first place. When those patents expire, generic drugs enter the marketplace and prices of brand name products fall, often precipitously, benefiting future generations of patients. Medications for hypertension, high cholesterol, HIV, diabetes, and other conditions have prolonged and improved the quality of lives of tens of millions of Americans, benefits that continue long after drug patents and exclusivity protections expire and generic copies enter the market. Generics now comprise 90% of all prescriptions in the United States (although high and increasing prices of some generic drugs have also come under scrutiny, an issue that further highlights the complexity of drug markets and the need for reforms).[25]

What policies will result in "acceptable" drug prices? Imposing federal controls on prescription drug prices, as is the practice in many countries, may seem an appealing and obvious solution, but it comes with trade-offs and questions. How should policymakers balance the benefits of lower prices against reductions in investment for future breakthroughs? How should appropriate incentives be set for drug companies to invest resources for different products across different diseases and populations? At what point are pharmaceutical industry profits "excessive"?

Permitting or requiring the government to negotiate drug prices raises the question of how prices should be set in the first place. On what basis does a price reflect "reasonable" or "fair" value? How should federal officials or private health insurers determine whether paying for a new medication for asthma or rheumatoid arthritis or childhood leukemia is worthwhile? For that matter, how should American physicians and their patients approach the matter, given ever-rising out-of-pocket spending on medications? Do drugs for cancer or rare diseases merit their exceptionally high prices? If so, why? What analytic methods should be used and what are their strengths and weaknesses? Are there examples in which American policymakers and their counterparts abroad have successfully applied pricing strategies to achieve fair value, while continuing to provide sufficient incentives to drug companies to innovate? What can we learn from them? The debate over these and related questions has profound consequences for the $500 billion US prescription drug industry, the $3.6 trillion healthcare sector, and for all of us as patients, caregivers, and taxpayers.

This book aims to provide a balanced and constructive view on the previously posed questions, focusing on the costs and benefits of pharmaceuticals, as well as valuation methods, and how public and private officials can take advantage of insights from these methods to inform policymaking. Such an inquiry involves delving into analytic approaches to measuring value, scrutinizing the experiences of organizations such as the Institute for Clinical and Economic Review (ICER) that are shaping the new landscape and addressing a host of related economic, ethical, and political issues.

Value measurement can be an esoteric topic. The goal here is a volume accessible to a broad readership, including health professionals, policymakers, managers, researchers, students, and interested lay readers. Presented appropriately, the question of whether drug benefits are worth the costs is a topic that should engage general audiences as well as experts. Toward that end, we illustrate concepts through the stories of recent high-profile drugs and gene therapies.

We have been examining such questions for many years. A formative experience for one of us (PJN) was a two-year stint in the 1990s working at the Health Care Financing Administration (since renamed the Centers for Medicare and Medicaid Services), the federal agency that administers the Medicare and Medicaid programs. Medicare at the time was trying to incorporate cost-effectiveness analysis formally into its procedures as a way of valuing new medical technology. The rationale seemed overwhelmingly sound, given escalating health spending, the diffusion of expensive new technologies, and the aging population. So did the timing: cost-effectiveness analysis was moving into leading medical journals and onto the minds of serious policymakers. And yet three decades later, the Medicare program has yet to include cost-effectiveness analysis formally in its procedures. Moreover, by law, Medicare is not permitted to use its leverage to negotiate the price of prescription drugs. Another influential episode was the opportunity to co-chair the Second Panel on Cost-Effectiveness in Health and Medicine, an update to the US guidelines for cost-effectiveness analysis.

Another of us (JTC) was influenced by his experience in the field of environmental risk assessment in the 1990s and early 2000s. The preceding decades had shaped a new awareness of the health risks posed by pollutants such as lead in gasoline exhaust and deteriorating house paint, dioxins deposited in soil, and particulate matter in the air. However, it also became apparent that eliminating all pollutant risks would be prohibitively expensive. Budget constraints motivated efforts to focus resources on measures that would most efficiently improve public health. The implication was that some risk mitigation measures, while beneficial, were not worth their cost. Similar thinking applies to medical care in general and to the evaluation of drugs and biologics in particular.

Finally, another of us (DAO) spent over a decade as Chief Scientific Officer at ICER, developing the approaches and processes that the organization uses in appraising the value of new and emerging pharmaceuticals and other technologies. While many facets of its approach are informed by health technology assessment agencies such as the United Kingdom's National Institute for Health and Care Excellence and the Canadian Agency for Drugs and Technologies in Health, ICER is the only US-based organization that regularly commissions cost-effectiveness analysis to examine the long-term value of prescription drugs and calculate a "value-based price" based on the results.

Over the years, the three of us have been addressing valuation methods for prescription drugs in research papers, reports, and commentaries. This book synthesizes, updates, and expands upon much of our earlier work into a comprehensive and—we hope—fresh, readable, and instructive treatment of the topic.

Some of the material has been adapted from articles and passages of books we have published previously and is included here with permission, including "Legislating against Use of Cost-Effectiveness Information"[26] (*NEJM*, 2010); "American Exceptionalism and American Health Care: Implications for the US Debate on Cost-Effectiveness Analysis"[27] (*OHE*, 2009); "Does the Institute for Clinical and Economic Review Revise Its Findings in Response to Industry Comments?[28] (*VIH*, 2019); "Should a Drug's Value Depend on the Disease or Population It Treats? Insights From ICER's Value Assessments"[29] (*Health Affairs'* blog, 2018); "QALYs in 2018—Advantages and Concerns"[30] (*JAMA*, 2018); "A Call for Open-Source Cost-Effectiveness Analysis"[31] (*Annals of Internal Medicine*, 2017); "Consideration Of Value-Based Pricing For Treatments And Vaccines Is Important, Even In The COVID-19 Pandemic" (*Health Affairs*, 2021)[32]. There are also passages adapted from *Using Cost-Effectiveness in Health and Medicine: Opportunities and Challenges*[33] (Neumann, Oxford University Press, 2005) and *Cost-Effectiveness in Health and Medicine*[34] (Neumann et al., Oxford University Press, 2017) again included with permission.

References

1. Kang, S.-Y., DiStefano, M.J., Socal, M.P., and Anderson, G.F. 2019. "Using external reference pricing in Medicare Part D to reduce drug price differentials with other countries." *Health Affairs* 38 (5): 804–811. https://doi.org/10.1377/hlthaff.2018.05207
2. Kavanos, P., Ferrario, A., Vandoros, S., and Anderson, G.F. 2013. "Higher US branded drug prices and spending compared to other countries may stem partly from quick uptake of new drugs." *Health Affairs* 32 (4): 753–761. https://doi.org/10.1377/hlthaff.2012.0920
3. Sarnak, D.O., Squires, D., Kuzmak, G., and Bishop, S. 2017. "Paying for prescription drugs around the world: Why is the U.S. an outlier?" *Issue Brief (Commonwealth Fund)* 2017: 1–14. https://www.ncbi.nlm.nih.gov/pubmed/28990747
4. Rimer, B.K. 2018. "The imperative of addressing cancer drug costs and value." *National Cancer Institute*. Accessed June 12, 2020. https://www.cancer.gov/news-events/cancer-currents-blog/2018/presidents-cancer-panel-drug-prices
5. Langreth, R. 2019. "Drug prices." *Bloomberg*. Accessed June 12, 2020. https://www.bloomberg.com/quicktake/drug-prices
6. Hilts, P.J. 2003. *Protecting America's health: The FDA, business, and one hundred years of regulation.* New York: Knopf.
7. Abramson, J. 2004. *Overdosed America: The broken promise of American medicine.* 1st ed. New York: Harper Collins.
8. Avorn, J. 2004. *Powerful medicines: The benefits, risks, and costs of prescription drugs.* New York: Knopf.
9. Angell, M. 2004. *The truth about drug companies: How they deceive us and what to do about it.* 1st ed. New York: Random House.

10. Moynihan, R., and Cassels, A. 2005. *Selling sickness: How the world's biggest pharmaceutical companies are turning us all into patients.* New York: Nation Books.
11. Goldacre, B. 2014. *Bad pharma: How drug companies mislead doctors and harm patients.* New York: Faber & Faber.
12. Prasad, V.K., and Cifu, A.S. 2015. *Ending medical reversal: Improving outcomes, saving lives.* Baltimore: Johns Hopkins University Press.
13. Rosenthal, E. 2017. *An American sickness: How healthcare became big business and how you can take it back.* New York: Penguin Press.
14. Posner, G. 2020. *Pharma: Greed, lies, and the poisoning of America.* New York: Avid Reader Press.
15. Kolchinsky, P. 2019. *The great American drug deal.* Boston: Evelexa Press.
16. Drummond, M.F., Sculpher, M.J., Claxton, K., Stoddart, G.L., and Torrance, G.W. 2015. *Methods for the economic evaluation of health care programmes.* 4th ed. Oxford: Oxford University Press.
17. Gold, M.E., Siegel, J.E., Russell, L.B., and Weinstein, M.C. 1996. *Cost-effectiveness in health and medicine.* 1st ed. New York: Oxford University Press.
18. Neumann, P.J., Sanders, G.D., Russell, L.B., Siegel, J.E., and Ganiats, T.G. 2017. *Cost-effectiveness in health and medicine.* 2nd ed. New York: Oxford University Press.
19. Drummond, M.F., and McGuire, A. 2001. *Economic evaluation in healthcare: Merging theory with practice.* New York: Oxford University Press.
20. Gray, A.M., Clarke, P.M., Wolstenholme, J., and Wordsworth, S. 2010. *Applied methods of cost-effectiveness analysis in health care.* New York: Oxford University Press.
21. Muennig, P., and Bounthavong, M. 2016. *Cost-effectiveness analysis in health: A practical approach.* 3rd ed. San Francisco: Jossey-Bass.
22. Dilokthorsakul, P., Thomas, D., Brown, L., and Chaiyakunapruk, N. 2019. "Interpreting Pharmacoeconomic Findings." In *Clinical pharmacy education, practice, and research: Clinical pharmacy, drug information, pharmacovigilance, pharmacoeconomics and clinical research*, edited by D. Thomas, 277–287. New York: Elsevier.
23. Rascati, K. 2014. *Essentials of pharmacoeconomics.* 2nd ed. Philadelphia: Lippincott Williams & Wilkins.
24. Danzon, P.M., and Nicholson, S. 2012. *The Oxford handbook of the economics of the bio-pharmaceutical industry.* New York: Oxford University Press.
25. The case for competition: 2019 generic drug & biosimilars access & savings in the U.S. report. 2019. *Association for Accessible Medicine.* Accessed January 19, 2021. https://accessiblemeds.org/sites/default/files/2019-09/AAM-2019-Generic-Biosimilars-Access-and-Savings-US-Report-WEB.pdf
26. Neumann, P.J., and Weinstein, M.C. 2010. "Legislating against use of cost-effectiveness information." *New England Journal of Medicine,* 363: 1495–1497.
27. Neumann, P.J. 2009, March. "American exceptionalism and American health care: Implications for the US debate on cost-effectiveness analysis." *Office of Health Economics.* Accessed January 19, 2021. https://www.ohe.org/publications/american-exceptionalism-and-american-health-care-implications-us-debate-cost
28. Cohen, J.T., Silver, M.C., Ollendorf, D.A., and Neumann, P.J. Does the Institute for Clinical and Economic Review revise its findings in response to industry comments? *Value in Health,* 22 (19): 1396–1401.
29. Neumann, P.J., Silver, M.C., and Cohen, J.T. 2018, November 6. "Should a drug's value depend on the disease or population it treats? Insights from ICER's value assessments." Health Affairs. Accessed January 19, 2021. https://www.healthaffairs.org/do/10.1377/hblog20181105.38350/full/
30. Neumann, P.J., and Cohen, J.T. 2018. "QALYs in 2018—advantages and concerns." *JAMA,* 319 (24): 2473–2474.

31. Cohen, J.T., Neumann, P.J., and Wong, J.B. 2017. "A call for open-source cost-effectiveness analysis." *Annals of Internal Medicine*, 167 (6): 432–433.
32. Neumann, P.J., Cohen, J.T., Kim, D.D., and Ollendorf, D.A. 2021. "Consideration of value-based pricing for treatments and vaccines is important, even in the COVID-19 pandemic." *Health Affairs*, 40 (1): 53–61.
33. Neumann, P.J. 2005. *Using cost-effectiveness in health and medicine: Opportunities and challenges.* New York: Oxford University Press.
34. Neumann, P.J., Ganiats, T.G., Russell, L.B., Sanders, G.D., and Siegel, J.E. 2017. *Cost-effectiveness in health and medicine.* New York: Oxford University Press.

PART I
THE ECONOMICS OF PRESCRIPTION DRUGS

1
Introduction

Emily's Story

Doctors feared the worst after 5-year old Emily Whitehead was diagnosed with acute lymphoblastic leukemia (ALL) in 2010. While pediatric ALL is one of the most common and curable childhood cancers, with a 5-year survival rate of roughly 90%, Emily's version proved resistant.[1,2] Despite standard chemotherapy, she suffered two relapses in a 5-month span. The prognosis for relapsed and refractory (resistant to treatment) ALL is poor.[2] According to her oncologists, her options were limited to a risky bone marrow transplant or hospice care.[3]

Emily's parents desperately searched for alternatives. They learned about an experimental technology at the University of Pennsylvania and a clinical study enrolling pediatric ALL patients at Children's Hospital of Philadelphia, where Emily had been transferred.[4] Chimeric antigen receptor T-cell (CAR-T) therapy involves harvesting a patient's T cells, the cells designed to detect and kill disease, and genetically engineering them to target a particular protein on the B cells that carry ALL. The engineered cells are then returned to the patient to attack and destroy the cancerous cells, with long-term remission or cure as the ultimate goal.[5]

As with the other aspects of Emily's treatment, the course of her CAR-T therapy was not without difficulties. She developed high fever, shock, and respiratory failure—a set of complications now better understood as cytokine release syndrome—which clinicians scrambled to address.[3] Serendipitously, one of Emily's doctors had a daughter taking a biologic, the interleukin-6 inhibitor tocilizumab, to control her juvenile rheumatoid arthritis. Emily had been expressing interleukin-6 at 1,000 times the normal level, but after a few doses of tocilizumab, her system returned more or less to normal.[3] Shortly thereafter, her ALL went into remission.

Clinical development of CAR-T therapies continued. In early 2017, drug companies filed the first CAR-T applications with the Food and Drug Administration for pediatric ALL and adult diffuse large cell B-cell lymphoma.[6] Given the poor prognosis and limited alternative

The Right Price. Peter J. Neumann, Joshua T. Cohen, and Daniel A. Ollendorf, Oxford University Press (2021).
© Peter J. Neumann, Joshua T. Cohen, and Daniel A. Ollendorf. DOI: 10.1093/oso/9780197512883.003.0001

treatment options for the refractory patients enrolled in the therapy's clinical trials, the results were astonishing. For example, in the pivotal study of Kymriah® (tisagenlecleucel; Novartis, Inc.), a CAR-T for pediatric ALL, 83% of 63 evaluable patients had no evidence of cancer three months after treatment.[7,8]

These developments generated considerable excitement but also concerns. For one, the published clinical studies had few patients and limited posttrial data. Estimates of the therapy's impact on survival and durability of remission remained decidedly uncertain.

And then there was the cost. Prior to approval, the product manufacturers did not divulge their pricing strategies, but mentioned the cost of bone marrow transplant, which can exceed $800,000, as one possibly relevant benchmark.[9] Following approval, Kymriah was priced at $475,000 per infusion, and the adult CAR-T, axicabtagene ciloleucel (Yescarta®; Gilead, Inc.) at $373,000. Even these prices seemed to reflect a lower bound for estimated treatment costs, which include inpatient treatment administration, bone marrow transplants in patients failing CAR-T, the potential for cytokine release syndrome and other complications, and the markup charged by hospitals on acquired drugs, all of which can push total treatment expenses above $1 million per case.[10,11] Perhaps unsurprisingly, public and private insurers have been slow to embrace CAR-T therapies, often negotiating agreements for patients on an ad hoc, case-by-case basis.[12]

Subsequent discussions around CAR-T's clinical effectiveness and costs have seemingly occurred as separate conversations, rather than an integrated one focused on the health benefits gained for the added costs. Ideally, one would like to know how the benefits and costs of CAR-T compare to last-resort (and also expensive) chemotherapy used in patients with refractory disease. Moreover, how does CAR-T compare to hospice treatment?

For many years that integrated dialogue did not occur in the United States, at least not broadly, formally, or publicly. The notion of explicitly evaluating a drug's "value for money," the concept of assessing whether the price of a new therapy was aligned with the benefits conferred, was equated by some to "rationing" by government bean counters in other countries.[13,14] Yet therapies like CAR-T have forced a reckoning in the United States.

The Institute for Clinical and Economic Review (ICER), a private, nonprofit organization that conducts independent economic evaluations to inform US drug pricing, has helped foster that integrated conversation. In its 2018 report on CAR-T therapies, ICER concluded that the two new treatments, even at their high prices, reflected reasonable value for money in comparison to either alternative chemotherapy or no treatment.[15,16]

As testament to the new drug's effectiveness, and a powerful reminder of the stakes involved for anyone attempting to place a value on new therapies, Emily Whitehead is now a thriving and precocious teenager who has been cancer-free since 2012.[1]

The Rising Cost of Prescription Drugs

Not long ago, advances such as CAR-T would have belonged in the realm of science fiction. Today, once deadly diseases like ALL can be managed or even cured. However, the progress has come at a cost. US retail prescription drug spending reached $335 billion in 2018, up from $258 billion in 2013,[17] rising faster in most years than other categories of health[18] and now comprising roughly one-sixth of health expenditures (Box 1.1).[19]

Spending on "specialty" drugs—generally defined as high-cost therapies for complex, chronic, and debilitating conditions with no known cures—has accelerated, rising 10% or more annually in some recent years, a trend expected to continue.[20-22] From 2010 to 2015, specialty drug spending rose from 13% to 31% of Medicare Part D drug spending, for example, and from 25% to 35% of Medicaid drug spending.[23] Although they accounted for only 3% of branded prescriptions filled, specialty drugs comprised 34% of branded drug spending in 2017.[21]

Driving these surges are increases in drug utilization and drug prices.[24] Between 2008 and 2015, prices for most commonly used brand-name drugs increased 164%, far in excess of the consumer price index (12%).[25,26] Between 1995 and 2013, the cancer drug launch prices rose by 10% annually, or $8,500 per year.[27] Median launch prices of cancer drugs have risen from $100 per month in the 1960s, for example, to more than $10,000 per month of treatment today.[28] Prices of many cancer drugs have increased considerably after their launch—by as much as 40%—often without any new evidence of effectiveness.[29]

Even some older, generic products have experienced dramatic price increases. The average price for insulin, for example, increased 300% from 2002 to 2013[30] and 55% from 2014 to 2019.[31] The annual insulin costs for a person with type 1 diabetes rose from $2,864 in 2012 to $5,705 in 2016.[32]

A 2018 study reported that prices increased faster than the medical price index for half of all generic products.[33] Another found that from 2008 to 2015, 400 generic drugs had price increases of more than 1,000%.[34]

Furthermore, drug spending and drug prices are considerably higher in the United States than in other countries. In 2013, US per capita prescription

Box 1.1 How Much Does the US Spend on Prescription Drugs?

Estimates of how much Americans spend on prescription drugs vary depending on whether estimates reflect manufacturer rebates, nonretail settings, patient out-of-pocket costs, and various markups added by retail pharmacies, physicians, clinics, or hospitals administering the drugs.[1-3] Many sources cite the US National Health Expenditure Accounts estimates—$335 billion in 2018; however, those estimates include only retail sales (net of rebates).[4,5] It excludes expenditures for drugs administered during a hospital visit, physician appointment, or home nursing stay (instead, the National Health Expenditure Accounts classifies these nonretail expenditures as part of physician, hospital, or nursing home costs). Altarum has estimated nonretail prescription drug sales (net of rebates) at $165 billion in 2018 yielding total drug spending of $500 billion, projected to grow to $725 billion in 2025.[6] Based on these estimates and projections, we note conservatively in various places in this book that Americans spend roughly $500 billion annually on prescription drugs.

Estimates of the fraction of total US health spending comprised of prescription drugs also vary, usually ranging from 10% to 17%, but sometimes as high as 28%, depending on the components included in the numerator and denominator.[1,19] As noted, the numerator may or may not include nonretail spending or various rebates, markups, and other items. Some estimates of total health spending (the denominator) include personal healthcare expenditures only (services or products used by patients, such as medications or durable medical equipment like hearing aids and eyeglasses) and amounted to $3.1 trillion in 2018.[17] Other estimates of total health spending also include administrative and investment costs (buildings, research, and capital equipment, such as X-ray machines, software, and hospital beds)[7] and amounted to $3.6 trillion in 2018.[4] Dividing our rough estimate of drug spending ($500 billion per year) by total health spending ($3.6 trillion) suggests drugs represent about 14% of this total. Dividing drug spending by personal health spending ($3.1 trillion per year) suggests drug spending is approximately 16% of this total.

[1] Kleinrock, M., Westrich, K., Buelt, L., Aitken, M., and Dubois, R.W. 2019. "Reconciling the seemingly irreconcilable: How much are we spending on drugs?" *Value Health* 22 (7): 792–798. https://doi.org/10.1016/j.jval.2018.11.009. https://www.ncbi.nlm.nih.gov/pubmed/31277826.

[2] IQVIA Institute. 2020, August. "Medicine spending and affordability in the United States." https://www.iqvia.com/insights/the-iqvia-institute/reports/medicine-spending-and-affordability-in-the-us#:~:text=Medicine%20Spending%20at%20Selected%20Reporting%20Levels%2C%20US%24Bn&text=Total%20net%20payer%20spending%20in,over%20the%20past%20five%20years.

[3] Roehrig, C. 2018, April. "The impact of prescription drug rebates on health plans and consumers." *Altarum.* https://altarum.org/sites/default/files/Altarum-Prescription-Drug-Rebate-Report_April-2018.pdf.

[4] CMS Office of the Actuary. 2019, December 5. "CMS Office of the Actuary releases 2018 national health expenditures." *Centers for Medicare & Medicaid Services.* https://www.cms.gov/newsroom/press-releases/cms-office-actuary-releases-2018-national-health-expenditures.

[5] CMS Office of the Actuary. 2018. "National health expenditure accounts: Methodology paper, 2018: Definitions, sources, and methods." https://www.cms.gov/files/document/definitions-sources-and-methods.pdf.

[6] Roehrig, C., and Turner, A. 2020. "Projections of the non-retail prescription drug share of national health expenditures." *Altarum.* https://altarum.org/sites/default/files/uploaded-publication-files/Altarum%20Projections%20of%20the%20Non-Retail%20Dru.pdf.

[7] Centers for Medicare & Medicaid Services. 2017. "National health expenditure accounts: Methodology paper, 2017, definitions, sources, and methods." https://www.cms.gov/Research-Statistics-Data-and-Systems/Statistics-Trends-and-Reports/NationalHealthExpendData/downloads/dsm-17.pdf.

drug spending was $858, for example, compared to $400 on average for 19 other industrialized nations, a phenomenon accounted for largely by price differences.[35] The list prices of the top 20 drugs are three times higher in the United States than the United Kingdom and substantially higher even after rebates.[36] Although the United States comprises only 4% of the world's population, US patients account for 46% of global cancer drug sales. In 2020, the US President's Council of Economic Advisors concluded that prices for top-selling patented drugs in other high-income countries cost 17% to 43% of what they cost in the United States.[37]

Rising drug spending has important consequences for already stretched public budgets. Medicare spends upwards of $100 billion on prescription drugs, while the Medicaid program spends over $30 billion.[17] Between 2010 and 2015 Medicare Part D spending on specialty drugs rose from $9 billion to $33 billion, while Medicaid spending increased from $4.8 billion to $9.9 billion.[23] In 2014, state Medicaid programs spent $1.1 billion (after discounts) on *a single drug*, Sovaldi (sofosbuvir), a treatment for hepatitis C. In 2015 spending on sofosbuvir and a follow-on product, Harvoni (ledipasvir/sofosbuvir) comprised almost 5% of all Medicaid drug spending.[38]

Rising out-of-pocket spending for deductibles and coinsurance has created financial difficulties for many individuals and their families, particularly among the sickest patients.[39,40] Over half of the US population routinely take a prescription drug, and 15% regularly take at least 5 prescribed medications.[41] But recent years have highlighted medication nonadherence and discontinuation altogether.[35,42] One study reported that almost 30% of adults did not take their drugs as prescribed in the past year because of costs.[43] A 2015 study found that "to save money, almost 8% of U.S. adults did not take their medication as prescribed, 15.1% asked a doctor for a lower-cost medication," and "1.6% bought prescription drugs from another country."[44p1]

The Value Imperative and the Organization of This Book

The dueling trends of scientific breakthroughs like CAR-T and ever-rising spending present an enduring challenge for American society. While policy recommendations vary, most everyone agrees that more attention should be paid to the health benefits achieved for the resources expended—that is, that a drug's price should reflect its value. If, as a society, we spend wastefully or inefficiently on drugs, we are diverting funds from other important areas of healthcare such as hospital and physician services, not to mention nonhealthcare needs such as education, the military, and public infrastructure. Next time you bemoan the state of US airports or crawl along on Amtrak from Boston to New York, consider that the United States spends 8% *more* of its gross domestic product on healthcare than do other industrialized countries—money that could be spent on other priorities.

But how to judge prescription drug value? As a 2018 National Academy of Medicine report on drug affordability emphasized, it is a contentious and confounding undertaking.[19p15] With that caution in mind, this book seeks to explore the matter.

Part I of the book (Chapters 2–4) describes the economic concepts that have led to the development of value assessment techniques for pharmaceuticals. Chapter 2 explains how the market for pharmaceuticals differs from the market for most other goods and how those differences—such as drug company monopolies, the role of insurance companies and doctors, and the incomplete knowledge that patients have—interfere with the normal mechanisms that automatically align prices with value.

Chapter 3 examines popular solutions that focus on restraining drug prices. Examples include linking prices to research and development costs, indexing prices to international benchmarks, or allowing the federal government to directly negotiate prices. We argue that these solutions have a limited impact or that they can work only if they are guided by value assessments for drugs.

With value assessment the key ingredient to establishing appropriate prices for drugs, Chapter 4 addresses the question of how to go about the task. It explores the history of valuing health, from early efforts that limited attention to the value of worker output and expressed health value in terms of its monetary equivalent, to later, more expansive efforts that developed measures that avoided direct monetization of improved health.

Part II of the book (Chapters 5–8) describes how researchers and policymakers have pursued drug valuation efforts. Chapter 5 reviews the experiences of policymakers overseas and in the United States in using economic evaluation to value prescription drugs. The chapter assesses the experience of the United Kingdom's National Institute for Health and Care Excellence, the health authority with a broad mandate to issue guidance on the effectiveness and cost-effectiveness of health technologies and the clinical management of specific conditions. The chapter also discusses the practices of public authorities in other nations including Australia, Canada, and Germany. In addition, the chapter considers not only the growing use of economic evaluation in certain quarters in the United States but also how opposition to the practice seemed to create an insurmountable obstacle to its widespread use.

Chapter 6 tells the story of how ICER, a private organization that evaluates the clinical and economic value of prescription drugs, has substantially increased the influence of cost-effectiveness analysis in the United States. We describe the key points of controversy over ICER's approach and how the organization substantially revised its methods in some cases but stuck to its guns in others.

In Chapter 7, we describe the other organizations that, like ICER, have tried to play a role in value assessment in the United States. These groups include the American Society of Clinical Oncology, the National Comprehensive Cancer Network, Memorial Sloan Kettering, the American College of Cardiology and the American Heart Association, Premera Health Plan, and Faster Cures/ Avalere. We argue that their approaches all had serious shortcomings and that it was largely these shortcomings that ultimately limited the influence of these groups. Chapter 8 considers valuation methods in the context of rare diseases and special populations. Should extra premium drug prices (and more lenient cost-effectiveness benchmarks) be allowed in certain areas (e.g., cancer or childhood diseases) and not in others—and, if so, on what basis? This question has provoked debates among economists, ethicists, and policymakers.

Part III of this book (Chapters 9–11) sets out a series of recommendations for how to further improve pharmaceutical value assessment in the United States and how to promote its influence. Chapter 9 considers strategies to improve value measurement. It discusses ways in which analysts can better frame and present studies, by considering all the elements that matter to society. It discusses the pros and cons of quality-adjusted life years, how cost-effectiveness analyses can better reflect the long term benefits of drug therapies by incorporating assumptions about a drug's genericization, and the role of uncertainty analysis. Finally, it takes up the issue of who should measure drug value in the United States.

Chapter 10 explores how to achieve value-based prices in the United States. It describes alternative methods for setting drug prices and steps that government and private sector decision makers can take, highlighting the most important and contentious issues that we believe must be addressed. Finally, Chapter 11 charts a path forward. If Americans are to enjoy better health and a more efficient healthcare system expended, leadership will be needed to provide the vision and to foster responsible reforms.

References

1. ASCO Post Staff. 2019, May 25. "Emily Whitehead, early recipient of CAR T-Cell Therapy for ALL, celebrates 7 years cancer-free." *The ASCO Post*. Accessed January 19, 2021. https://www.ascopost.com/issues/may-25-2019/emily-whitehead-celebrates-7-years-cancer-free/.
2. Martin, A., Morgan, E., and Hijiya, N. 2012. "Relapsed or refractory pediatric acute lymphoblastic leukemia." *Pediatric Drugs* 14 (6): 377–387. https://doi.org/10.1007/BF03262418.
3. Rosenbaum, L. 2017. "Tragedy, perseverance, and chance—the story of CAR-T therapy." *New England Journal of Medicine* 377 (14): 1313–1315. https://doi.org/10.1056/NEJMp1711886.
4. Children's Hospital of Pennsylvania. 2012, December. "Relapsed leukemia: Emily's story." Last modified July 2017. Accessed June 22, 2020. https://www.chop.edu/stories/relapsed-leukemia-emilys-story.
5. Kochenderfer, J.N., Dudley, M.E., Kassim, S.H., Somerville, R.P.T., Carpenter, R.O., Stetler-Stevenson, M., Yang, J.C., Phan, G.Q., Hughes, M.S., Sherry, R.M., Raffeld, M., Feldman, S., Lu, L., Li, Y.F., Ngo, L.T., Goy, A., Feldman, T., Spaner, D.E., Wang, M.L., Chen, C.C., Kranick, S.M., Nath, A., Nathan, D.-A.N., Morton, K.E., Toomey, M.A., and Rosenberg, S.A. 2015. "Chemotherapy-refractory diffuse large B-Cell lymphoma and Indolent B-Cell malignancies can be effectively treated with autologous T Cells expressing an anti-CD19 chimeric antigen receptor." *Journal of Clinical Oncology* 33 (6): 540–549. https://doi.org/10.1200/jco.2014.56.2025.
6. US Food and Drug Administration. 2017. "KYMRIAH (tisagenlecleucel)." Last modified May 2018. Accessed January 19, 2021. https://www.fda.gov/vaccines-blood-biologics/cellular-gene-therapy-products/kymriah-tisagenlecleucel.
7. Buechner, J., Kersten, M.J., Fuchs, M., Salmon, F., and Jäger, U. 2018. "Chimeric antigen receptor-T cell therapy: Practical considerations for implementation in Europe." *HemaSphere* 2 (1): e18–e18. https://doi.org/10.1097/HS9.0000000000000018.
8. "Novartis receives first ever FDA approval for therapy, Kymriah™ (tisagenlecleucel, CTL019), for children and young adults with B-cell ALL that is refractory or has relapsed at least twice." 2017, August 30. *Novartis*. Accessed January 19, 2021. https://novartis.gcs-web.com/novartis-receives-fda-approval-for-KymriahTM.
9. Palmer, E. 2017, June 9. "Manufacturing costs loom large for personalized CAR-T cancer meds and their need for speed." *Fierce Pharma*. Accessed January 19, 2021. https://www.fiercepharma.com/pharma/manufacturing-costs-loom-large-as-car-t-cancer-meds-march-toward-approval.
10. Whittington, M.D., Ollendorf, D.A., and Campbell, J.D. 2018. "Accounting for all costs in the total cost of chimeric antigen receptor t-cell immunotherapy." *JAMA Oncology* 4 (12): 1784–1785. https://doi.org/10.1001/jamaoncol.2018.4625.
11. Whittington, M.D., McQueen, R.B., Ollendorf, D.A., Kumar, V.M., Chapman, R.H., Tice, J.A., Pearson, S.D., and Campbell, J.D. 2018. "Long-term survival and value of chimeric

antigen receptor t-cell therapy for pediatric patients with relapsed or refractory leukemia." *JAMA Pediatrics* 172 (12): 1161–1168. https://doi.org/10.1001/jamapediatrics.2018.2530.

12. Swetlitz, I. 2019. "Hospitals are saving lives with CAR-T: Getting paid is another story." *STAT.* Accessed January 19, 2021. https://www.statnews.com/2019/03/12/hospitals-arent-getting-paid-for-car-t/.

13. Singer, P. 2009, July 15. Why we must ration healthcare. *The New York Times.* Accessed January 19, 2021. https://archive.nytimes.com/www.nytimes.com/2009/07/19/magazine/19healthcare-t.html.

14. Lopert, R., and Elshaug, A.G. 2013. "Australia's 'fourth hurdle' drug review comparing costs and benefits holds lessons for the United States." *Health Affairs* 32 (4): 778–787. https://doi.org/10.1377/hlthaff.2012.1058.

15. Tice, J.A., Walsh, J.M.E., Otuonye, I., Chapman, R., Kumar, V., Seidner, M., Ollendorf, D.A., and Pearson, S.D. 2018, March 23. "Chimeric antigen receptor T-cell therapy for B-Cell cancers: Effectiveness and value." *Institute for Clinical and Economic Review.* https://icer.org/wp-content/uploads/2020/10/ICER_CAR_T_Final_Evidence_Report_032318.pdf.

16. Whittington, M.D., McQueen, R.B., Ollendorf, D.A., Kumar, V.M., Chapman, R.H., Tice, J.A., Pearson, S.D., and Campbell, J.D. 2019. "Long-term survival and cost-effectiveness associated with axicabtagene ciloleucel vs chemotherapy for treatment of b-cell lymphoma." *JAMA Network Open* 2 (2): e190035–e190035. https://doi.org/10.1001/jamanetworkopen.2019.0035.

17. Centers for Medicare and Medicaid Services. 2019. "National health expenditure data: Historical." Page last modified December 16, 2020 Accessed January 19, 2021. https://www.cms.gov/Research-Statistics-Data-and-Systems/Statistics-Trends-and-Reports/NationalHealthExpendData/NationalHealthAccountsHistorical.

18. Centers for Medicare and Medicaid Services. 2018, February 14. "CMS Office of the Actuary releases 2017–2026 projections of national health expenditures." Accessed January 19, 2021. https://www.cms.gov/newsroom/press-releases/cms-office-actuary-releases-2017-2026-projections-national-health-expenditures.

19. Augustine, N.R., Madhavan, G., and Nass, S.J., eds. 2018. *Making medicines affordable: A national imperative.* Washington, DC: The National Academies Press.

20. Pharmaceutical Care Management Association. n.d. "What is a specialty drug?" Accessed January 19, 2021. https://www.pcmanet.org/pcma-cardstack/what-is-a-specialty-drug/.

21. Blue Cross Blue Shield Association. 2018, November 14. "Prescription drug costs: Trend update." *The Health of America Report.* Accessed January 19, 2021. https://www.bcbs.com/sites/default/files/file-attachments/health-of-america-report/HoA-Rx-Costs-Trend-Update.pdf.

22. Aitken, M., and Kleinrock, M. 2018. "Medicine use and spending in the U.S.: A review of 2017 and outlook to 2022." *IQVIA Institute for Human Data Science.* Accessed January 19, 2021. https://www.iqvia.com/insights/the-iqvia-institute/reports/medicine-use-and-spending-in-the-us-review-of-2017-outlook-to-2022.

23. Anderson-Cook, A., Maeda, J., Ding, R., Patel, Y.M., and Nelson, L. 2019, March. "Prices for and spending on specialty drugs in Medicare Part D and Medicaid." *Congressional Budget Office.* Accessed January 19, 2021. https://www.cbo.gov/system/files/2019-03/54964-Specialty_Drugs.pdf.

24. Kamal, R., Cox, C., and McDermott, D. 2019, February 20. "What are the recent and forecasted trends in prescription drug spending?" *Peterson-Kaiser Family Foundation.* Accessed January 19, 2021. https://www.healthsystemtracker.org/chart-collection/recent-forecasted-trends-prescription-drug-spending/#item-start.

25. Express Scripts. 2015, March. "The 2015 drug trend report." Accessed January 19, 2021. https://corporate-site-labs-dev.s3.amazonaws.com/2019-09/Express%20Scripts%20 2015%20Drug%20Trend%20Report.pdf.
26. US Bureau of Labor Statistics. n.d. "Databases, tables and calculators by subject." Accessed January 19, 2021. https://www.bls.gov/data/.
27. Howard, D.H., Bach, P.B., Berndt, E.R., and Conti, R.M. 2015. "Pricing in the market for anticancer drugs." *Journal of Economic Perspectives* 29 (1): 139–162. https://doi.org/ 10.1257/jep.29.1.139.
28. Bach, P.B. 2009. "Limits on Medicare's ability to control rising spending on cancer drugs." *New England Journal of Medicine* 360 (6): 626–633. https://doi.org/10.1056/ NEJMhpr0807774.
29. Gordon, N., Stemmer, S.M., Greenberg, D., and Goldstein, D.A. 2018. "Trajectories of in-jectable cancer drug costs after launch in the United States." *Journal of Clinical Oncology* 36 (4): 319–325. https://doi.org/10.1200/JCO.2016.72.2124.
30. Hua, X., Carvalho, N., Tew, M., Huang, E.S., Herman, W.H., and Clarke, P. 2016. "Expenditures and prices of antihyperglycemic medications in the United States: 2002–2013." *JAMA* 315 (13): 1400–1402. https://doi.org/10.1001/jama.2016.0126.
31. Lee, B. 2020, November 6. "How much does insulin cost? Here's how 23 brands compare." *GoodRx.* Accessed January 19, 2021. https://www.goodrx.com/blog/how-much-does-insulin-cost-compare-brands/.
32. Biniek, J.F., and Johnson, W. 2019, January 21. "Spending on individuals with type 1 dia-betes and the role of rapidly increasing insulin prices." *Health Care Cost Institute.* Accessed January 19, 2021. https://healthcostinstitute.org/diabetes-and-insulin/spending-on-individuals-with-type-1-diabetes-and-the-role-of-rapidly-increasing-insulin-prices.
33. Conti, R.M., Nguyen, K.H., and Rosenthal, M.B. 2018. "Generic prescription drug price increases: Which products will be affected by proposed anti-gouging legisla-tion?" *Journal of Pharmaceutical Policy and Practice* 11: 29–29. https://doi.org/10.1186/ s40545-018-0156-8.
34. O'Brien, E. 2015, September 21. "Why drug prices remain insanely high and 6 things you can do to save." *MarketWatch.* Accessed January 19, 2021. https://www.marketwatch.com/ story/six-tips-for-fighting-rising-prescription-drug-costs-2015-09-15.
35. Kesselheim, A.S., Avorn, J., and Sarpatwari, A. 2016. "The high cost of prescription drugs in the United States: Origins and prospects for reform." *JAMA* 316 (8): 858–871. https:// doi.org/10.1001/jama.2016.11237.
36. Hirschler, B. 2015, October 12. "Exclusive—transatlantic divide: How US pays three times more for drugs." *Reuters.* Accessed January 19, 2021. https://www.reuters.com/article/ us-pharmaceuticals-usa-comparison/exclusive-transatlantic-divide-how-u-s-pays-three-times-more-for-drugs-idUSKCN0S61KU20151012.
37. The Council of Economic Advisers. 2020, February. Funding the global benefits to bio-pharmaceutical innovation. *Executive Office of the President of the United States.* Accessed January 19, 2021. https://www.whitehouse.gov/wp-content/uploads/2020/02/Funding-the-Global-Benefits-to-Biopharmaceutical-Innovation.pdf.
38. Centers for Medicare & Medicaid Services. 2016, November 14. "Medicaid drug spending dashboard." Accessed January 19, 2021. https://www.cms.gov/newsroom/fact-sheets/medicaid-drug-spending-dashboard.
39. Claxton, G., Levitt, L., Rae, M., and Sawyer, B. 2018. "Increases in cost-sharing payments continue to outpace wage growth." *Peterson-Kaiser Family Foundation.* Accessed January 19, 2021. https://www.healthsystemtracker.org/brief/increases-in-cost-sharing-payments-have-far-outpaced-wage-growth/#item-start.

40. Dusetzina, S.B., Huskamp, H.A., and Keating, N.L. 2019. "Specialty drug pricing and out-of-pocket spending on orally administered anticancer drugs in Medicare part D, 2010 to 2019." *JAMA* 321 (20): 2025–2028. https://doi.org/10.1001/jama.2019.4492.

41. Kantor, E.D., Rehm, C.D., Haas, J.S., Chan, A.T., and Giovannucci, E.L. 2015. "Trends in prescription drug use among adults in the United States from 1999–2012." *JAMA* 314 (17): 1818–1830. https://doi.org/10.1001/jama.2015.13766.

42. Ramsey, S., Blough, D., Kirchhoff, A., Kreizenbeck, K., Fedorenko, C., Snell, K., Newcomb, P., Hollingworth, W., and Overstreet, K. 2013. "Washington state cancer patients found to be at greater risk for bankruptcy than people without a cancer diagnosis." *Health Affairs* 32 (6): 1143–1152. https://doi.org/10.1377/hlthaff.2012.1263.

43. Kirzinger, A., Lopes, L., Wu, B., and Brodie, M. 2019. "KFF health tracking poll: February 2019: Prescription drugs." *Kaiser Family Foundation*. Accessed January 19, 2021. https://www.kff.org/health-costs/poll-finding/kff-health-tracking-poll-february-2019-prescription-drugs/.

44. Cohen, R.A., and Villaroel, M.A. 2015. "Strategies used by adults to reduce their prescription drug costs: United States, 2013." *National Center for Health Statistics*. https://www.cdc.gov/nchs/data/databriefs/db184.pdf.

2

The Prescription Drug Market

One of These Products Is Not Like the Others

Go to Walgreens.com, click on "Shop," and you will find a wide range of product categories, including beauty, personal care, vitamins and supplements, household goods, and groceries. The experience of purchasing the displayed products—either online or in the store—is ordinary and familiar. Consider a decision to purchase toothpaste (in economists' parlance, the demand side of the market). You can select an item based on the product's slick packaging and advertised features (e.g., "tartar-fighting," "enamel protection," "non-irritating, safe ingredients," or "taste and consistency," and, of course, on the price, which you consider carefully because you will pay for the product yourself).[1] With knowledge and choices, you and other shoppers collectively influence the production of toothpaste through your preferences, enjoying what economists refer to as "consumer sovereignty."

The "supply side" of the toothpaste market (which refers to decisions by manufacturers about how much product to provide at different prices) is relatively uncomplicated, although to be sure, there are certain hurdles for sellers, such as Food and Drug Administration (FDA) regulations governing fluoride-containing toothpaste to prevent dental cavities.[2] There is a wide variety of items available. We found 39 toothpaste brands listed in Wikipedia and 217 different toothpastes on the Walgreens website.[3,4]

Considering the many knowledgeable and cost-conscious consumers on the demand side, and the abundance of manufacturers on the supply side, economists would characterize the toothpaste market as "highly competitive." Well-informed and rational consumers can readily judge the costs and benefits of alternative products and make optimal choices given their preferences and budgets. Firms seek to maximize profits, but competition among many firms, who can readily enter and exit the marketplace, keeps prices reasonably close to production costs. Under these conditions, prices satisfy buyers and sellers and, in turn, reflect the value of goods and services to society.[5]

Although markets for most products at Walgreens may be reasonably competitive, they deviate from this ideal to various degrees. Even the toothpaste

The Right Price. Peter J. Neumann, Joshua T. Cohen, and Daniel A. Ollendorf, Oxford University Press (2021).
© Peter J. Neumann, Joshua T. Cohen, and Daniel A. Ollendorf. DOI: 10.1093/oso/9780197512883.003.0002

market diverges from "perfect" competition. For example, few consumers know precisely how well different toothpastes protect against cavities, fight tartar, and protect enamel. The market is also somewhat "concentrated": of the 217 types of toothpaste available from Walgreens, Crest (produced by Procter and Gamble) accounts for 61 and Colgate (produced by Colgate Palmolive) for 52. Such concentration can reduce competition because a few firms predominate and thus have greater leverage in terms of their pricing power.

However, those deviations—"market imperfections" or "market failures" in economist-speak—are relatively minor. Although they do not possess detailed knowledge about different toothpastes' cavity-fighting potential, consumers develop a familiarity and comfort with their choices through repeated purchases. On the supply side, while Procter and Gamble and Colgate Palmolive dominate, there is sufficient competition from the other 37 brands available at Walgreens.com. If you Google "market failure" and "toothpaste," few results emerge. You will not find news headlines suggesting toothpaste prices are unreasonable. The same is true for most other items at Walgreens, with one glaring exception: prescription drugs. Google "market failure" and "prescription drugs," and over 50 million results appear. Why? The reasons pertain to both the demand and supply sides of the market and are central to any effort to understand the valuation of prescription drugs.

The Demand Side: Consumer Sovereignty—Not So Much

It's Complicated

Suppose (in the pre-COVID-19 era, anyway) you had recently recovered from an upper respiratory virus (a "cold") but had developed a cough. You suspect you might have a secondary bacterial infection for which you would need an antibiotic. What to do? First, your cough may have been viral rather than bacterial, and if so, antibiotics would have conferred no benefit (indeed, inappropriate antibiotic use can induce bacteria to evolve into treatment-resistant forms). Second, even if bacteria caused the cough, which antibiotic should you have used? Not every antibiotic treats every bacterium. Third, what would have been the appropriate treatment duration? Fourth, what about side effects? Antibiotics can kill helpful bacteria in your gut, causing stomach upset, for example. They might even cause more serious problems if you have other health conditions, such as liver or kidney disease. Antibiotics can also change the way other drugs work. For example, they can boost the potency of a common anticoagulant, warfarin, causing bleeding in some patients. For these reasons and others, the patient information sheet published by the drug manufacturer Pfizer for Zithromax (azithromycin), an antibiotic sometimes used to treat coughs, runs to more than 1,400 words, equivalent to about four pages in this book.[6] Even with all that information, Pfizer concludes, "If you would like more information, talk with your healthcare provider."

Because of the products' risks and potential harms, you cannot walk into Walgreens, select an antibiotic off the shelf, and proceed to the cash register. You do not choose such drugs yourself. Instead, your physician selects and prescribes one for you (ideally after an informative discussion with you about your options).

While patients suffering from a wide range of conditions often have an array of potential products available, the government does not permit their purchase without a prescription. As Nobel-Prize winning economist Kenneth Arrow observed in a seminal 1963 paper, healthcare markets deviate from "normal" competitive markets in their "adaptations to the existence of uncertainty in the incidence of disease and in the efficacy of treatments."[7p851] Economists also characterize the market as having "information asymmetry," meaning that buyers have much less information than sellers and thus cannot appropriately value products.

Physicians, of course, tend to their patients' best interests, but they are unavoidably influenced by their own interests as well, including the financial incentives confronting them. For example, for some drugs (e.g., certain medications to treat cancer or rheumatoid arthritis) the federal Medicare program pays physicians a fee that depends on the drug's price: the more expensive the drug, the greater the fee and thus the greater the inducement to prescribe.[8-10] Prescribers also vary in terms of training and education about specific diseases and treatments, preferences and practice styles, and the degree to which they are influenced by drug marketing and advertising.[11]

To be sure, the FDA does permit consumers to purchase medications without a prescription if it finds a drug "to be safe and effective for direct consumer use based on the label instructions and warnings."[12,13] Purchasing drugs in the "over-the-counter" category feels more like purchasing toothpaste. The category even includes drugs, such as ibuprofen, that the FDA once considered too risky for consumers to select and use on their own. However, for many drugs, including some that treat common conditions with limited symptoms (e.g., high blood pressure or high cholesterol levels) and others that treat less common or severe conditions (e.g., multiple sclerosis or cancer), you need a prescription. You depend on your doctor to represent your interests because you lack the knowledge necessary to make informed choices yourself—and because the government insists on it. But interjecting someone else's judgment into decisions disrupts signals from consumers' own preferences on what the market should produce. In short, consumer sovereignty is limited.

Moreover, your physician is not the only party with a say in what medications you can use. Medications must gain regulatory approval by the FDA before they can be marketed. The FDA interprets and enforces laws requiring that drugs undergo extensive testing before entering the marketplace. The agency also oversees manufacturing practices and postmarket commitments, as well as drug company labeling and promotional activities.

Numerous books and scholarly papers provide excellent histories and analyses of all aspects of these laws and regulations (see Box 2.1).[14–16] These accounts highlight the lack of federal oversight before the 20th century and the evolution of government requirements, punctuated by the 1906 Food and Drug Act (prohibiting the interstate transport and misbranding of "adulterated" drugs), the 1938 Food, Drug and Cosmetic Act (requiring that new drugs were safe before they entered the market), and the 1962 Amendments to the Food, Drug and Cosmetic Act (requiring companies to demonstrate the safety and effectiveness of their products prior to market entry). Many laws and regulations along the way have added other conditions.

State laws can also influence whether patients receive brand-name drugs—the original formulation marketed by the company that invented a medication—or a typically much less expensive copy (a "generic") that other companies can market after the brand-name manufacturer's exclusivity period has expired. Some states permit, but do not require, pharmacists to substitute generic for brand name drugs, although in others pharmacists must first obtain patients' consent.[15,16] Physicians in all states can issue "dispense as written" prescriptions, stipulating that pharmacists cannot substitute generic products on their own.[15]

Who Decides, and Who Pays?

The previously discussed elements suggest that consumers' role in choosing prescription drugs is, at best, a shared one. There is another way in which the selection of drugs is a shared decision. Unlike the case for toothpaste, consumers generally do not pay directly for their prescriptions.[17pxx] Roughly 92% of Americans have health insurance, which almost always covers pharmaceuticals to some degree. But because they do not pay the full cost at the point of purchase, consumers are much less sensitive to a drug's price.[18,19]

Box 2.1 How Much Premarket Testing of Drugs Should Be Required?

In 1937, more than 100 Americans, including 71 adults and 34 children, died after taking Elixer Sulfanilamide, a drug sold to treat various infections.[1] At the time, formal approval of drugs was not required before a company could market them; instead, a company simply had to reveal the product's ingredients on the label. The uproar that followed led to passage of the 1938 Food, Drug, and Cosmetic Act, requiring drugs to be tested for safety before they are marketed. Laws passed in 1962 made premarket demonstration of a drug's effectiveness mandatory.

While mandating rigorous premarket testing of drugs helped to ensure that approved drugs were safe and effective, they also led to charges that it unreasonably increased drug development costs and thus led to higher drug prices and impeded innovation. In striving for an appropriate balance between rigorous testing and access to essential new medicines, Congress and the FDA have drawn fire from all sides. Some critics have complained about an overly lenient agency, captive of industry influence, that has allowed drugs with poor risk–benefit ratios to enter or linger in the marketplace.[2] On the other hand, some economists, including luminaries such as Milton Friedman (1912–2006) and Gary Becker (1930–2014), have argued that FDA requirements are onerous and largely unnecessary, resulting in higher prices and lives lost because of delays in drug approvals. Friedman, for example, warned: "Considerable evidence has accumulated that indicates that FDA regulation is counterproductive, that it has done more harm by retarding progress in the production and distribution of valuable drugs than it has done good by preventing the distribution of harmful or ineffective drugs."[3pp205-206]Becker argued, "Eliminating all requirements except a reasonable safety standard would vastly reduce drug prices in the U.S., as companies would be encouraged to develop additional compounds to compete for customers."[4]

Concerns about delays in drug approval by patient advocacy groups—perhaps most notably from organizations supporting faster reviews for drugs for HIV/AIDS in the early 1990s—led to provisions for FDA-expedited reviews. Other laws have sought to ease drug approval pathways. The 21st Century Cures Act of 2016 promoted expedited review by permitting companies to use real-world data rather than complete clinical trial results for new indications of existing drugs and by easing approval requirements for drugs to treat rare diseases.[5] Nonetheless, critics on both sides continue to complain, some arguing that the industry has unwisely loosened its standards while others contending that seeking approval for a novel drug remains inordinately time-consuming and expensive. Policymakers have offered a wide variety of proposed solutions, including levers affecting market entry, monopoly protections, and payer requirements, as well as tax policy and direct financial incentives (see Chapters 3 and 10 of this volume).[16]

[1] Akst, J. 2013. "The elixir tragedy, 1937." *The Scientist*. Accessed January 19, 2021. https://www.the-scientist.com/foundations/the-elixir-tragedy-1937-39231.

[2] Light, D.W., Lexchin, J., and Darrow, J.J. 2013. "Institutional corruption of pharmaceuticals and the myth of safe and effective drugs." *Journal of Law, Medicine, and Ethics* 14 (3): 590–610. https://papers.ssrn.com/sol3/papers.cfm?abstract_id=2282014.

[3] Friedman, M., and Friedman, R. 1980. *Free to choose: A personal statement*. New York: Harcourt Brace Jovanovich.

[4] Becker, G.S. 2002, September 15. "Get the FDA out of the way, and drug prices will drop." *Bloomberg*. Accessed January 19, 2021. https://www.bloomberg.com/news/articles/2002-09-15/get-the-fda-out-of-the-way-and-drug-prices-will-drop.

[5] H.R.34, 21st Century Cures Act, 114th Congr. (2015–2016). https://www.congress.gov/bill/114th-congress/house-bill/34.

Studies find that patients—and even their prescribing physicians—are often unaware of the actual costs of pharmaceuticals.[17p116]

While insurance protects consumers from a prescription drug's full price, insurance companies also influence how much consumers pay. A drug's affordability depends on one's type of coverage and benefit design.[17p116] Consumers can face very different insurance design features as plans vary in their premiums, deductibles, copayments, lifetime caps on payments, and other dimensions.[20] One individual may face a $7,900 deductible and pay nothing after that level is reached, while another has a $2,500 deductible, but is responsible for 30% of costs above that amount.

To limit access to expensive therapies, health insurers frequently impose coverage restrictions, such as prior authorization requirements, or criteria based on a patient's age or degree of disease severity, and step edits, which require patients to try cheaper alternatives before gaining access to pricier options. As an example, some insurers have required that to gain access to a costly medication for ankylosing spondylitis, an inflammatory disease affecting the spine, patients must first fail to achieve clinical benefit or experience adverse effects on *five* less expensive alternatives.[21] Limiting access to expensive drugs helps insurers maintain lower premiums, but this benefits healthy plan enrollees who infrequently use prescription drugs while disadvantaging those in need of the medications.

Insurance companies also influence pharmaceutical prices because of their purchasing power (i.e., their share of the market), which enables them to demand concessions from drug manufacturers. Roughly 180 million Americans have private or "commercial" insurance.[22] Insurers who cover these individuals negotiate prices with drug companies and typically bargain for discounts—as much as 30% or more—on the list or wholesale prices.[17pp15,67] The bargaining power of any individual insurer is limited by marketplace fragmentation—there are hundreds of insurers in the United States, although several large ones control the lion's share of the market—and by the limited number of alternative drugs in certain therapeutic classes.[23]

Health insurers may favor one drug company's medication in return for favorable pricing. For example, some insurers require rheumatoid arthritis patients to first try Humira (adalimumab), a widely used drug produced by Abbvie, before they can gain access to other (and sometimes more effective) medications. That may seem a minor imposition, but forcing rheumatoid arthritis patients to "step through" drugs that may not work for them can put their health at risk. Insurers may counter that the favorable pricing they receive on Humira for making it a "first-line" therapy lowers overall costs, improving patient access and affordability. As this example illustrates, insurers can leverage their market power to achieve lower drug prices, but it can disadvantage certain groups of patients, thus further compromising consumer sovereignty.

The pharmaceutical market is further complicated by pharmacy benefit managers (PBMs), entities that negotiate with drug manufacturers on behalf of insurers and manage high-cost specialty medications. Developed in the 1990s to help employers manage (and reduce) pharmaceutical costs, PBMs have attracted controversy because their revenues and profits depend on the size of the rebates they negotiate.[15] By supplying the drug with the highest rebate, a PBM can gain more profit, even if customers pay a higher price.[24] Three PBMs—Express Scripts, CVS Health, and United Healthcare (Optum Rx)—dominate the marketplace, a concentration that allows them to negotiate larger rebates but that also enables them to retain more of those discounts for themselves, rather than passing them on to patients.[25p51,17p168] Moreover, because patient copayments for drugs typically reflect *list* and not *rebated* prices, rebates negotiated by PBMs may not reduce the patients' share of the financial burden.[17p59]

There is little transparency about the tactics of PBMs, or other middlemen or intermediaries, such as drug wholesalers and distributors. Some researchers have found that intermediaries retain as much as $41 of every $100 spent on prescription drugs.[26] Further muddying the picture (for privately insured and Medicare Part D patients) is the presence of drug company-provided "patient assistance programs," under which companies pay for patients' cost-sharing for a period of time, often steering them to the most expensive drugs and further raising costs.[17p106]

Over 100 million Americans have prescription drug coverage through government programs, such as Medicare, Medicaid, and the Veterans Administration, each with their own rules and reimbursement policies.[27] That would seem to put the government in a powerful position to negotiate favorable terms with drug companies. However, even here, the fragmentation of public payers and agency-specific rules limit the government's ability to influence drug prices. For example, the Medicare program, which covers some 60 million, mostly older individuals and accounts for 30% of all retail prescription drug spending,[28,29] is not permitted to use its leverage to negotiate prices or to exclude drugs from the formulary (see Box 2.2). As of this writing, Congress continues to debate proposed legislation that would enable the Department of Health and Human Services to negotiate prices, particularly for high-priced drugs for which there is little or no competition (see Chapter 10 of this volume). The Veterans Administration, subject to its own rules, can set relatively low drug prices for eligible recipients, in part because it has the power to exclude drugs from its formulary. However, the program covers only 9 million Americans, roughly 3% of the population.[30-32] Medicaid programs, administered by individual states and subject to federal rules, cover 66 million people for a wide range of health and nonhealth services, including prescription drugs, but have separate laws governing drug prices, some of which limit their own bargaining power.[33,34]

In summary, when it comes to prescription drugs, the complexity and risks mean that consumers do not have sovereignty. Instead, their physicians and insurance companies play a major role in the selections. Moreover, most consumers do not pay directly for their drugs and hence are not directly exposed to their prices. While insurers assemble large groups of consumers to achieve better terms with drug manufacturers, they prioritize the interests of some consumers over others, are somewhat fragmented in their ability to leverage bargaining power, and, in the case of government payers, are limited by rules and regulations. Requirements that government programs such as Medicare and Medicaid cover certain classes of drugs further boost demand for some products, regardless of their price.[15]

The Supply Side

Just as the experience of purchasing a drug differs from the experience of purchasing most everyday products so does the process of developing and

Box 2.2 Prescription Drugs Under Medicare and Medicaid

Medicare

Even in the fragmented public–private US health insurance market, certain entities have a large footprint. Notably, the Medicare program provides health insurance for some 60 million Americans, including most individuals over the age of 65 and others who qualify based on their disability status. By virtue of its size and the fact that older and disabled individuals are disproportionately heavy users of prescription drugs, the program's policies exert a hefty influence on the US pharmaceutical market. At the same time, various legislative restrictions limit Medicare's leverage over drug prices.

Medicare covers prescription drugs through several component programs. Medicare Part A pays for drugs used during hospital visits as part of bundled payments for the covered stay.[1] On occasion, the rules allow for add-on payments for costly new products (see Chapter 10 of this volume).

Medicare Part B pays for drugs administered in a physician's office or hospital out-patient setting—drugs "you wouldn't usually give to yourself"[2]—such as infused or injectable drugs dispensed by licensed medical providers. Part B drugs are paid for on the basis of average sales prices plus a markup of several percentage points (the magnitude has varied over time).[3] The upshot is that Medicare cannot bargain for Part B drug prices itself; instead it must accept prevailing prices in the marketplace (although in a few settings, Medicare Part B bundles drug payments with other services).[4] Moreover, by law, Medicare Part B must cover cancer treatments approved by the FDA or included in several published compendia. Because many physicians receive reimbursement for Part B drugs plus a markup, they have an incentive to prescribe costlier products. Medicare Part B spending growth has averaged 9% per year recently.[4] Beneficiaries are responsible for paying premiums ($144.60 per month in 2020), as well as an annual deductible ($198 in 2020) and 20% of the cost of services. (Many individuals also have supplemental insurance that helps pay for these and other out-of-pocket costs.)

Medicare Part D covers outpatient prescription drugs. Enrollees pay a deductible up to a certain amount ($415 in 2019 for the standard Part D benefit) and then pay 25% coinsurance up to a coverage limit ($3,820 in 2019), above which a different formula for cost-sharing applies for brand and generic drugs, until enrollee out-of-pocket spending reaches (in 2020) $5,100. Above that amount, another formula applies: enrollees pay either 5% of drug costs or a set dollar amount for each generic and brand-name drug. Roughly 25% of enrollees receive financial assistance through a low-income subsidy program. Some plans waive the deductible or do not charge the full standard amount. Part D plans frequently use tiered copayments (higher payments for more expensive products) or coinsurance for covered drugs, particularly high-cost specialty drugs, instead of charging the 25% coinsurance rate.[5]

A range of private companies offer Part D plans and enrollees can choose which plan they wish to enroll in. The plans differ in terms of their premiums and the details of the coverage offered. By law, Medicare cannot negotiate prices or interfere with negotiations between private Part D plans and drug companies. Instead, individual plans negotiate discounts with each drug company and employ various management techniques—tiered copayments, prior authorization, and step therapy requirements—to control utilization. Part D also has six "protected" drug classes for which health insurers must cover products—antidepressants, antipsychotics, anticonvulsants, immunosuppressants for treatment of transplant rejection, antiretrovirals, and antineoplastics—which further limits the ability of the plans to bargain.[6]

Medicaid

The joint federal–state Medicaid program—managed by states but subject to federal oversight and certain requirements—provides healthcare to over 70 million low-income Americans. The federal government does not require states to cover prescription drugs, although all states do provide this coverage. A company's drug prices must conform to the Medicaid Drug Rebate Program, which requires the company to maintain national rebate agreements with the Department of Health and Human Services in exchange for coverage of the company's drugs by state Medicaid programs.[7] The rebate corresponds to a discount of at least 23.1% on a drug company's "best price" to other customers and is adjusted in response to changes in the Consumer Price Index–Urban. (The rebate differs somewhat for certain drugs such as blood clotting factors and drugs approved exclusively for pediatric indications.)

Because they operate under fixed budgets and are required to balance budgets annually, states have attempted to limit Medicaid drug spending in various ways, sometimes applying to the Centers for Medicare & Medicaid Services for waivers to authorize state-level "demonstration" or pilot projects. In 2001, for example, Michigan established a preferred drug list requiring providers to obtain authorization before prescribing drugs not on the list and allowing companies with drugs not on the list to offer supplemental rebates to attain preferred listing.[8] In 2018, Oklahoma received a waiver to negotiate rebates based on how well a drug achieved particular outcomes.[9] States can establish rules regarding cost-sharing for Medicaid recipients, subject to certain limits (e.g., they can charge a co-payment up to 20% for recipients with incomes exceeding 150% of the federal poverty line).[10]

¹ U.S. Centers for Medicare & Medicaid Services. n.d. "What Part A covers." Accessed January 19, 2021. https://www.medicare.gov/what-medicare-covers/what-part-a-covers.

² U.S. Centers for Medicare & Medicaid Services. n.d. "What part B covers." Accessed January 19, 2021. https://www.medicare.gov/what-medicare-covers/what-part-b-covers.

³ Werble, C. 2017, August 10. "Medicare Part B." *Health Affairs.* https://doi.org/10.1377/hpb20171008.000171.

⁴ Medpac. 2019. "Part B drugs payment systems." http://www.medpac.gov/docs/default-source/payment-basics/medpac_payment_basics_19_partb_final_sec.pdf?sfvrsn=0.

⁵ Hoadley, J., Cubanski, J., and Neuman, T. 2015. "Medicare Part D at ten years: The 2015 marketplace and key trends, 2006–2015." *Kaiser Family Foundation.* Accessed January 19, 2021. https://www.kff.org/report-section/medicare-part-d-at-ten-years-section-3-part-d-benefit-design-and-cost-sharing/.

⁶ "Medicare advantage and Part D drug pricing final rule (CMS–4180- F)." 2019. *Centers for Medicare & Medicaid Services.* https://www.cms.gov/newsroom/fact-sheets/medicare-advantage-and-part-d-drug-pricing-final-rule-cms-4180-f.

⁷ "Medicaid payment for outpatient prescription drugs." 2018. *Medicaid and CHIP Payment and Access Commission.* https://www.macpac.gov/wp-content/uploads/2015/09/Medicaid-Payment-for-Outpatient-Prescription-Drugs.pdf.

⁸ Bernasek, C., Farkas, J., and Felman, H. *Case study: Michigan's Medicaid prescription drug benefit.* Washington, DC: Kaiser Commission on Medicaid and the Uninsured.

⁹ Centers for Medicare and Medicaid Services. 2018, June 27. "CMS approves state proposal to advance specific Medicaid value-based arrangements with drug makers." https://www.cms.gov/newsroom/press-releases/cms-approves-state-proposal-advance-specific-medicaid-value-based-arrangements-drug-makers.

¹⁰ "Medicaid eligibility information, by state." 2017. *Eligibility.com.* Accessed January 19, 2021. https://eligibility.com/medicaid.

bringing a drug to market. The differences generate distinctive incentives for companies that develop "brand-name" drugs and those that produce "generic" copies. These differences necessitate special intellectual property protections from the government. Establishing appropriate protections—so that they promote innovation in the drug industry, while at the same time avoiding their unwanted effects—proves challenging.

The First Pill Costs a Fortune but the Second Costs Pennies

Inventing a new drug and achieving regulatory approval for its use is difficult and time consuming. The process starts with discovery and development, during which researchers identify compounds that appear to be promising because, for example, they interact chemically with pertinent physiological pathways or have effects that may be beneficial. At this step, researchers investigate how the body absorbs, metabolizes, and excretes the compound, as well as the chemical mechanisms by which it might influence disease and its potential side effects. Once identified, a promising compound undergoes testing in a test tube or in animals to determine its toxicity.[17,35pp161–162]

If it appears to be relatively safe, the compound can then proceed to a series of human clinical trials. A Phase 1 clinical trial typically lasts several months, involves a small number of people, and aims to characterize the appropriate dose range and assess the compound's safety in healthy volunteers. A Phase 2 trial typically lasts from two months to two years, can enroll up to several hundred people, and seeks to assess efficacy (whether the drug works as intended), appropriate dosing, and side effects. Finally, a Phase 3 trial, which aims to measure more rigorously the drug's efficacy and adverse effects, can last from one to four years (depending on the nature of the treated disease) and enroll from hundreds to thousands of individuals. Phase 2 and 3 studies are typically "randomized," meaning that based on a coin flip (conducted by a computer these days), patients with a condition receive either the drug under investigation or an older drug or placebo (an inert substance with no therapeutic effect). Often, studies are "double-blinded," meaning that neither participating patients nor their physicians know whether they received the new drug until the study's completion. Assuming all of these trials go well, the FDA will review the evidence, consider the drug's benefits and risks, and decide if it warrants approval for routine use in humans. Even after a drug's approval, the testing process continues with postmarketing surveillance and often requirements for additional follow on studies.

Unsurprisingly, the process takes time. Drug discovery and preclinical testing may last from three to six years and clinical trials from six to seven years.[17p.37] Even after a drug receives approval, scaling up manufacturing can take another two years. There is also a high degree of risk. Although it varies by disease, trial design and other factors, a drug discovery process that starts with 5,000 to 10,000 compounds typically yields 250 compounds that survive to preclinical trials. Of those 250, only about 5 make it to clinical trials, and only about 1 of those 5 receives FDA approval.[36]

The prolonged time periods and high failure rates make drug research and development expensive, although just how expensive remains controversial. A series of widely cited papers have reported that pharmaceutical research and development (R&D) spending has increased dramatically over time, even accounting for inflation, rising to $2.8 billion per approved drug in 2013.[37,38] This research points to high preclinical costs, particularly for biologic products or "biologics" (entities grown in cell cultures, rather than synthesized chemically), long development times, increasing protocol complexity, technical risks, and high failure rates (which have increased over time). Because the process can take years, companies must tie up capital for extended periods before they can earn a return on their investment—even for drugs that are ultimately approved. The investments that drug companies forgo while they await their gamble to pay off (the "opportunity cost of capital") can be substantial.[37,39]

Other studies on the costs of drug development using different methods have found lower costs for drug development.[38,40] Although virtually all observers agree that R&D costs have increased steadily, it is difficult to compare estimates and to pinpoint the true costs because methods, data, and assumptions vary across studies. Every swing of the researcher's bat at this question lands the result in a different place, depending on the sample and assumptions used. The methodology underlying the $2.8 billion per drug cost estimate is faulted for relying on confidential business data and aggressive assumptions about how well companies would have done if they could have invested that money in other opportunities.[40,41] Another study that relied on publicly available data reported a median estimate of about $1 billion per approved drug for R&D costs.[38] But that study also had limitations: it is tilted more toward smaller biotech firms, which may run more efficient operations than larger pharma companies; it relies on drug company reported R&D, which vary in quality and accounting practices across firms; and while larger than previous efforts, still only comprises one fifth of drugs approved by the FDA between 2009 and 2018. To further complicate matters, the federal government helps to foot the bill for drug R&D (see Chapter 10 of this volume). In any case, although there is considerable uncertainty about how much it costs drug companies to develop new drugs, their outlays are substantial.

While the fixed costs of discovering, testing, and gaining approval for a new drug is expensive, for many medications—especially those comprised of relatively small, simple molecules—actual production costs are often characterized as "pennies per pill."[42] That makes the role of "generic manufacturers" attractive. To be sure, even "generic" drug manufacturers must spend resources to gain FDA approval, including demonstrating that their manufacturing processes are adequate, that any inactive ingredients are safe, that their container labels are correct, and so on. But these tasks are far simpler, faster, and cheaper than inventing and achieving regulatory approval for new medications. For tablets and capsules, one study found the cost of regulatory approval to range from $2 million to $5 million.[43]

Drug Company Monopolies as a System Feature, Not a "Bug"

Left to their own devices, companies would gladly enter a drug market as generic suppliers virtually every time an innovator developed a new drug and won approval for its use. As in any market, the participation of competitors would lower prices. In theory, all competitors would continue to reduce their prices to capture market share from other firms—and to avoid relinquishing the market entirely and continue doing so until drug prices neared the marginal costs of production.

The problem is that the "at-cost" pricing that would result would cover only the marginal cost of producing the next pill; it would fail to include the fixed cost of developing and introducing the drug in the first place, leaving no incentive for any company to "go first" and play the role of innovator. But there is a fix for that. High prices for brand-name drugs—rather than reflecting a policy flaw or "bug" in the system—is an expected and even intentional outcome. Monopolistic pricing is a system "feature," designed to incentivize companies to invest in expensive and risky drug discovery by providing the prospect of a big payoff if the investment succeeds. Rather than allowing generic producers to drive prices down immediately, the government grants firms that develop new drugs exclusive, although temporary, rights (through legally protected patents and market exclusivity) to sell their products and thus recoup their investments and earn profits. Companies with new drugs can thus charge what the market will bear without worrying that a generic manufacturer will undercut their pricing.[44]

The incentive for drug companies to innovate is driven by expected gains from discovery, gains that are tied to the size of potential markets and profit expectations. The rationale for patents hinges on a "pull" mechanism—the idea that the lure of temporary monopolies and their promise of revenue generation will encourage innovation that addresses the needs and preferences of patients.

The idea of intellectual property rights or patent protection dates to the US Constitution to encourage inventions that are "novel, useful and nonobvious."[45] The US Patent and Trademark Office issues patents lasting 20 years or more.[46] Pharmaceutical companies typically obtain patents when they first synthesize a drug.[15] Over the years, various laws have modified patents for pharmaceuticals. The 1984 Patent Protection and Restoration Act (known as "Hatch–Waxman," after the lawmakers who championed it), for example, extended the life of patents to account for some of the time a drug is under FDA regulatory review. Because drug development and FDA review can take many years, thus eroding the effective patent life, companies can receive market exclusivity, granted by the Patent and Trademark Office and FDA, thus establishing a minimum duration for their legal protection.[15] Companies can obtain exclusivity for five to seven years after receiving FDA approval for small molecule drugs (i.e., drugs that can be synthesized chemically).

For biologics, the competitive landscape is somewhat different. Unlike small molecule drugs, which manufacturers typically synthesize using chemical processes, biologics are large, complex molecules generally produced in a biological system such as a cell culture or a plant.[47] Because biologics can differ in small ways as a result of differences in manufacturing processes, the FDA does not require that subsequent competitors produce chemically identical copies of the originally approved drug. Instead, companies need only show that their product is as safe and effective as the original approved drug.[47] Rather than referring to the near copies as "generics," they are termed "biosimilars," meaning "biological products that are highly similar to and have no clinically meaningful differences from an existing FDA-approved reference product."[47] Whereas the FDA maintains 5 to 7 years of exclusivity before other companies can sell generic copies of a small molecule drug, it maintains 12 years of exclusivity for biologics after first licensure before competitors can sell biosimilars.[13,48]

Congress has enhanced these exclusivity provisions to encourage certain policy goals. For example, a 1997 law grants drug companies an additional six months of market exclusivity if they test products in children. The Orphan Drug Act of 1983 promotes the development of drugs to treat diseases afflicting small numbers of patients. In addition to providing federal funding and tax breaks for research into conditions that affect no more than 200,000 people in the United States, the act extends the period of exclusivity for treatments indicated for so-called orphan diseases (see Box 2.3 and Chapter 8 of this volume).

Drug Company Monopolies: Too Much of a Good Thing?

Patents and market exclusivity confer a powerful incentive, restricting competition and providing drug developers considerable pricing power.[43] The Orphan Drug Act has encouraged drug companies to develop more products for rare diseases, for example, and to charge more for each treatment (see Box 2.3).

Compared to the situation in most countries in which governments negotiate or set drug prices (and exclude drugs from national formularies if prices are too high), drug companies in the United States are largely free to set their own prices. In an important, although qualified way, US drug pricing reflects what the market will bear.[15] Patents and exclusivity provide government-protected monopoly and pricing power, and certain government coverage mandates (requirements that government healthcare programs pay for certain

Box 2.3 The Orphan Drug Act of 1983

Medications for rare diseases, termed "orphan drugs" given the limited markets and the historic absence of drug companies willing to develop them, have occupied their own corner of legislative and regulatory drug policy.[1] In the decades before the 1980s, few drugs for rare diseases were developed as drug firms targeted products for more common diseases and larger revenue potential.

Incentives changed with passage of the 1983 Orphan Drug Act, directed at diseases affecting fewer than 200,000 persons. Spurred by grassroots efforts from patient advocacy groups that ultimately formed the National Organization for Rare Disorders, the act included federal funding of clinical trials to support orphan drug development, tax credits to defray clinical development costs, and an extended market exclusivity period (seven years versus the typical three to five years for most other drugs) following a drug's FDA approval.[2] The orphan drug regulatory pathway was further eased by closer coordination and consultation between drug companies and the FDA on trial protocols, priority and/or accelerated drug review status, and a waiver of drug application fees.[2] Japan and the European Union (EU Regulation 141/2000) enacted similar legislation and incentives in 1993 and 1999, respectively. The act's impact was immediate. In the 17 years prior to its passage, the FDA approved 34 orphan drugs versus 42 in the 7 years after enactment.[3]

While the act accelerated the development and approval of drugs to treat rare conditions, its exclusivity provisions have also contributed to higher prices. For the first few decades after the act's passage, an unwritten understanding of sorts existed between manufacturers and payers that the small patient populations and modest number of approved drugs would allow public and private insurers to offer generous access to orphan products, despite annual prices that often ranged from $200,000 to $400,000 or higher.[4]

The market dynamics have shifted markedly in recent years, however, as such orphan drugs have proliferated. In 2018, 58% of the novel compounds approved by the FDA had an orphan designation.[5] Worldwide sales of orphan drugs are expected to top $240 billion by 2024, representing one fifth of global pharmaceutical sales.[6] Average annual prices for the top 100 orphan drugs in 2017 were estimated to be $147,300.[7] Payers have begun actively monitoring the orphan drug pipeline and expressing alarm about the budget implications. As one recent example, the Canadian province of British Columbia noted that year-over-year increases in budget expenditures for its public drug plan were being consumed entirely by orphan drugs that were benefiting only 100 or so of the province's 5 million residents.[8]

Given high orphan drug prices and strained budgets, as well as perceived abuses of the act's provisions, many observers have called for reforms (see Chapter 3 of this volume).[7] Drug companies have frequently sought to expand the set of conditions treated by orphan drugs to include broader populations after a drug's approval, for example (although orphan designations are indication-specific).[7] Nearly one quarter of orphan drugs approved since 1983 have at least one indication for a common condition.[9] Critics have also pointed to the manufacturer practice of "salami slicing"—that is, identifying narrow, biomarker-defined subsets of common diseases to receive orphan status, with an ultimate goal of broadening the indication to larger populations,[10] and submitting older drugs that have been marketed outside the United States at much lower prices for orphan status in the United States.[9] Among the proposed solutions are removal of the extended exclusivity period (i.e., retaining only the tax credit incentive), subjecting tax credits to "clawbacks" for drugs when it appears ex post that they did not need incentives to be developed, and requiring agreement from firms receiving tax credits to price regulations after patent expiry.[7]

[1] Aronson, J.K. 2006. "Rare diseases and orphan drugs." *British Journal of Clinical Pharmacology* 61 (3): 243–245. https://doi.org/10.1111/j.1365-2125.2006.02617.x.

[2] Kesselheim, A.S. 2011. "An empirical review of major legislation affecting drug development: Past experiences, effects, and unintended consequences." *The Milbank Quarterly* 89 (3): 450–502. https://doi.org/10.1111/j.1468-0009.2011.00636.x.

[3] Asbury, C.H. 1991. "The orphan drug act: The first 7 years." *JAMA* 265 (7): 893–897. https://doi.org/10.1001/jama.1991.03460070075046.

[4] Ollendorf, D.A., Chapman, R.H., and Pearson, S.D. 2018. "Evaluating and valuing drugs for rare conditions: No easy answers." *Value in Health* 21 (5): 547–552. https://doi.org/10.1016/j.jval.2018.01.008.

[5] "Novel drug approvals for 2018." 2019. *U.S. Food & Drug Administration.* Last modified November 15, 2019. Accessed January 19, 2021. https://www.fda.gov/drugs/new-drugs-fda-cders-new-molecular-entities-and-new-therapeutic-biological-products/novel-drug-approvals-2018.

[6] "EvaluatePharma orphan drug report 2019." 2019. *EvaluatePharma.* Accessed January 19, 2021. https://www.evaluate.com/thought-leadership/pharma/evaluatepharma-orphan-drug-report-2019#:~:text=The%20EvaluatePharma%20Orphan%20Drug%20Report%202019%20arrives%20at,FDA%E2%80%99s%20approval%20of%20the%20first%20gene%20therapy%20product.

[7] Bagley, N., Chandra, A., Garthwaite, C., and Stern, A.D. 2018, December 19. "It's time to reform the Orphan Drug Act." *New England Journal of Medicine Catalyst.* https://catalyst.nejm.org/doi/full/10.1056/CAT.18.0032.

[8] Lun, E. 2019. "Managing the "expense" in expensive drugs for rare diseases (EDRD)." CADTH Symposium, Edmonton, Canada. https://cadth.ca/sites/default/files/symp-2019/presentations/april15-2019/A1-presentation-elun.pdf.

[9] Sarpatwari, A., and Kesselheim, A.S. 2019. "Reforming the orphan drug act for the 21st century." *New England Journal of Medicine* 381 (2): 106–108. https://doi.org/10.1056/NEJMp1902943.

[10] Kesselheim, A.S., Treasure, C.L., and Joffe, S. 2017. "Biomarker-defined subsets of common diseases: Policy and economic implications of orphan drug act coverage." *PLOS Medicine* 14 (1): e1002190. https://doi.org/10.1371/journal.pmed.1002190.

classes of drugs) provide further protection.[15] For certain drugs, pharmaceutical companies enjoy substantial leverage that persists for many years. Many companies have launched drugs with high prices, only to increase them over time, even when alternative therapies that might be expected to exert downward pressure on prices become available.[15,17p17] The price of a brand name statin, Rosuvastatin, for example, increased from 2007 to 2012 even as the price of a competing product, atorvastatin, declined. The price of Copaxone (glatiramer acetate) for multiple sclerosis increased from roughly $8,000 per year in 1996 at its launch to $90,000 in 2015, without any material changes or product improvements.[49]

However, the idea that the drug industry is relatively free to set prices does not mean that their pricing power is unconstrained, nor does it describe other ways in which prices are controlled. Many factors influence a company's pricing power, including the degree of competition from other brand-name products in a therapeutic class, and physician and patient demand for a product.[17p47] Even sole source, brand-name drugs with no competitors face limits on what the market can afford, as well as concerns about the "court of public opinion"—the idea that overly aggressive pricing will attract unwanted government intervention.

What one means by a drug's "price" also requires some elaboration. Prescription drugs have an official "list" or published price. PBMs, hired by health insurers, typically negotiate rebates on drug prices. Because these negotiated prices are confidential, it is difficult to know the actual price any particular insurer pays. List prices are still important: they represent the starting point for payer negotiations, may determine the patient's copayment, and reflect the price that uninsured patients pay.[17p74] In setting prices for its customers, drug companies commonly "price discriminate" (i.e., charge different payers different prices).[50]

Because of their influence, it is reasonable to ask how much protection patents and market exclusivity *should* offer. How much is enough to incentivize drug development? At what point do high drug prices become an unnecessary and excessive windfall for the industry? Moreover, can monopolies translate into *insufficient* industry-wide innovation and dissemination of the new goods discovered, because they stifle new firms from investing? [51]

The answers depend on factors that vary across drugs.[52] For example, for diseases that are more challenging and expensive to investigate, longer exclusivity helps firms compensate for the added risks and costs. For rare diseases, longer exclusivity can compensate for the limited number of patients companies can count on for revenue.

Moreover, the patent system may be subject to manipulation. Drug companies sometimes extend the protection conferred by patents, for example, by delaying the entry of generics into the marketplace, thus retaining their monopolies and high prices. Manufacturers have employed various "ever-greening" approaches, such as obtaining additional patents for drugs (e.g., on the method of administration) or patenting minor reformulations while discontinuing older versions.[15,17p38] One study found that drug companies successfully extended patents protecting almost 80% of the 100 best-selling drugs at least once and did so more than once for almost 50% of these drugs.[53] Because of such tactics, the overall monopoly periods of best-selling drugs Humira (adalimumab) and Enbrel (etanercept) have exceeded 20 years.[16] Humira alone has over 70 patents.[16] Drug firms have also sometimes manipulated the rules by, for example, paying generic drug manufacturers to delay their product entry (so called pay-for-delay tactics), withholding samples of brand name drugs, or exploiting FDA-required risk mitigation strategies of their own products to impede generic products.[15p39,17,54] Backlogs at the FDA have contributed to the delayed entry of generics.

Nor is it clear that there is sufficient competition for biologics. The FDA approved the first biosimilar, filgrastim-sndz, in the United States in 2015. As of 2019, there were 16 biosimilars approved in the United States, but only 6 were commercially available.[55] In contrast, the European Medicines Agency approved its first biosimilar in 2006, and over two dozen biosimilars have been approved and used widely in Europe since then.[17p80,56] Several reasons underlie these discrepancies. The FDA requires human efficacy and safety trials of biosimilars (rather than trials that focus on pharmacodynamics as the European Medicines Agency requires), for example, and manufacturers of originator products often increase rebates or introduce patent-infringement litigation in the United States to slow or reduce biosimilar competition, all of which serve to reduce incentives for biosimilar development.[57,58]

Some have argued that patents are a crude tool for the purpose of incentivizing drug research because the period of market exclusivity they afford does not align well with the time in which the drugs are sold.[59] On one hand, patents must be sought early in the scientific discovery process. Otherwise, information about a candidate drug may be considered ineligible for patent protection. The more information that emerges about a candidate drug before it receives a patent, the less secure the innovation is against copycats even after patent is awarded. On the other hand, because the duration of patent protection is limited, the protection may be largely exhausted before a new drug can be marketed. This makes investment returns uncertain.

Many observers have pointed to outsized profits in the drug industry as a clear sign of inflated and unfair prices and the resulting need to curb existing protections against competition.[60-62] One study found, for example, that between 2000 and 2018 large pharmaceutical company profitability substantially exceeded profitability at other large public companies.[62] The reality around industry profits is more complicated, however. For one, the pharmaceutical industry generally invests a greater percentage of its revenues (about 17%) into R&D than do other industries.[63,64] For another, the share of drug spending as a percentage of total health spending has been relatively constant; for example, according to one estimate in both 1960 and 2017, retail drug spending comprised 10% of national health spending (see Box 1.1),[65] although, of course, this proportion has remained stable in part because of rapid increases in other categories of healthcare spending. On the other hand, it excludes the rapid escalation of costs for hospital-based drugs and other medicines supplied outside the retail sector.

Importantly, drug company profitability is uncertain. In part, that is because the concentration of profits from a limited number of highly successful drugs means that many companies are not as successful as average results would suggest.[39] Moreover, the effectiveness of R&D in terms of high-quality patents seems to be falling,[66,67] and returns on investments (along with net prices) may be declining (page 64).[17,68p64,69,70] Still, venture capital funding—at least in the biotechnology space—has remained robust in recent years, suggesting that financial returns in the sector remain strong.[71] The debates will go on. *The Economist* perhaps put it best in a recent piece, noting, "Everyone hates pharmaceutical firms, but their share of health-care rent-seeking is relatively trivial, especially once you include the many midsized and small firms that are investing heavily."[72] Some research has even shown that if one wants to find outsized profits in the healthcare industry, they tend to come from health insurers and PBMs, who face limited competition and low costs (e.g., PBMs have little to no physical plant or R&D costs), rather than drug companies. That analysis suggests the gains of insurers and PBMs represent two thirds of the excess profits in the healthcare industry per year.[72]

Although patents and market exclusivity create the revenue and profits that incentivize the investments needed to discover and develop drugs, they are rather crude tools. The duration of a drug's market exclusivity is uncertain, and during that period, drug companies can charge what the market will bear. Whether the system produces sufficient or excessive profits is unclear, but it does facilitate prices that strike many people as excessive. That, in turn, has led to numerous proposals to rein in drug prices.

References

1. Deleon, M. 2020. "The best toothpaste for a healthy and sparkling smile." *ConsumerSearch*. Accessed January 19, 2021. https://www.consumersearch.com/toothpaste/how-to-buy-toothpaste.

2. Sandier, M. 1997. "The regulation of toothpaste." *Harvard University*. https://dash.harvard.edu/handle/1/8846762.

3. "List of toothpaste brands." *Wikipedia*. Last modified June 28, 2020. Accessed January 19, 2021. https://en.wikipedia.org/wiki/List_of_toothpaste_brands.

4. "'Toothpaste.'" *Walgreens*. Accessed January 19, 2021. https://www.walgreens.com/search/results.jsp?Ntt=toothpaste.

5. Gruber, J. 2020. *Valuing rare pediatric drugs: An economics perspective*. Working paper, MIT.

6. Pfizer. 2020. "ZITHROMAX (azithromycin dihydrate)." Accessed January 19, 2021. https://www.pfizermedicalinformation.com/en-us/patient/zithromax.

7. Arrow, K.J. 1963. "Uncertainty and the welfare economics of medical care." *The American Economic Review* 53 (5): 941–973. www.jstor.org/stable/1812044.

8. Elliott, S.P., Jarosek, S.L., Wilt, T.J., and Virnig, B.A. 2010. "Reduction in physician reimbursement and use of hormone therapy in prostate cancer." *JNCI* 102 (24): 1826–1834. https://doi.org/10.1093/jnci/djq417.

9. Jacobson, M., Earle, C.C., Price, M., and Newhouse, J.P. 2010. "How Medicare's payment cuts for cancer chemotherapy drugs changed patterns of treatment." *Health Affairs* 29 (7): 1391–1399. https://doi.org/10.1377/hlthaff.2009.0563.

10. Conti, R.M., Rosenthal, M.B., Polite, B.N., Bach, P.B., and Shih, Y.-C.T. 2012. "Infused chemotherapy use in the elderly after patent expiration." *Journal of Oncology Practice* 8 (3S): e18s–e23s. https://doi.org/10.1200/JOP.2012.000541.

11. Llamas, M. 2016. "Selling side effects: Big Pharma's marketing machine." *Drug Watch*. Last modified July 28, 2020. Accessed January 19, 2021. https://www.drugwatch.com/featured/big-pharma-marketing/.

12. "FAQs about drug distribution in the United States." *Consumer Healthcare Products Association*. Accessed January 19, 2021. https://www.chpa.org/about-consumer-healthcare/faqs/FAQs-drug-distribution-in-US.

13. FDA. "CFR – code of federal regulations Title 21." U.S. Food & Drug Administration. Last modified April 1, 2020. Accessed January 19, 2021. https://www.accessdata.fda.gov/scripts/cdrh/cfdocs/cfcfr/CFRSearch.cfm?CFRPart=201&showFR=1.

14. Hilts, P.J. 2003. *Protecting America's health: The FDA, business, and one hundred years of regulation*. New York: Alfred A. Knopf.

15. Kesselheim, A.S., Avorn, J., and Sarpatwari, A. 2016. "The high cost of prescription drugs in the United States: Origins and prospects for reform." *JAMA* 316 (8): 858–871. https://doi.org/10.1001/jama.2016.11237.

16. Khullar, D., Ohn, J.A., Trusheim, M., and Bach, P.B. 2020. "Understanding the rewards of successful drug development—thinking inside the box." *New England Journal of Medicine* 382 (5): 473–480. https://doi.org/10.1056/NEJMhpr1911004.

17. National Academies of Sciences Engineering, and Medicine. 2018. *Making medicines affordable: A national imperative*. Edited by N.R. Augustine, G. Madhavan, and S.J. Nass. Washington, DC: The National Academies Press.

18. Berchick, E.R., Hood, E., and Barnett, J.C. 2018. *Health insurance coverage in the United States: 2017*. United States Census Bureau. https://www.census.gov/library/publications/2018/demo/p60-264.html.

19. Collins, S.R., Bhupal, H.K., and Doty, M.M. 2019. "Health insurance coverage eight years after the ACA." The Commonwealth Fund. Accessed January 19, 2021. https://www.commonwealthfund.org/publications/issue-briefs/2019/feb/health-insurance-coverage-eight-years-after-aca.

20. "Compare Obamacare health plans." 2020. HealthInsurance. Accessed January 19, 2021. https://www.healthinsurance.com/obamacare/quotes.

21. Chambers, J.D., Panzer, A.D., and Neumann, P.J. 2018. "Variation in the use of step therapy protocols across US health plans." *Health Affairs*. https://www.healthaffairs.org/do/10.1377/hblog20180912.391231/full/.

22. Klein, P. 2019. "Elizabeth Warren leaves no doubt: She's 'with Bernie' on kicking 180 million people off of private insurance." Washington Examiner. Accessed January 19, 2021. https://www.washingtonexaminer.com/opinion/elizabeth-warren-leaves-no-doubt-shes-with-bernie-on-kicking-180-million-people-off-of-private-insurance.

23. "Facts + statistics: Industry overview." *Insurance Information Institute*. Accessed January 19, 2021. https://www.iii.org/fact-statistic/facts-statistics-industry-overview.

24. Arnold, J. 2018. "John Arnold: Are pharmacy benefit managers the good guys or bad guys of drug pricing?" *STAT*. Accessed January 19, 2021. https://www.statnews.com/2018/08/27/pharmacy-benefit-managers-good-or-bad/.

25. Bai, G., Sen, A.P., and Anderson, G.F. 2018. "Pharmacy benefit managers, brand-name drug prices, and patient cost sharing." *Annals of Internal Medicine* 168 (6): 436–437. https://doi.org/10.7326/M17-2506.

26. Sood, N., Shih, T., Van Nuys, K., and Goldman, D. 2017. "Flow of money through the pharmaceutical distribution system." *University of Southern California, Leonard D. Schaeffer Center for Health Policy & Economics*. https://healthpolicy.usc.edu/research/flow-of-money-through-the-pharmaceutical-distribution-system/.

27. Cubanski, J., Damico, A., and Neuman, T. 2018. "Medicare part D in 2018: The latest on enrollment, premiums, and cost sharing." *Kaiser Family Foundation*. https://www.kff.org/medicare/issue-brief/medicare-part-d-in-2018-the-latest-on-enrollment-premiums-and-cost-sharing/.

28. "An overview of Medicare." 2019. *Kaiser Family Foundation*. https://www.kff.org/medicare/issue-brief/an-overview-of-medicare/.

29. "10 essential facts about Medicare and prescription drug spending." 2019. *Kaiser Family Foundation*. https://www.kff.org/infographic/10-essential-facts-about-medicare-and-prescription-drug-spending/.

30. Golding, H., Mosher, D., and Keating, E.G. 2018. "Possible higher spending paths for veterans' benefits." *Congressional Budget Office*. https://www.cbo.gov/publication/54881

31. McCaughan, M. 2017, August 10. "Veterans Health Administration." *Health Affairs*. https://www.healthaffairs.org/do/10.1377/hpb20171008.000174/full/.

32. President's budget. 2019. *Office of Management and Budget*. https://www.whitehouse.gov/wp-content/uploads/2018/02/budget-fy2019.pdf.

33. Young, K. 2019. "Utilization and spending trends in Medicaid outpatient prescription drugs." *Kaiser Family Foundation*. https://www.kff.org/medicaid/issue-brief/utilization-and-spending-trends-in-medicaid-outpatient-prescription-drugs/.

34. "March 2020 Medicaid & CHIP enrollment data highlights." 2020. *Medicaid.gov*. https://www.medicaid.gov/medicaid/program-information/medicaid-and-chip-enrollment-data/report-highlights/index.html.

35. US Food and Drug Administration. "The drug development process." Last modified January 4, 2018. Accessed January 19, 2021. https://www.fda.gov/patients/learn-about-drug-and-device-approvals/drug-development-process.

36. Dailey, J.W. 2018. "Pharmaceutical industry: Drug discovery and development." *Encyclopaedia Britannica*. Accessed January 19, 2021. https://www.britannica.com/technology/pharmaceutical-industry.

37. DiMasi, J.A., Grabowski, H.G., and Hansen, R.W. 2016. "Innovation in the pharmaceutical industry: New estimates of R&D costs." *Journal of Health Economics* 47: 20–33. https://doi.org/10.1016/j.jhealeco.2016.01.012.

38. Wouters, O.J., McKee, M., and Luyten, J. 2020. "Estimated research and development investment needed to bring a new medicine to market, 2009–2018." *JAMA* 323 (9): 844–853. https://doi.org/10.1001/jama.2020.1166.

39. DiMasi, J.A., and Grabowski, H.G. 2012. "R&D costs and returns to new drug development: A review of the evidence." In *The Oxford Handbook of the Economics of the Biopharmaceutical Industry*, edited by P.M. Danzon and S. Nicholson, 34–46. New York: Oxford University Press.

40. Prasad, V., and Mailankody, S. 2017. "Research and development spending to bring a single cancer drug to market and revenues after approval." *JAMA Internal Medicine* 177 (11): 1569–1575. https://doi.org/10.1001/jamainternmed.2017.3601.

41. Angell, M. 2004. *The truth about drug companies: How they deceive us and what to do about it* (1st ed.). New York: Random House.

42. Frank, R.G., and Ginsburg, P.B. 2017, November 13. "Pharmaceutical industry profits and research and development." *Health Affairs*. Accessed January 19, 2021. https://www.healthaffairs.org/do/10.1377/hblog20171113.880918/full/.

43. Berndt, E.R., and Newhouse, J.P. 2012. "Pricing and reimbursement in US pharmaceutical markets." In *The Oxford Handbook of the Economics of the Biopharmaceutical Industry*, edited by P.M. Danzon and S. Nicholson, 201–265. New York: Oxford University Press.

44. Lupkin, S. 2016. "Government-protected 'monopolies' drive drug prices higher, study says." *Kaiser Health News*. Accessed January 19, 2021. https://khn.org/news/government-protected-monopolies-drive-drug-prices-higher-study-says/.

45. Conditions for patentability: Novelty and non-obvious subject matter. US Code §103. https://uscode.house.gov/view.xhtml?req=granuleid:USC-prelim-title35-section103&num=0&edition=prelim#sourcecredit.

46. Contents and term of patent: Provisional rights, 35 U.S.C. 154. Department of Commerce, US Patent and Trademark Office. https://www.uspto.gov/web/offices/pac/mpep/s2701.html#:~:text=S.C.%20154%20Contents%20and%20term%20of%20patent%3B%20provisional,%28c%29%2C%20or%20386%20%28c%29%20from%20the%20date%20.

47. US Food and Drug Administration. 2017. "Biosimilar and interchangeable products." Last modified October 23, 2017. Accessed January 19, 2021. https://www.fda.gov/drugs/biosimilars/biosimilar-and-interchangeable-products.

48. Regulation of biological products, 42 USC 262.

49. Cohen, J. 2018, September 12. "The curious case of Gleevec pricing." *Forbes*. Accessed January 19, 2021. https://www.forbes.com/sites/joshuacohen/2018/09/12/the-curious-case-of-gleevec-pricing/#3f8182e4543.

50. Danzon, P.M., and Nicholson, S. 2012. *The Oxford handbook of the economics of the biopharmaceutical industry*. New York: Oxford University Press.

51. Lakdawalla, D.N., and Sood, N. 2012. "Incentives to Innovate." In *The Oxford handbook of the economics of the biopharmaceutical industry*, edited by P.M. Danzon and S. Nicholson, 143–166. New York: Oxford University Press.

52. Sampat, B.N., and Lichtenberg, F.R. 2011. "What are the respective roles of the public and private sectors in pharmaceutical innovation?" *Health Affairs* 30 (2): 332–339. https://doi.org/10.1377/hlthaff.2009.0917.

53. Feldman, R. 2018. "May your drug price be evergreen." *Journal of Law and the Biosciences* 5 (3): 590–647. https://doi.org/10.1093/jlb/lsy022.

54. Dave, C.V., Sinha, M.S., Beall, R.F., and Kesselheim, A.S. 2020. "Estimating the cost of delayed generic drug entry to Medicaid." *Health Affairs* 39 (6): 1011–1017. https://doi.org/10.1377/hlthaff.2019.00673.

55. Peterson, C. 2019. "Biosimilars in the U.S.: More approvals but not more access." *Express Scripts*. Accessed January 19, 2021. https://express-scripts.com/corporate/articles/biosimilars-us-more-approvals-not-more-access.

56. Mehr, S. 2020, April 23. "An interesting comparison: The latest data on US and EU biosimilar uptake." *Biosimilars Review & Report*. https://biosimilarsrr.com/2020/04/23/an-interesting-comparison-the-latest-data-on-us-and-eu-biosimilar-uptake/.

57. Bach, P.B., and Trusheim, M. 2019, August 21. "Time to throw in the towel on biosimilars." *Wall Street Journal*. Accessed January 19, 2021. https://www.wsj.com/articles/time-to-throw-in-the-towel-on-biosimilars-11566428299.

58. Chambers, J.D., Lai, R.C., Margaretos, N.M., Panzer, A.D., Cohen, J.T., and Neumann, P.J. 2020. "Coverage for biosimilars vs reference products among US commercial health plans." *JAMA* 323 (19): 1972–1973. https://doi.org/10.1001/jama.2020.2229.

59. Eisenberg, R.S. 2012. "Patents and regulatory exclusivity." In *The Oxford handbook of the economics of the biopharmaceutical industry*, edited by P.M. Danzon and S. Nicholson, 167–200. New York: Oxford University Press.

60. Chen, L. 2015, December 21. "The most profitable industries in 2016." *Forbes*. Accessed January 19, 2021. https://www.forbes.com/sites/liyanchen/2015/12/21/the-most-profitable-industries-in-2016/#1f3628265716.

61. Herman, B. 2017. "Health care profits concentrated at drug companies." *Axios*. Accessed January 19, 2021. https://www.axios.com/health-care-profits-concentrated-at-drug-companies-1513306919-821dd691-cc16-49d8-bdc0-fb5eb8832906.html.

62. Ledley, F.D., McCoy, S.S., Vaughan, G., and Cleary, E.G. 2020. "Profitability of large pharmaceutical companies compared with other large public companies." *JAMA* 323 (9): 834–843. https://doi.org/10.1001/jama.2020.0442.

63. Nicholson, S. 2012. "Financing research and development." In *The Oxford handbook of the economics of the biopharmaceutical industry*, edited by P.M. Danzon and S. Nicholson, 47–74. New York: Oxford University Press.

64. "Average research & development costs for pharmaceutical companies." 2018. *Investopedia*. Last modified August 8, 2019. Accessed January 19, 2021. https://www.investopedia.com/ask/answers/060115/how-much-drug-companys-spending-allocated-research-and-development-average.asp.

65. Glied, S., and Kim, G. 2018. "Health spending in 2017: What policy can do, and what it can't." *Health Affairs*. https://doi.org/10.1377/hblog20181205.543905.

66. Jack, A. 2012. "Fall in number of patents filed by big pharma." *Financial Times*. Accessed January 19, 2021. https://www.ft.com/content/0912c0ea-70f9-11e1-a7f1-00144feab49a.

67. National Academies of Sciences, Engineering, and Medicine. Policy and Global Affairs. 2017. *Beyond patents: Assessing the value and impact of research investments*. Government–University–Industry Research Roundtable. Washington, DC: National Academies Press. https://www.ncbi.nlm.nih.gov/books/NBK458648/.

68. Stott, K. 2017. "Pharma's broken business model—Part 1: An industry on the brink of terminal decline." *LinkedIn*. Accessed January 19, 2021. https://www.linkedin.com/pulse/pharmas-broken-business-model-industry-brink-terminal-kelvin-stott/.

69. Thaxter, M. 2018, December 20. "Unlocking R&D productivity—the state of pharmaceutical innovation in 2018." *Center for Health Solutions, Deloitte*. https://blogs.deloitte.co.uk/health/2018/12/unlocking-rd-productivity-the-state-of-pharmaceutical-innovation-in-2018.html.

70. Berndt, E.R., Nass, D., Kleinrock, M., and Aitken, M. 2015. "Decline in economic returns from new drugs raises questions about sustaining innovations." *Health Affairs* 34 (2): 245–252. https://doi.org/10.1377/hlthaff.2014.1029.

71. Cutler, D.M. 2020. "Are pharmaceutical companies earning too much?" *JAMA* 323 (9): 829–830. https://doi.org/10.1001/jama.2020.0351.

72. "Which firms profit most from America's health-care system." 2018, March 15. *The Economist*. https://www.economist.com/business/2018/03/15/which-firms-profit-most-from-americas-health-care-system.

3

Proposed Solutions for Rising Drug Prices

Finally, Something We Can All Agree On

> *The drug industry is "getting away with murder. . . . Pharma has a lot of lobbies, a lot of lobbyists, a lot of power. And there's very little bidding on drugs."*[1]
>
> **—President-Elect Donald Trump, 2017**

President Trump was not alone in his frustration about drug prices, even in the traditionally business-friendly Republican Party. In 2019, Senator Chuck Grassley, a Republican from Iowa and the powerful chairman of the Senate Finance Committee, referred to "skyrocketing prescription drug costs."[2] Joining forces with Democrat Ron Wyden of Oregon, he hosted a series of hearings on the issue.[3]

Democrats have, perhaps unsurprisingly, given the party's historically less favorable views toward large corporations, expressed more uniform outrage. Senator Wyden called the pharmaceutical industry "morally repugnant" and labeled its behavior "unacceptable."[4] Democratic Senator from Massachusetts, Elizabeth Warren, then running for president, declared that drug companies were lining "their pockets at the expense of American families."[5] Fellow candidate Bernie Sanders, Democratic Senator from Vermont, pledged, "If the pharmaceutical industry will not end its greed, which is literally killing Americans, then we will end it for them." Former Vice President Joe Biden, the reputed standard bearer of his party's more moderate wing in the 2020 presidential primary, promised to "stand up to abuse of power by prescription drug corporations if elected."[6]

State officials have joined the chorus of critics and are taking or proposing action. Charlie Baker, the popular Republican governor of Massachusetts—a state that has benefited enormously from its pharmaceutical/biotech cluster—has backed plans to limit drug prices in the state's Medicaid program.[7,8] Gavin

The Right Price. Peter J. Neumann, Joshua T. Cohen, and Daniel A. Ollendorf, Oxford University Press (2021).
© Peter J. Neumann, Joshua T. Cohen, and Daniel A. Ollendorf. DOI: 10.1093/oso/9780197512883.003.0003

Newsom, the Democratic governor of California—another state that is home to prominent biotechnology companies—stated, "California is leading the nation in holding drug companies accountable and fighting prescription drug prices," adding that "taxpayers are tired of being 'screwed.'"[9]

This foment is not new. Frustration about drug prices has been mounting for years. A Google News search limited to stories prior to 2010 yields the following headlines, among others: "Co-Payments for Expensive Drugs Soar"[10] and "Why We Pay So Much for Drugs."[11] The frustration has spawned the idea that action is essential.

This chapter explores proposed solutions for high drug prices. They include measures to rein in the "middlemen" pharmacy benefit managers (PBMs) highlighted in Chapter 2 of this volume; increase generic drug competition to prevent price spikes for older, off-patent drugs; enhance competition for new drugs after brand-name products reach the intended period of market protection; align US drug prices with the lower prices available in other wealthy countries; and leverage the collective bargaining power of government payers to compel drug companies to accept lower prices for their products.

We explore whether and how these measures might substantially address the problems posed by high drug prices and which strategy would affect a sufficient share of drugs to meaningfully reduce drug costs incurred by America's healthcare system. We also question whether the measures might introduce unintended consequences that could interfere with the delivery of desired care. Spoiler alert: we find the proposed solutions inadequate.

Cutting Out the Middleman

The drug price debate can sometimes seem a contest between hostile camps—one arguing that drug firms are awash in profits and the other contending that companies require high prices to support further innovation to improve population health. However, the sides agree on certain issues—in particular, the need to address the role of PBMs.

PBMs, introduced in Chapter 2 of this volume, have been described as "key participants in the administration of drug benefits for more than 266 million Americans with health insurance, using volume-buying leverage to negotiate discounts from manufacturers, generally delivered in the form of rebates."[12] The explanations add that "PBMs subsequently share these rebates with their customers—the payers." That sounds like a useful function—one that should help consumers boost their purchasing power. Indeed, the Centers for Medicare and Medicaid Services (CMS) credits PBMs with reducing drug prices and moderating growth in Medicare Part D spending.[13] Some researchers have estimated substantial savings from PBM actions for commercial insurers.[14] Even for newly approved products, when drugs have little or no competition, PBMs have achieved substantial price reductions. For example, Express Scripts tightly restricted access to drugs to treat hepatitis C (Sovaldi/Harvoni) and high cholesterol (PCSK9 inhibitors, Repatha and Praluent).[12]

However, critics also *blame* PBMs for contributing to high and increasing drug prices. The problem arises because PBMs do not simply pressure drug companies to reduce prices. Instead, they seek to induce companies to return revenue in the form of "rebates." The distinction between lower prices and higher rebates may seem inconsequential, but it matters for two reasons. First, as noted in Chapter 2 of this volume, because patient co-payments can depend on a drug's list price (not the net price after rebates), those co-payments often remain elevated even if the PBM negotiates a substantial discount from the list price.[13] While the rebates could be returned to patients to defray high cost-sharing requirements, payers often use them to defray the costs of other medications or even to reduce premiums for their general enrollees. In short, patients who consume expensive medications may generate large rebates that payers then use to subsidize others.

Second, payer contracts call for PBMs to receive a portion of the negotiated rebates. That may seem reasonable: larger rebates mean more savings, so contracts should incentivize PBMs to achieve them. However, greater rebates do not necessarily translate into savings for payers or consumers. PBMs can increase rebates by raising the list price, rather than by negotiating a reduction of the price paid to the manufacturer. For example, a PBM that increases the rebate paid by the drug company on a $100 drug from $20 to $30 has saved the payer or patient money, as the drug company's revenue drops from $80 to $70. But if the drug's list price instead increases from $100 to $200 and the rebate remains fixed at, say, 20% of the list price, the rebate will again increase—this time, from $20 to $40. If the PBM pockets a fixed fraction of the rebate, it ends up benefiting from the higher drug price, even if payers and consumers pay more.

As the National Academy of Medicine observes, "the interaction between rebates and list prices can be complicated... market price negotiations based on a drug's list price can even induce drug manufacturers to further increase their drug prices."[15p60] If payments to PBMs depend on the size of the rebate, the payments going to PBMs can grow while, simultaneously, list price increases can be kept sufficiently high to cover the rebates that drug companies must pay. With PBMs and drug manufacturers both gaining, it follows that payers—and consumers, whose premiums cover the payer costs—must lose.

The effectiveness of the PBM industry depends on its concentration (i.e., how much of the market is controlled by the largest firms). The more concentrated the industry, the greater the negotiating power of those large PBMs. As the National Academy of Medicine explains, the high concentration can cut both ways:

> While some PBMs act as agents for payers, receiving a fee for their services, in many case [sic] PBMs act as principals, retaining a share of the discount they have negotiated from the manufacturer. In a sense, the market concentration of PBMs can be seen as a double-edged sword from the patient and the payer perspective: it enhances the ability of the PBMs to extract bigger discounts from the manufacturer, and also the ability to pass on less of these discounts to the patients than would be the case if they were less concentrated.[15pp51-52]

As noted in Chapter 2 of this volume, the three largest firms (Express Scripts, CVS Health, and United Health-OptumRx) comprise over 80% of the market.[16p51,17] Financial success has followed. Examining industry-wide income above levels considered normal in terms of incurred risk and invested capital, *The Economist* estimated that PBMs have "excess profits" of $126 per American annually (amounting to around $40 billion for the entire country).[18] Of even greater note (as pointed out in Chapter 2 of this volume), *The Economist* estimated that PBMs capture two-thirds of the excess profits in the entire healthcare sector.

With that backdrop, it is unsurprising that proposals to reform the PBM industry have ensued. A 2019 review of the Ohio Medicaid program revealed that although PBMs saved the state $145 million per year, they earned profits of $224 million on the difference between their payments to drug manufacturers and the reimbursements they received from the state.[19] Proposed remedies have included "pass-through" pricing, which awards the PBM administrative and dispensing fees rather than a profit based on the price spread. As the same article noted, other states have pursued measures such as direct regulation of price spreads, prohibitions on levying co-payments that exceed the total cost of the drug, and requirements that rebates be returned to states rather than getting pocketed by PBMs.

The Trump administration took notice. In 2018, the president opined on PBMs, declaring, "We're very much eliminating the middlemen. . . . The middlemen became very, very rich. Whoever those middlemen were, and a lot of people never even figured it out, they're rich. They won't be so rich anymore."[20] A January 2019 Trump administration proposal called for a prohibition on arrangements that tied manufacturers-to-PBMs rebates to favorable formulary treatment of drugs by PBMs and instead allowed for discounts to be provided directly to consumers at the point of sale.[21] The Congressional Budget Office (CBO) characterized the rule's objective, stating, "When announcing the rule, HHS [the US Department of Health and Human Services] indicated that its intention was for manufacturers to lower their list prices, replace rebates with discounts, or do both."[22p2] Lowering list prices would reduce consumer co-payments. Eliminating rebates to PBMs would remove incentives for PBMs to include high-priced brand name drugs on formularies and instead encourage them to favor generics with the same clinical benefit.[23]

In July 2019, the Trump administration withdrew its proposal (and PBM stock prices soared).[24] However, even if that plan had advanced, there are reasons to believe its impact on reducing drug prices would have been limited. First, eliminating rebates received by the PBMs has its downsides. Those rebates can be thought of as payments from manufacturers to PBMs in exchange for favorable formulary placement. The PBMs retain some of those rebates, but they pass along some of the gains to their own customers to retain them.

CBO estimated that the proposed rule would have *increased* costs to Medicare and Medicaid by approximately $177 billion over a decade.[22] CBO estimated that in "converting" PBM rebates to consumer discounts, drug manufacturers would reduce their refunds by 15% because they would no longer be receiving a service (favorable formulary placement) in return. Moreover, without the rebate "income," they had been receiving from PBMs and using to reduce beneficiary premiums, insurers would in turn raise premiums. Because the federal government subsidizes premiums, its cost would also rise.

Another way to view this problem is by re-examining *The Economist*'s estimates of PBM's "excess profits." Recall that those profits (which *The Economist* estimated at $40 billion annually) represent what the PBM industry earns above what one would expect in light of the risks and the capital it ties up. In theory, a perfectly crafted rule would recover those excess profits and return them to consumers without a corresponding loss of the benefits now conferred by PBMs. Savings of $40 billion per year are not trivial, but still pale relative to the $500 billion or so that Americans spend on prescription drugs. Even if the middlemen could be removed, it would make a relatively modest dent in drug prices.

Lower Prices Through Competition

Chief executives of small drug companies that market a handful of decades-old medications do not usually receive mention in the opening monologue of Stephen Colbert's *The Late Show*. But, in June 2017, Martin Shkreli, CEO of Turing Pharmaceuticals, managed that feat. Colbert spent more than two minutes skewering Shkreli, who had gained infamy by raising the price of Daraprim (pyrimethamine), a medication for HIV patients infected with toxoplasmosis, from $13.50 to $750 per pill. (Shkreli was later back in the news for his trial and conviction for securities fraud unrelated to Daraprim.)

Beyond the moral outrage was a policy puzzle. High prices for new, brand-name products generate anger, but there is at least an argument that such prices reflect temporary exclusive marketing rights for companies and are needed to incentivize research and development. But Daraprim was approved by the US Food and Drug Administration (FDA) during the Eisenhower administration. For a drug that old, there should be no patent protection. Competition among firms should have made Shkreli's expected profits for Daraprim impossible.

Competition from and among generics has effectively reduced prices for many drugs. Data from the FDA show that while drug prices fall (39%) following the entry of a single generic manufacturer, a second generic manufacturer causes prices to fall by around half (54%), and four entries reduce prices by 79% or more.[25] For that reason, generics accounted for 9 in 10 prescriptions in the United States in 2018[26] (incidentally, a fraction much higher than France [30%], Spain [47%], or Germany [80%], although those countries tend to have price controls, which lowers brand-name prices.[27p32,28] Annual savings (estimated by comparing generic to brand name drug prices) have reached nearly $300 billion.[26]

However, as the Daraprim example illustrates, generics are not a perfect remedy, in part because competition can be hampered by regulatory delays.[29] Under the Drug Price Competition and Patent Term Restoration Act of 1984 (the Hatch–Waxman Act), gaining approval for a generic copy of a brand-name product involves demonstrating "therapeutic equivalence" to a product—that is, it contains the "same active ingredient(s), dosage form and route of administration, same strength"[30] and it is "bioequivalent" (i.e., absorbed into the body at the same rate and distributed to tissues in the same way). This requirement for an Abbreviated New Drug Application (ANDA) is substantially less expensive than a New Drug Application (NDA,) requiring clinical trials to demonstrate that an "innovative" drug is safe and effective. But the ANDA is still not costless. Moreover, even if a competitor wants to pursue an ANDA, the FDA's review backlog imposes a delay. Indeed, one report noted that "none of the approximately 1500 applications for generic drugs submitted in fiscal 2014 had been approved by the end of that year."[31]

Nor is Daraprim an isolated example. The price for 500 tablets of the antibiotic doxycycline increased from $20 to nearly $2,000 between October 2013 and April 2014. A one-year supply of pravastatin, a medication to treat "bad" cholesterol, increased from $27 to nearly $200 over the same period of time.[32] In its study of 1,441 generic drugs covering the period 2010 to 2015, the General Accounting Office found that prices increased by 100% or more for 315 drugs.[33]

Why is generic competition more effective in some cases than in others? An investigation by Senators Susan Collins of Maine and Claire McCaskill of Missouri considered five case studies of old, off-patent drugs that experienced price spikes: Turing Pharmaceutical's Daraprim; Retrophin's Thiola (tipronin, first marketed in 1988 to treat cystinuria, a genetic condition that affects the kidneys); Rodelis Pharmaceutical's Seromycin (cycloserine, first marketed in 1964 to treat drug-resistant tuberculosis); Valeant Pharmaceutical's Cuprimine and Syprine (penicillamine and trientine approved by the FDA in 1965 and 1988, respectively, to treat Wilson's disease, a genetic condition that causes copper poisoning); and Valeant Pharmaceutical's Nitropress (nitroprusside) and Isuprel (isoproterenol) isolated in the 19th century, patented in 1956, and used in cardiac emergencies.[34]

In all five cases, Collins and McCaskill concluded that although the drugs in question were off-patent and thus lacked government protection from generic duplication, they enjoyed at least temporary de facto monopoly status because of factors including (i) the existence of a single manufacturer and hence no possibility of immediate competition; (ii) "gold standard" status that meant physicians would tend to continue to prescribe the drug even when its price increases substantially; (iii) small market size that does not attract large generic manufacturers or organized opposition by large patient groups (e.g., Daraprim is used by 2,000 people per year in the United States)[35]; and (iv) a closed distribution system that limits options for acquiring the drug through other market channels.

Policymakers have proposed various measures to open these types of cases to competition, such as increasing FDA funding for generic drug application reviews, allowing the agency to rely on data from other industrialized countries, and expediting reviews for products with limited competition (e.g., three or fewer manufacturers).[36,37] One challenge is that greater competition that reduces generic prices can sometimes have the perverse effect of forcing weaker manufacturers out of business and giving rise to "sole source" (or near sole source) generics that make shortages and price gouging more likely. While there are, no doubt, de facto monopoly cases that would benefit from regulatory adjustments to increase competition, this dynamic raises questions about how much further generic drug prices can be reduced by promoting competition in general.

Preventing generic drug price spikes would certainly benefit the patients who depend on these medications. But that positive outcome should not be confused with addressing high drug prices in the aggregate. That is because the drugs most likely to lack real generic competition tend to serve small markets and hence add little to overall drug spending. For example, the US Department of Health and Human Services (HHS) observed that between July 1, 2013 and June 30, 2014, less than one-eighth of expenditures were for drugs for which prices increased substantially (more than 20%).[38] Because generic drugs account for less than one-fourth of all US drug costs,[15pxviii] cases like Shkreli's Daraprim, while outrageous, do not explain the drug cost problem in the aggregate. Referring to stories like Daraprim, HHS summed up their findings by noting, "These spikes are on one hand troubling in that they disadvantage particular patient groups but also sufficiently limited so they exert no sizable influence on overall drug spending."[38p1]

Lower Prices Through Even More Competition

In part, improving competition in pharmaceutical markets means encouraging competition among branded products, and some proposals attempt to do so with ideas, such as more efficient trial designs to accelerate the drug approval process (see Chapter 10 of this volume). But because brand-name drug companies may retain considerable leverage before their products lose exclusivity—even in cases where there exists competition from other brands (see Chapter 2 of this volume)—proposals to address drug costs often focus on what critics see as unnecessary obstacles to the introduction of generic competition. We consider three areas of controversy.

Pay for Delay

As the *New York Times* remarked, "the pharmaceutical company Cephalon had a cash cow on its hands" to the tune of around $900 million a year by 2007 for its drug, Provigil, used to treat excessive sleepiness.[39] But Cephalon had a problem: the patents protecting Provigil's market exclusivity were approaching expiration. In the old days, before passage of the 1984 Hatch–Waxman Act, that would have posed little worry to the manufacturer. Before the act, each generic drug manufacturer had to conduct the same long, expensive clinical trials (described in Chapter 2 of this volume) to establish the safety and efficacy of their copy of a drug. Hatch–Waxman eased matters for generic manufacturers by requiring that they only demonstrate therapeutic equivalence with the original drug. With potential profits looming, it was a good bet that companies would market generic versions of Provigil as soon as its patent protection expired.

With this threat approaching, Cephalon's leadership saw an opportunity for a win–win solution for itself and generic drug companies. They realized that the money to be earned collectively by Cephalon and the copycats would be much diminished by open competition because prices for everyone's version of the drug would be decimated. What if, instead, the monopolistic prices could be preserved and the resulting revenues shared between Cephalon and its aspiring competitors?

That reasoning produced a series of arrangements between Cephalon and the generic manufacturers whereby Cephalon paid them $300 million for the "intellectual property" they had created in developing therapeutically equivalent versions of Provigil. In return, the generic companies agreed to withhold their versions until 2012. Cephalon continued to enjoy monopoly pricing power (minus the $300 million it had to pay to the copycats), and the generic manufacturers, having developed generic Provigil, could collect a check with no further effort.

Consumers, on the other hand, suffered because they continued to pay monopolistic prices for Provigil. The Federal Trade Commission (FTC) sued Cephalon for impeding consumer choice, and ultimately (in 2015, after a seven-year law suit) the company settled with the government, agreeing to pay $1.2 billion to parties (e.g., insurance companies) that had "overpaid" for Provigil in the interim. In a similar case that the FTC did not settle, the Supreme Court ruled that outlays from brand-name to generic manufacturers can usually be regarded as "reverse payments" to block competition and that FTC findings that the payments reflect violations of anti-trust laws are justified.

After those cases, such reverse payments greatly diminished, suggesting that the FTC has largely addressed this problem.[40] Still, the impact was modest. The FTC argued that these arrangements cost American consumers $3.5 billion each year[41]—real money to be sure, but quite small relative to the $500 billion annual spend on prescription drugs.

Complex Generics

A year before the outbreak of America's Civil War, Henry Salter, a physician in England, wrote, "Asthma is immediately cured in situations of either sudden alarm or violent fleeting excitements." That observation suggested a possible therapeutic intervention (i.e., natural adrenaline) to reverse asthma attacks and, more generally, potentially fatal anaphylaxis attacks in which victims find it difficult to breathe following exposure to an allergen (like peanuts). Chemical company Parke-Davis filed for a patent for adrenaline (known chemically as epinephrine) in 1901 and therapeutic use by hypodermic administration began by 1909.[42]

More than a century later, in 2016, a single dose of epinephrine, its patent long-expired, costs about one dollar to manufacturer.[43] It had been available in a popular dispenser called the "EpiPen" at under $100 for a two-pack. In that year, its manufacturer, Mylan, increased the two-pack price to $600. After the ensuing outcry, it produced a generic version available for $300 per two-pack, a price still three times higher than previous one.[44] Teva Pharmaceuticals announced it would introduce its own generic EpiPen, also at $300 per two-pack. Once again, effective generic competition seemed absent, despite US EpiPen sales of $750 million per year.[45]

In this case, the "barrier to market entry" was not duplication of an active ingredient but development of a competing delivery mechanism. Although epinephrine's patent has long expired, the patent for the EpiPen's auto-injector delivery device protects Mylan until 2025.[46] Competitors are working on EpiPen alternatives, but with customers placing a premium on reliability, no company has yet created an acceptable substitute.[46]

Epinephrine illustrates how the expedited pathway for generics provided by the 1984 Hatch–Waxman Act can become congested. For epinephrine, safety and effectiveness also depend on how the product is delivered. A simple demonstration of "bioequivalence"—that is, that the generic copy is absorbed and distributed throughout the body as it does in the original—does not establish that generic epinephrine matches the originator's safety and effectiveness.[47] If a generic manufacturer could copy the EpiPen, they could piggyback on its prior FDA approval. However, patent protection on the EpiPen (rather than epinephrine itself) makes that impossible until those patents expire (in 2025). Generic manufacturers must instead develop and receive FDA approval for their own epinephrine delivery devices, a far more time-consuming and expensive undertaking than a conventional demonstration of bioequivalence.

Nor is epinephrine a unique case. Former FDA Commissioner Scott Gottlieb considers it an example of "complex generic medicines"—that is, products for which bioequivalence alone fails to establish safety and efficacy equivalence to an originator drug because the medicine's performance depends on delivery by a patented device (as in the EpiPen case) or because it acts in the gut rather than the bloodstream (where bioequivalence is measured). As Gottlieb has observed, complex medicines are relatively common among injectable drugs, noting, "It's many of these old 'parenteral' medicines that have recently been in shortage, and have seen some enormous price increases."[47]

Gottlieb's proposed solution includes granting FDA authority to examine data beyond bioequivalence when evaluating complex generic drugs. For epinephrine, for example, the FDA could investigate whether patients can use a new delivery device as safely and reliably as they use an EpiPen, rather than insisting on either an equivalent device (which is prohibited by patents) or complete regulatory review required for a novel design. Gottlieb also suggests allowing generic versions of complex generic medicines to include usage instructions that differ in minor ways from the instructions for the original drug, thus facilitating the introduction of new competing delivery devices.

The EpiPen case, while well known, is but one example of the challenge posed by complex generic medicines. Although there are others, the total value of products in this category is unclear, as is how much total drug costs might be reduced if the problem were addressed. Moreover, technical challenges hinder any path forward. Mylan's EpiPen patents protect its innovative technology—as evidenced by the difficulty competitors are having in developing alternatives. What is the proper duration for protection of that technology? For drugs not administered via the typical pathway (i.e., gut intake, blood stream absorption) regulators need approaches to measure the analog to bioequivalence. Otherwise, they cannot know if a copy is therapeutically similar to the original.

Biosimilars

In terms of its contribution to US health costs, Abbvie's Humira (adalimunab), a drug used to treat a host of immune system conditions including rheumatoid arthritis, Crohn's disease, and psoriasis, is a clear champion. At revenues exceeding $18 billion annually in 2017, it topped the runner up—Rituxan (rituximab), a cancer drug sold by Genentech and Biogen—by a factor of nearly two.[48] By way of comparison, Humira's sales exceed the EpiPen's ($750 million per year)[49] by a factor of nearly 25 and peak annual revenues of Turing Pharmaceutical's Daraprim ($78.5 million)[50] by more than 230.

Humira is a biologic, a large, complex molecule generally produced by a biological system, such as a cell culture or plant (see Chapter 2 of this volume). Biologics include both older drugs (e.g., insulin) and new ones. According to reports, less than 2% of Americans are prescribed biologics, but those biologics comprise 35% of drug spending.[51] As noted in Chapter 2 of this volume, Congress enacted laws to promote competition for biologics by allowing their exclusivity to expire 12 years after the FDA first licenses a product.

Although rules for biosimilars took effect in 2010, their uptake in the United States has been sluggish.[52] As of November 2019, the FDA had approved 25 biosimilars that could, in theory, be substituted for nine different "reference" biologics,[53] but manufacturers had made biosimilars available for only four.[54p5] Estimated savings from biosimilars in the United States amounted to only $250 million annually, roughly 1% of Humira's sales. The future promises greater returns. The RAND Corporation projected potential savings of $54 billion over 10 years from biosimilars or $5.4 billion per year. The Pacific Research Institute estimated savings of $7.2 billion per year if the biosimilars market grows to 75% of total sales.[54(p.5)] Even these figures are relatively small, however, compared to total US biologic sales of $120 billion annually.[55]

Why such limited savings for biologics when generic copies of small molecule drugs save some $300 billion each year (see previous discussion)? Industry watchers have identified multiple intertwined factors, including (i) a slow regulatory process; (ii) vigorous protection of (often complex and overlapping) patents by the brand-name biologic originators (the so-called patent thicket problem)[56]; (iii) difficulty establishing that biosimilars can readily substitute for originator biologics; and (iv) inadequate education of physicians to promote substitutions.[57] The first two factors slow the introduction of biosimilar competitors. The remaining factors hamper uptake even after biosimilars receive FDA approval because pharmacies need approval from prescribing physicians to substitute biosimilars if the biosimilar has not been designated interchangeable, and US physicians have limited incentives to make substitutions. Marketing campaigns promoting the idea that biosimilars are inferior to originator biologics may further impede uptake. Yet another barrier may be the power of brand-name drug companies to engage in aggressive price reductions to cause biosimilar manufacturers with large start-up costs to lose money.[58] Whatever the cause, there are fewer approved biosimilars in the US as compared to Europe, and even fewer that have been marketed. Moreover, existing biosimilars tend to have a smaller market share of each biologic class, and downward pressures on originator biologics are much less pronounced.[57]

Because of the various obstacles, some have argued that biosimilars will never achieve much success in reducing prices for biologics.[59] Indeed, some critics contend that the barriers bestow "natural monopoly" characteristics for biologics. Rather than continuing to promote biosimilars in the face of those obstacles, they instead suggest that the US government should simply mandate the desired outcome—that is, low prices once the 12-year exclusivity period for the originator biologic expires. Bach and Trusheim argue that the idea would have collateral benefits in speeding innovation by precluding the costly and time-consuming testing requirements that biosimilar manufacturers have to undertake and by freeing up patients who would otherwise be diverted for biosimilar clinical trials from other clinical studies.[60] Investor, author, and virologist Peter Kolchinsky has argued more generally that we should employ price controls "for drugs that appear to be immune to genericization after their patents expire."[28p103] He would have the government set prices close to the cost of production, regulating such products as one would a public utility or the biodefense industry.

Even so, the savings would likely be modest. Kolchinsky has estimated that 96% of the US government's branded drug spending (approximately $148 billion in 2018) is on drugs that will drop in price as generics or biosimilars come to market (leaving only 4% or roughly $6 billion of this spending on drugs that cannot go generic).[28pp96–97,61] Trusheim et al. (2019) estimate that if biologic prices after exclusivity expiration were capped at 10% to 30% of the original price, savings would amount to $50 to $60 billion annually between 2018 and 2022.[59] Setting aside arguments about whether price controls on biologics are the best response to the issues identified, the estimates suggest that $50 and $60 billion might be an upper bound for annual savings that biosimilars (or price controls) might achieve. Those savings are substantial, representing roughly half of current US spending on biologics. However, it would reduce overall drug costs of roughly $500 billion in the United States by 12% to 15%—important to be sure, but not enough to eliminate the problem posed by high drug prices. Crucially, new biologics would continue to enjoy market exclusivity and hence monopoly pricing power for 12 years following licensure.

Why Can't the US Get Canada's (or England's) Drug Prices?

The evening's news footage was dramatic. On a Sunday in July 2019, as the presidential preprimary season ground on, Vermont senator and presidential candidate Bernie Sanders crossed the Canadian border with a busload of individuals with diabetes, television camera crews in tow. Their destination: a drug store in Windsor, Ontario. Their mission: to purchase insulin.[62]

The media entourage may have been unusual, but the purchase of prescription drugs from abroad was not. Eight percent of respondents to a 2016 Kaiser Family Foundation poll reported that they or a household family member had purchased prescription drugs from another country to save money.[63] It is not difficult to see why. Insulin prices in the United States tripled between 2002 and 2013; for patients with type 1 diabetes, the annual cost of life-saving insulin treatment increased from roughly $12,000 in 2012 to $18,000 in 2016.[64] Some news outlets have reported that north of the border, insulin sells for one-tenth its US price.[65]

Insulin may present a particularly egregious case, but broader surveys comparing US drug prices to those abroad also reveal striking disparities. HIS Markit POLI, a global pharmaceutical pricing database estimated that prescription drug prices in Canada were 65% lower than in the United States. Other studies show that average prices across other high-income countries—including Australia, Canada, France, Germany, Japan, Italy, Spain, and the United Kingdom—were 56% of those in the United States.[66]

Unsurprisingly, 80% of Americans favor legalizing prescription drug imports from Canada.[67] Lawmakers have responded, with 30 bills filed in 17 states as of August 2019—although absent federal government legalization of such imports (most drug importation remains illegal because of concerns about the safety and efficacy of such products), these proposals will have little real effect.[68] The Trump administration has expressed interest in the idea, with Health and Human Services (HHS) Secretary Alex Azar declaring in July 2019, "for the first time in HHS's history, we are open to importation."[69] Prospects for action remain unclear, however. As of August 2019, laws beginning the process to permit prescription drug imports had passed in only two states: Florida and Vermont. Even if enacted, President Trump's plan could take years of regulatory review before implementation.[70] In the meantime, importation of many drugs—including insulin—would remain illegal.

Nor is the Canadian government excited about the idea of exporting its prescription drugs to the United States. Officials there have cited a 2010 study concluding that Canadian drug supplies would be exhausted in under eight months if the United States imported even 10% of its prescription drugs from its northern neighbor.[71] An April 2019 briefing for Canadian government officials stated bluntly, "Canada does not support actions that could adversely affect the supply of prescription drugs in Canada and potentially raise costs of prescription drugs for Canadians."[71]

The call to legalize prescription drug imports is something of a red herring. When it comes to pricing drugs, Canada and other countries do not possess inherent advantages, such as more efficient drug manufacturing facilities, compared to the United States. Instead, drugs are more expensive in the United States because, as highlighted in Chapter 2 of this volume, the US government purposely grants companies that develop new drugs a monopoly (which is similar to what happens in Canada and Europe) and allows them to charge what the market will bear (which is not similar to Canada and Europe). As the Canadian government helpfully offered, "importing drugs from Canada is probably not your silver bullet."[71] Rather, it suggested to US officials that other solutions existed for restraining drug costs.[71] They advised that Americans could enjoy Canadian prices by adopting Canadian policies. In other words, a US resident need not board Bernie Sanders's bus, or even bother with cross-border mail-order delivery, to receive those benefits.

Even adoption of Canadian policies may be unnecessary. Instead of mimicking their policies, the United States need only mimic Canadian prices. So-called reference pricing or index pricing dictates that drug companies charge no more for their products in the United States than a benchmark reflecting what they charge elsewhere (e.g., in selected European countries).

In 2018, the Trump administration proposed reference pricing for Medicare Part B drugs (medications administered in a doctor's office or outpatient hospital setting).[72,73] Under existing rules, Medicare reimburses doctors for drugs and tops off payments with a 6% commission. Drug companies are paid whatever price they choose to charge (accounting for what they perceive the market can bear) and, through the commission, the doctor's pay grows along with the drug's price. For example, a physician receives $60 to administer a drug that costs $1,000, and $120 to administer one that costs $2,000. Trump's proposal holds the doctor's commission constant, so he or she gains no advantage from administering more expensive drugs. Most strikingly, the proposal sets the drug's price based on an index reflecting prices in 16 countries: Austria, Belgium, Canada, Czech Republic, Finland, France, Germany, Greece, Ireland, Italy, Japan, Portugal, Slovakia, Spain, Sweden, and the United Kingdom.

In a policy brief, HHS estimated that the proposal would reduce Medicare Part B prices by 30%, saving American tax payers $17.2 billion over five years; individuals would see out-of-pocket costs fall by $3.4 billion over that time period.[74] While those savings are modest in the context of Medicare and Medicaid's $1 trillion annual budget, they would certainly be welcome and perhaps, if expanded, could help meaningfully narrow the gap between American and other countries' drug prices. A 2019 Johns Hopkins study estimated that if Medicare paid what other countries pay for Part D drugs (medications purchased over the counter in pharmacies), it would save $73 billion annually.[75]

The HHS brief on the Trump administration proposal suggested such savings were achievable at essentially no cost, noting there would be "no changes to the Medicare benefit, just more discounts from drug companies."[74] It added that the proposal's "free-market approach seeks the same type of discounts that drug makers already voluntarily negotiate with economically-similar countries"[74] and that "the Trump Administration will only pursue drug pricing solutions that will protect the incentives for inventing new cures and protect patient access."[74]

In fact, the likely outcome is much less clear. In response to the Trump administration's proposal, a coalition of medical associations, patient advocates, drug companies, and other groups[76] submitted a letter to Congress arguing that the proposal could deny US residents access to treatments and would threaten incentives for innovation.[77] The letter suggests that the US would "import" those adverse impacts experienced in other countries.

Even if those resulting impacts were minor (and conceivably they could be substantial), by adopting other countries' prices, the United States would implicitly embrace the preferences and trade-offs made by their decision makers and hence *their* notions of value. Possibly, US residents would find those trade-offs acceptable, but the United States would defer its value assessment to 16 other countries—chosen not because of a due diligence review of their decisions but because they are often "reference priced" by other higher-income countries, and because they make their drug pricing data readily available.[72,78] In other words, the United States would simply "outsource" its policy-making and absolve itself of responsibility to review drug value itself.

Taking Control Through Negotiation

"Congress should focus on price negotiations on key drugs for the same reason that bank robbers rob banks: Because that's where all the money is," said Ben Wakana, executive director of Patients for Affordable Drugs in June 2019.[79] Given its prescription drug spending, the US Medicare program would have strong leverage to achieve favorable prices. For example, Medicare Part D spent $101 billion in 2017, roughly 30% of the nation's total retail prescription drug spending.[80]

In a sense, Medicare negotiates Part D drug prices, but only indirectly, through the efforts of the many private insurance companies and PBMs that administer the program. As a practical matter, those companies have limited leverage because no one company has broad coverage of the Medicare population; the largest covers little more than one in five Medicare beneficiaries.[81] While negotiations on behalf of the entire program would no doubt achieve greater leverage, the Medicare Modernization Act of 2003 states that the HHS secretary "may not interfere with the negotiations between drug manufacturers and pharmacies and [Part D Plan] sponsors, and may not require a particular formulary or institute a price structure for the reimbursement of covered Part D drugs."[82]

Some federal lawmakers urge preservation of this prohibition. Senator Chuck Grassley of Iowa has argued that "the non-interference clause ensures that plan sponsors create plan options that respond to what beneficiaries want" and prevents the establishment of a "one-size-fits-all list of covered drugs."[83] That view, coupled with Republican control of the Senate and lower-than-expected Part D drug costs due to a substantial number of brand name drug patent expirations, has kept price negotiation legislation on Congress's back burner.[84]

But others have kept the idea alive. In 2019, California governor Gavin Newsom issued an executive order calling for the use of California's purchasing power "to create significant negotiating leverage on behalf of over 13 million Californians and generate substantial annual [medication cost] savings."[85] Some members of Congress have introduced their own bills. The proposals differ in detail—for example, some eliminate Medicare's noninterference clause while others remove the clause while also requiring the secretary of HHS to negotiate to reduce drug prices.[84]

Achieving lower prices through direct Medicare negotiation has its own trade-offs. Any credible negotiator must be willing to walk away from the table—in other words, deny access to a drug if its price is not acceptable. As the Congressional Budget Office noted,

> for HHS to use the greater market share of the entire Medicare population as a source of leverage to secure deeper price discounts and greater cost savings, it would probably have to threaten similar exclusions and limitations on coverage for that entire population—a threat that could be difficult to make credible given the potential impact on stakeholders.[86]

Various proposals offer tactics that ostensibly avoid the need to threaten such outright denials. These tactics include competitive licensing (granting the government authority to remove a drug manufacturer's exclusivity privileges) or fallback pricing (allowing the government to impose a "default price"—e.g., pricing from another country). Another idea is binding arbitration (granting a neutral third party the power to choose between the drug company's proposed pricing and the government's recommended terms).[87] The hope is that the chance of "losing" a binding arbitration case would compel drug manufacturers to issue moderate, "reasonable" proposals in the first place.[87]

Even these tactics pose a risk to government interests, however. All of these measures make future drug company profits less certain, a prospect that reduces the expected return on investment and hence the incentives for drug companies to invest in research and development.[84] The eventual consequence is less innovation and foregone benefits in the form of reduced patient health. Estimating these foregone benefits is challenging, but the trade-offs cannot be dismissed. Kolchinsky has estimated that if branded drug spending could somehow fall by 90%, it would result in a one-time reduction of 6.7% of healthcare spending, reflecting about 1.2% of US gross domestic product; however, it would grind the "innovation conveyer belt" to a halt, depriving future generations of advances for migraine, bone fracture, cancer, diabetes and many other diseases.[28p26] Ideally, negotiators would maximize benefits by focusing on drugs that would yield the greatest savings (e.g., products lacking competition and hence having inordinately high prices).[87] At the same time, negotiators should signal to drug companies the type of innovation that will be rewarded. Effective signaling will best guide future industry spending, but will depend on an ability to characterize each drug's value so that manufacturers can be appropriately compensated.

Houston, We Still Have a Problem

There is no shortage of suggested fixes to high drug prices. And yet, as this chapter highlights, an effective solution remains elusive.

The policy puzzle is intrinsic to the prescription drug market (Chapter 2, this volume). On the supply side, the challenge is to protect revenue streams so that manufacturers have incentives to make the substantial, risky investments needed to develop those drugs in the first place.

That leaves incremental solutions. Eliminating the PBM "middlemen" that tap into drug company revenues would save at most 10% on prescription drug spending. Moreover, PBMs play a useful role by achieving hard-to-win concessions from drug companies. Bolstering generic competition in markets for older drugs with expired patents would help—and would mitigate the behavior of a few shameless actors who have exploited market imperfections. However, the total savings would be miniscule relative to the nation's annual drug spend. Ensuring generic competition—or at least lower prices—following expiration of market exclusivity and patent protections for brand-name drugs could conceivably have a larger impact—especially for biologics. But even these measures would produce a modest dent in the nation's $500 billion annual drug bill.

Proposed "demand-side" solutions have greater potential. If the United States "imported" drug prices imposed in other wealthy countries or allowed the federal government to leverage its own purchasing power, drug prices in the United States would decrease. But would the new, lower prices be *better*? As we previously argued, the government's leverage to force drug prices down, saving patients money, could choke off development of new drugs, limiting patient access to their health benefits. Whether reduced drug access hurts the population depends on how a drug's price compares to the value of its health benefits. *Paying more for a drug than the value of its health benefits clearly leaves the population worse off.* On the other hand, *insisting on a lower price might discourage drug industry innovation, foreclosing access to new drugs.* The point is that estimating the value of a drug's health benefits is crucial to establishing appropriate pricing. Characterizing the value of a drug's health benefits presents myriad challenges. We turn to these next.

References

1. Karlin-Smith, S. 2017, January 11. "Trump says drug industry 'getting away with murder.'" *Politico.* Accessed January 25, 2021. https://www.politico.com/story/2017/01/trump-press-conference-drug-industry-233475.
2. Grassley, C. 2019. "Grassley op-ed: Top priority is reducing health care costs." Accessed January 25, 2021. https://www.grassley.senate.gov/news/news-releases/grassley-op-ed-top-priority-reducing-health-care-costs.
3. Grassley, C. 2019. "Grassley, Wyden invite 7 major pharmaceutical companies to drug pricing hearing." January 25, 2021. https://www.grassley.senate.gov/news/news-releases/grassley-wyden-invite-7-major-pharmaceutical-companies-drug-pricing-hearing.
4. Drash, W. 2019. "Senator: Big pharma is 'morally repugnant.'" *CNN.* Accessed January 25, 2021. https://www.cnn.com/2019/02/26/health/senate-hearing-skyrocketing-drug-prices/index.html.
5. Jaffa, E. 2019. "Bernie Sanders and Elizabeth Warren team up to lower prescription drug prices." *Common Dreams.* Accessed January 25, 2021. https://www.commondreams.org/views/2019/02/02/bernie-sanders-and-elizabeth-warren-team-lower-prescription-drug-prices.
6. Facher, L. 2019. "Biden puts forth an elaborate—and aggressive—plan to lower drug prices." *STAT.* Accessed January 25, 2021. https://www.statnews.com/2019/07/15/biden-drug-pricing-plan/.

7. Whyte, D. 2016. "Top 10 pharmaceutical hubs in the USA." *Proclinical.* Accessed January 25, 2021. https://www.proclinical.com/blogs/2016-3/top-10-pharmaceutical-hubs-in-the-usa.

8. Bebinger, M. 2019. "Baker outlines steps to lower Medicaid drug prices." *CommonHealth.* Accessed January 25, 2021. https://www.wbur.org/commonhealth/2019/01/24/baker-steps-lower-medicaid-drug-prices.

9. Young, S. 2019. "Newson: California leads on prescription drugs." *Kaiser Health News.* Accessed January 25, 2021. https://khn.org/news/newsom-california-leads-on-prescription-drugs/.

10. Kolata, G. 2008, April 14. "Co-payments soar for drugs with high prices." *The New York Times.* Accessed January 25, 2021. https://www.nytimes.com/2008/04/14/us/14drug.html?mtrref=www.google.com&gwh=8A2E2317A7B1F110F341CC7AEB3B9383&gwt=pay&assetType=REGIWALL.

11. Bartlett, D.L., and Steele, J.B. 2004. "Why we pay so much for drugs." *CNN.* Accessed January 25, 2021. https://www.cnn.com/2004/ALLPOLITICS/01/27/timep.drugs.tm/.

12. Werble, C. 2017, September 14. "Pharmacy benefit managers." *Health Affairs.* https://doi.org/10.1377/hpb20171409.000178.

13. "Pharmacy benefit managers and their role in drug spending." 2019. *Commonwealth Fund.* Accessed January 25, 2021. https://www.commonwealthfund.org/publications/explainer/2019/apr/pharmacy-benefit-managers-and-their-role-drug-spending.

14. Roehrig, C. 2018. "The impact of prescription drug rebates on health plans and consumers." *Altarum.* https://altarum.org/sites/default/files/Altarum-Prescription-Drug-Rebate-Report_April-2018.pdf.

15. National Academies of Sciences Engineering, and Medicine. 2018. "Complexity in Action." In *Making medicines affordable: A national imperative,* edited by N.R. Augustine, G. Madhavan, and S.J. Nass, 31–72. Washington, DC: The National Academies Press.

16. Paavola, A. 2019. "Top PBMs by market share." *Becker Hospital Review.* Accessed January 25, 2021. https://www.beckershospitalreview.com/pharmacy/top-pbms-by-market-share.html.

17. Sood, N., Shih, T., Van Nuys, K., and Goldman, D.P. 2017. "Follow the money: The flow of funds in the pharmaceutical distribution system." *Health Affairs Blog.* https://www.healthaffairs.org/do/10.1377/hblog20170613.060557/full/.

18. "Which firms profit most from America's health-care system." 2018, March 15. *The Economist.* https://www.economist.com/business/2018/03/15/which-firms-profit-most-from-americas-health-care-system.

19. Royce, T.J., Kircher, S., and Conti, R.M. 2019. "Pharmacy benefit manager reform: Lessons from Ohio." *JAMA* 322 (4): 299–300. https://doi.org/10.1001/jama.2019.7104.

20. Mershon, E., and Swetlitz, I. 2018. "Trump denounces 'middlemen' and largely spares pharma in drug pricing speech." *STAT Medicine.* Accessed January 25, 2021. https://www.scientificamerican.com/article/trump-denounces-middlemen-and-largely-spares-pharma-in-drug-pricing-speech/.

21. Department of Health & Human Services. 2019. *Fact sheet: Trump administration proposes to lower drug costs by targeting backdoor rebates and encouraging direct discounts to patients.*

22. Congressional Budget Office. 2019. *Incorporating the effects of the proposed rule on safe harbors for pharmaceutical rebates in CBO's budget projections—supplemental material for updates budget projections: 2019 to 2029.*

23. Sullivan, T. 2019. "Trump backs away from plan to ban rebates to PBMs." *Policy & Medicine.* Accessed January 25, 2021. https://www.policymed.com/2019/08/trump-backs-away-from-plan-to-ban-rebates-to-pbms.html.

24. Toy, S. 2019. "Stocks of drug distributors and PBM-owners surge after Trump administration pulls rebate proposal." *Market Watch.* Accessed January 25, 2021. https://www.

marketwatch.com/story/stocks-of-drug-distributors-and-pbm-owners-surge-after-trump-administration-pulls-rebate-proposal-2019-07-11.

25. "Generic competition and drug prices." 2017. *U.S. Food & Drug Administration.* Last Modified December 13, 2019. Accessed January 25, 2021. https://www.fda.gov/about-fda/center-drug-evaluation-and-research-cder/generic-competition-and-drug-prices.

26. Association for Accessible Medicines. 2019. *The case for competition: 2019 generic drug & biosimilars access & savings in the U.S. report.*

27. "Generic drugs." 2019. *U.S. Food & Drug Administration.* Accessed January 25, 2021. https://www.fda.gov/drugs/buying-using-medicine-safely/generic-drugs.

28. Kolchinsky, P. 2019. *The great American drug deal.* Boston: Evelexa Press.

29. Gupta, R., Kesselheim, A.S., Downing, N., Greene, J., and Ross, J.S. 2016. "Generic drug approvals since the 1984 Hatch-Waxman Act." *JAMA Internal Medicine* 176 (9): 1391–1393. https://doi.org/10.1001/jamainternmed.2016.3411.

30. US Food and Drug Administration. 2017. "Drugs@FDA glossary of terms." Accessed January 25, 2021. https://www.fda.gov/drugs/drug-approvals-and-databases/drugsfda-glossary-terms#B.

31. Greene, J.A., Anderson, G., and Sharfstein, J.M. 2016. "Role of the FDA in affordability of off-patent pharmaceuticals." *JAMA* 315 (5): 461–462. https://doi.org/10.1001/jama.2015.18720.

32. Jaret, P. 2015. "Prices spike for some generic drugs." *AARP Bulletin.* https://www.aarp.org/health/drugs-supplements/info-2015/prices-spike-for-generic-drugs.html.

33. US Government Accountability Office. 2016. *Generic drugs under Medicare: Part D generic drug prices declined overall, but some had extraordinary price increases.*

34. Sudden price spikes in off-patent prescription drugs: The monopoly business model that harms patients, taxpayers, and the U.S. health care system. S. Rept. 114-429, 114th Congr. (2015–2016) (S.M. Collins and C. McCaskill).

35. Luthra, S. 2018. "'Pharma bro' Shkreli is in prison, but Daraprim's price is still high." *Kaiser Health News.* Accessed January 25, 2021. https://khn.org/news/for-shame-pharma-bro-shkreli-is-in-prison-but-daraprims-price-is-still-high/.

36. Wouters, O.J., Kanavos, P.G., and McKee, K.M. 2017. "Comparing generic drug markets in Europe and the United States: Prices, volumes, and spending." *Milbank Q* 95 (3): 554–601. https://doi.org/10.1111/1468-0009.12279.

37. Engelberg, A.B., Avorn, J., and Kesselheim, A.S. 2016, February 26. "Addressing generic drug unaffordability and shortages by globalizing the market for old drugs." *Health Affairs.* https://doi.org/10.1377/hblog20160223.053266.

38. US Department of Health and Human Services, Office of the Assistant Secretary for Planning and Evaluation. 2016. *Understanding recent trends in generic drug prices.* ASPE issue brief.

39. Ruiz, R.R., and Thomas, K. 2015. "Teva settles Cephalon generics case with F.T.C for $1.2 Billion." *The New York Times.* Accessed January 25, 2021. https://www.nytimes.com/2015/05/29/business/teva-cephalon-provigil-ftc-settlement.html?_r=0.

40. Barlas, S. 2019. "FTC gives generics victory on 'pay for delay': Reverse payments crimped, patent thickets untouched." *P T* 44 (5): 234–266. https://doi.org/10.3390/ph3082470.

41. Silverman, E. 2016. "Supreme Court lets pay-to-delay ruling against pharma stand." *STAT.* Accessed January 25, 2021. https://www.statnews.com/pharmalot/2016/11/07/supreme-court-pay-delay-glaxo-teva/.

42. Arthur, G. 2015. "Epinephrine: A short history." *Lancet Respiratory Medicine* 3 (5): 350–351. https://doi.org/10.1016/S2213-2600(15)00087-9.

43. Donachie, R. 2016, August 24. "The price explosion for EpiPen's is linked to one key gov't decision." *Daily Caller.* Accessed January 25, 2021. https://dailycaller.com/2016/08/24/the-price-explosion-for-epipens-is-linked-to-one-key-govt-decision/.

44. Kokosky, G. 2019, January. "Newly approved generic version of EpiPen is not cheaper than available option." *Pharmacy Times*. Accessed January 25, 2021. https://www.pharmacytimes.com/publications/issue/2019/january2019/newly-approved-generic-version-of-epipen-is-not-cheaper-than-available-option.

45. Cohen, T. 2019. "Teva expects sales injection from U.S. EpiPen market." *Reuters*. Accessed January 25, 2021. https://www.reuters.com/article/us-teva-pharm-ind-outlook/teva-expects-sales-injection-from-u-s-epipen-market-idUSKCN1Q80TH.

46. Keshavan, M. 2016. "5 reasons why no one has built a better EpiPen." *STAT*. Accessed January 25, 2021. https://www.statnews.com/2016/09/09/epipen-lack-of-innovation/.

47. Gottlieb, S. 2016, October 24. "EpiPen shows a path to solve the bigger drug pricing challenge." *Forbes*. Accessed January 25, 2021. https://www.forbes.com/sites/scottgottlieb/2016/10/24/epipen-drug-pricing-challenge/#6aa9719858a6.

48. Philippidis, A. 2018. "The top 15 best-selling drugs of 2017." *Genetic Engineering & Biotechnology News*. Accessed January 25, 2021. https://www.genengnews.com/a-lists/the-top-15-best-selling-drugs-of-2017/.

49. Keown, A. 2019. "Teva eyes 25 percent of the $750 million EpiPen market by year's end." *BioSpace*. Accessed January 25, 2021. https://www.biospace.com/article/teva-eyes-25-percent-of-the-750-million-epipen-market-by-year-s-end/.

50. Mole, B. 2018. "The 5,000% price hike that made Martin Shkreli infamous is no longer paying off." *arsTechnica*. Accessed January 25, 2021. https://arstechnica.com/tech-policy/2018/07/shkrelis-former-company-is-now-losing-money-even-with-the-5000-price-hike/.

51. "Biosimilar drugs promise to slash health-care costs in rich countries." 2018, November 10. *The Economist*. Accessed January 25, 2021. https://www.economist.com/business/2018/11/10/biosimilar-drugs-promise-to-slash-health-care-costs-in-rich-countries.

52. Baghdadi, R. 2017, July 21. "Biosimilars." *Health Affairs*. https://doi.org/10.1377/hpb20170721.487227.

53. US Food and Drug Administration. 2019. "Biosimilar product information." Last modified December 17, 2020. Accessed January 25, 2021. https://www.fda.gov/drugs/biosimilars/biosimilar-product-information.

54. Winegarden, W. 2019. "The biosimilar opportunity: A state breakdown." *Pacific Research Institute, Center for Medical Economics and Innovation*. https://www.pacificresearch.org/wp-content/uploads/2019/10/BiosimilarSavings_web.pdf.

55. IQVIA. 2018. "Medicine use and spending in the U.S.: A review of 2017 and outlook to 2022." https://www.iqvia.com/-/media/iqvia/pdfs/institute-reports/medicine-use-and-spending-in-the-us-a-review-of-2017-and-outlook-to-2022.pdf?_=1600097137961.

56. Brennan, Z. 2019. "Biologic patent thickets: New bill aims to publicize info." *Regulatory Affairs Professionals Society*. Accessed January 25, 2021. https://www.raps.org/news-and-articles/news-articles/2019/3/biologic-patent-thickets-new-bill-aims-to-publici.

57. Cohen, J. 2018, June 20. "What's holding back market uptake of biosimilars?" *Forbes*. Accessed January 25, 2021. https://www.forbes.com/sites/joshuacohen/2018/06/20/whats-holding-back-market-uptake-of-biosimilars/#1f28a987691a.

58. Chambers, J.D., Lai, R.C., Margaretos, N.M., Panzer, A.D., Cohen, J.T., and Neumann, P.J. 2020. "Coverage for biosimilars vs reference products among US commercial health plans." *JAMA* 323 (19): 1972–1973. https://doi.org/10.1001/jama.2020.2229.

59. Trusheim, M.R., Atteberry, P., Ohn, J.A., and Bach, P.B. 2019, April 15. "Biologics are natural monopolies (Part 2): A proposal for post-exclusivity price regulation of biologics." *Health Affairs*. https://doi.org/10.1377/hblog20190405.839549.

60. Bach, P.B., and Trusheim, M. 2019, August 21. "Time to throw in the towel on biosimilars." *Wall Street Journal*. Accessed January 25, 2021. https://www.wsj.com/articles/time-to-throw-in-the-towel-on-biosimilars-11566428299.

61. Centers for Medicare & Medicaid Services. 2020. "NHE fact sheet." Last modified December 17, 2020. Accessed January 25, 2021. https://www.cms.gov/Research-Statistics-Data-and-Systems/Statistics-Trends-and-Reports/NationalHealthExpendData/NHE-Fact-Sheet#:~:text=Historical%20NHE%2C%202018%3A,16%20percent%20of%20total%20NHE.

62. Spalding, D. 2019. "Bernie Sanders visits Canadian pharmacy, talks drug prices." *Reuters*. Accessed January 25, 2021. https://www.reuters.com/article/us-usa-election-sanders-canada/bernie-sanders-visits-canadian-pharmacy-talks-drug-prices-idUSKCN1UN0SV.

63. Kaiser Family Foundation. 2016. "Kaiser health tracking poll: November 2016." http://files.kff.org/attachment/Kaiser-Health-Tracking-Poll-November-2016-Topline.

64. Rappold, R.S. 2019. "Families cross borders in search for affordable insulin." *WebMD*. Accessed January 25, 2021. https://www.webmd.com/diabetes/news/20190718/spiking-insulin-costs-put-patients-in-brutal-bind.

65. Harrop, F. 2019. "Drug price gouging: An American story." *RealClear Politics*. Accessed January 25, 2021. https://www.realclearpolitics.com/articles/2019/07/16/drug_price_gouging_an_american_story_140785.html.

66. Miller, E. 2018. "U.S. drug prices vs the world." *DrugWatch*. Last modified July 27, 2020. Accessed January 25, 2021. https://www.drugwatch.com/featured/us-drug-prices-higher-vs-world/.

67. Kirzinger, A., Lopes, L., Wu, B., and Brodie, M. 2019. "KFF health tracking poll: February 2019: Prescription drugs." *Kaiser Family Foundation*. Accessed January 25, 2021. https://www.kff.org/health-costs/poll-finding/kff-health-tracking-poll-february-2019-prescription-drugs/.

68. National Academy for State Health Policy. 2020. "2020 state legislative action to lower pharmaceutical costs." Accessed January 25, 2021. https://www.nashp.org/rx-legislative-tracker/.

69. Azar II, A.M., 2019. "Remarks on the safe importation of certain prescription drugs." Accessed January 25, 2021. https://www.hhs.gov/about/leadership/secretary/speeches/2019-speeches/remarks-safe-importation-certain-prescription-drugs.html.

70. Florko, N. 2019. "Trump administration unveils plan to allow drug importation from Canada." *STAT*. Accessed January 25, 2021. https://www.statnews.com/2019/07/31/trump-importation-plan/.

71. Martell, A. 2019. "Exclusive: Canada warns U.S. against drug import plans, citing shortage concerns." *Reuters*. Accessed January 25, 2021. https://www.reuters.com/article/us-canada-pharmaceuticals-exports-exclus/exclusive-canada-warns-us-against-drug-import-plans-citing-shortage-concerns-idUSKCN1UD2LN.

72. Roy, A. 2018, October 26. "Trump's dramatic new proposal to lower Medicare drug prices by linking to an international index." *Forbes*. Accessed January 25, 2021. https://www.forbes.com/sites/theapothecary/2018/10/26/trumps-dramatic-new-proposal-to-lower-medicare-drug-prices-by-linking-to-an-international-index/#71494474c3a1.

73. Centers for Medicare & Medicaid Services. 2018. "ANPRM international pricing index model for Medicare Part B drugs." Accessed January 25, 2021. https://www.cms.gov/newsroom/fact-sheets/anprm-international-pricing-index-model-medicare-part-b-drugs.

74. U.S. Department of Health & Human Services. 2018. "What you need to know about President Trump cutting down on foreign freeloading." Accessed January 25, 2021. https://www.hhs.gov/about/news/2018/10/25/ipi-policy-brief.html.

75. Kang, S.Y., DiStefano, M.J., Socal, M.P., and Anderson, G.F. 2019. "Using external reference pricing in Medicare Part D to reduce drug price differentials with other countries." *Health Affairs (Millwood)* 38 (5): 804–811. https://doi.org/10.1377/hlthaff.2018.05207.

76. Inserro, A. 2018, December 10. "More than 300 groups seek halt to CMS' plans for global drug pricing index." *American Journal of Managed Care*. Accessed January 25, 2021.

https://www.ajmc.com/newsroom/more-than-300-groups-seek-halt-to-cms-plans-for-global-drug-pricing-index.

77. Part B Access for Seniors and Physicians Coalition. 2018, December 10. "Letter to Mitch McConnell, Charles Schumer, Paul Ryan, and Nancy Pelosi." https://www.partbaccess.org/wp-content/uploads/2017/06/12.10.18-ASP-Coalition-letter.pdf.

78. U.S. Department of Health & Human Services, Office of the Assistant Secretary for Planning and Evaluation. 2018. "Comparison of U.S. and international prices for top Medicare Part B drugs by total expenditures." Accessed January 25, 2021. https://aspe.hhs.gov/system/files/pdf/259996/ComparisonUSInternationalPricesTopSpendingPartBDrugs.pdf.

79. Cancryn, A. 2019, June 6. "Liberals fight their own party over drug prices." *Politico.* Accessed January 25, 2021. https://www.politico.com/story/2019/06/06/democrats-prescription-drug-prices-1497676.

80. Cubanski, J., Rae, M., Young, K., and Damico, A. 2019. "How does prescription drug spending and use compare across large employer plans, Medicare Part D, and Medicaid?" *Kaiser Family Foundation.* Accessed January 25, 2021. https://www.kff.org/medicare/issue-brief/how-does-prescription-drug-spending-and-use-compare-across-large-employer-plans-medicare-part-d-and-medicaid/.

81. McCaughan, M. 2017, August 10. "Health policy brief, prescription drug pricing #6: Medicare Part D." *Health Affairs.* https://doi.org/10.1377/hpb20171008.000172.

82. Medicare Prescription Drug, Improvement, and Modernization Act of 2003. Public Law 108–173, 108th Congr. (2003).

83. Grassley, C. 2019. "Grassley on Medicare Part D price negotiation." Accessed January 25, 2021. https://www.grassley.senate.gov/news/news-releases/grassley-medicare-part-d-price-negotiation.

84. Cubanski, J., Neuman, T., True, S., and Freed, M. 2019. "What's the latest on Medicare drug price negotiations." *Kaiser Family Foundation.* Accessed January 25, 2021. https://www.kff.org/medicare/issue-brief/whats-the-latest-on-medicare-drug-price-negotiations/.

85. Executive Order N-01-19, Executive Department, State of California, 2019.

86. Congressional Budget Office. "A detailed description of CBO's cost estimate for the Medicare prescription drug benefit." 2004.

87. Frank, R.G., and Nichols, L.M. 2019. "Medicare drug-price negotiation—why now . . . and how." *New England Journal of Medicine* 381 (15): 1404–1406. https://doi.org/10.1056/NEJMp1909798.

4
Measuring the Value of Prescription Drugs

Automated external defibrillators (AEDs) are ubiquitous. You see them in restaurants and libraries, and on airplanes. But has the money spent on them been a wise investment? How to balance the resources invested in their development, installation, and maintenance against the lives saved and any untoward effects (e.g., shocking someone not actually in cardiac arrest)? Researchers have examined the question using standard tools of economic evaluation and—spoiler alert—multiple studies have determined that AEDs are in fact "worth it."[1-4]

The formula for measuring the value of health interventions like AEDs is applicable to prescription drugs, and as discussed in Chapter 5 of this volume, institutions have emerged to conduct such evaluations. Examples include the National Institute for Health and Care Excellence (NICE) in England and Wales, the Institute for Clinical and Economic Review in the United States, the Canadian Agency for Drugs and Technologies in Health, and the Pharmaceutical Benefits Advisory Committee in Australia. These and similar entities have related missions: to develop and use economic analyses to measure the value of prescription drugs (and other medical technologies). The rationale, as described in Chapter 3 of this volume, is that drug value must be understood for society to spend resources on medications sensibly.

Spending wisely on other goods, such as toothpaste, also depends on assessing their value. And yet there are no agencies charged with developing and using economic techniques to do so. As we saw in Chapter 2 of this volume, toothpaste sells in a competitive market: relatively informed consumers choose items based on their preferences, and producers compete for customers. Hence, toothpaste prices reasonably reflect "value"—that is, how much consumers will forego to acquire a product. For prescription drugs, the market distortions described in Chapter 2 of this volume mean that prices do *not* reasonably represent value. As a consequence, economists have developed value assessment techniques for medications.

The Right Price. Peter J. Neumann, Joshua T. Cohen, and Daniel A. Ollendorf, Oxford University Press (2021).
© Peter J. Neumann, Joshua T. Cohen, and Daniel A. Ollendorf. DOI: 10.1093/oso/9780197512883.003.0004

The Value of a Life: Cost–Benefit Analysis

Human Capital: You're Worth What You Earn

William Petty (1623–1687), a 17th-century Englishman who had ascended from an unremarkable background to acquire substantial landholdings, faced a problem: the high taxes levied by the English government to pay for a series of wars with the Netherlands between 1652 and 1674. Not that Petty opposed the idea of paying taxes; he just thought that he and his fellow landowners had been asked to pay more than their fair share.[5] To convince others, he quantified national income contributions from different sectors of the economy. Estimating England's total annual income to be £40 million and income from houses, land and ships to total £15 million, he estimated labor earnings to be the difference (i.e., £25 million). Petty argued that the tax burden should be apportioned according to the source of income (presumably reducing his tax bill). Summing labor earnings stretching into the future, Petty also estimated the value of "human capital." This allowed Petty to estimate the monetary value of a life lost in war as equivalent to the deceased individual's lost future earnings.[6] He further argued that medical care (such as it was in the 17th century) was "worthwhile" in that the value of the lives saved exceeded the cost of that care.[7]

Petty's calculations omitted some important details. For example, from his estimated labor income stream, he did not deduct food or housing expenses. Two hundred years later, in 1853, another Englishman, William Farr (1807–1883), a founder of medical statistics and modern epidemiology, argued that one could estimate the value of human capital by subtracting living expenses from the value of future earnings.[6] Americans Louis Dublin (1882–1969) and Alfred Lotka (1880–1949) would later use the idea that human capital reflected the difference between earnings and consumption to estimate life insurance payouts.[6]

A succession of economists continued to refine the human capital approach and eventually some began to compare the monetized value of a program's or intervention's benefits (valued as the consequence to people's future earnings minus consumption) to the program's or intervention's costs. The basic idea of such a "cost–benefit analysis" is straightforward: if an intervention's monetized benefits exceed its costs, then the intervention is worthwhile (i.e., it has a "positive net benefit").

An early example, published in 1921, examined a program to improve worker health through "periodic physical examination."[8pp368-369] The analysis used Farr's human capital approach to estimate the value of the life of a typical worker (aged 31) to be $8,000, and the care costs for one day of illness (described as "medical, nursing and other sickness costs") to be $3. The analysis estimated that periodic physical examination would prevent four deaths and avert 2,920 days of illness for every 1,000 workers examined. Applied to America's labor force at the time (42 million workers), the benefit amounted to about $1.3 billion for the saved lives and a savings of $368 million for the averted days of illness, yielding a total benefit of approximately $1.7 billion. The analysis estimated the medical exam cost to be $5 per worker, or $210 million for the population, with follow-up care costs amounting to $500 million. Subtracting total medical costs of $710 million from the monetized health benefits of $1.7 billion yielded a net benefit of approximately $1 billion.[8p370]

You Work to Live; You Don't Just Live to Work: Willingness to Pay

While the human capital approach provides an objective and straightforward calculation, it ignores valued aspects of life beyond productive capacity. As critics have noted, the approach implies that "unproductive" periods, like leisure time and retirement, have no value. Ethical problems escalate as one considers that the approach places no value on people with conditions that prevent them from working.[9,10]

Because we are interested in the total value that people place on life (not just the value derived from productive capacity), it makes sense to ask how much people would be willing to pay to save a life. Of course, posing this "willingness-to-pay" question is fraught. It might be considered infinite—at least for the person whose life is in the balance. But placing an infinite value on each life would make priority setting impossible, as all measures would seem to be worthwhile, no matter their cost. A key refinement to the willingness-to-pay framework asks respondents to consider not the value of saving a *specific* life, but instead the value of reducing *small risks* of death. Anyone who doubts the reasonableness of placing a *finite* value on avoiding (or even accepting) small fatality risks should consider the following thought experiment. Suppose you learn that there is a bag containing $10,000 at an address 10 miles from you (say, a 15-minute ride). To claim the money, you simply need to drive to that address (or take an Uber or Lyft). Most people would accept this exchange—and would not change their mind even upon learning that traveling 10 miles in a motor vehicle means incurring a small but nonzero fatality risk.

If people can place a value on reducing or eliminating a small risk, we can estimate the value of a life by summing the values placed on these small risks. Suppose, for example, an optional car safety feature reduces the owner's fatality risk by 1 in 50,000 (but does not improve safety for anyone else). Now imagine that buyers each place an average value of $100 on this feature. If 50,000 people buy the feature at $100 per car, they have collectively spent 50,000 × $100, or $5 million. Installed in those 50,000 cars, the safety feature can be expected "statistically" to save one life—although we do not know beforehand *whose* life will be saved. For these car buyers, economists would conclude that the "value of a *statistical* life" is $5 million. Critically, it does not mean that people would exchange an *identifiable* person's life for $5 million. Rather, it means that the value they place on eliminating small risks adds up to $5 million for each *nonidentifiable* life saved. The "value of a statistical life" is economist short-hand for characterizing how much people are willing to pay to avoid small fatality risks.[11] Similar approaches can be used to calculate the value of a statistical heart attack, case of cancer, and so forth.

Still, how in practice does one determine the value individuals place on small fatality and illness risks? People do not typically buy and sell risks to their health. There are no published prices to avoid a 1 in 1,000 fatality risk, for example. Instead, economists employ two approaches to estimate these values.

The first exploits the fact that although consumers do not buy risk reductions explicitly, they do purchase goods (and make other decisions, like accepting jobs) that involve assorted features, including risk levels. Consider the choice between two cars: one a large, luxury model and the other, a compact. By virtue of its size, the larger car is safer. The difference in the sales price (the amount people are willing to pay) reflects, in part, the safety disparity. It also reflects other features, such as extra seats, cup holders, the moon roof, and so forth. While the safety difference is "bundled" with other attributes, economists use statistical techniques (such as regression analysis) and data describing lots of different cars to isolate how much the added safety contributes to a car's price. In similar fashion, economists examine housing data to estimate how much a second bathroom, central air conditioning, or proximity to an elementary school each add to a house's value. Because it uses statistics to *reveal* consumer preferences, economists refer to the technique as a "revealed preference" approach.[12]

There are limitations to the method. First, it assumes that the different features do not always appear in the same combinations. For example, if air conditioning and a second bathroom are essentially a "package deal" (i.e., if all houses with central air conditioning also include a second bathroom, and all houses with a second bathroom also have air conditioning), we cannot determine how much the bathroom and air-conditioning *individually* contribute to the house price. If people are willing to pay $20,000 more for a luxury house, we cannot know whether that extra $20,000 reflects their distaste for being hot in the summer or their aversion to waiting to use the bathroom. Likely, it reflects some combination of value for each of these features.

Economists confront a similar problem when using wage data to estimate the value people place on occupational risks.[13] Riskier jobs (e.g., roofing or mining) often come with more physically demanding conditions. The statistical techniques economists use can erroneously attribute a portion of the wage premium demanded for roofing and mining to their added risk, when in reality workers demand higher pay for these occupations because they prefer to work in comfortable, climate-controlled, indoor settings. Similarly, in automobile and other product markets, risk is often "confounded" with other product features, complicating statistical estimation of the value of risk reduction alone.

Even if economists could statistically isolate the influence of risk on wages or a product's price, revealed preferences are based on the assumption that consumers and workers know (and understand) the size of the risks and the trade-offs involved. If people do not realize the benefits they are purchasing, it makes little sense to use market data to estimate the value they place on them. The knowledge that workers and consumers possess about risk magnitude is unclear.

In light of these challenges, some economists have employed a different approach. Instead of inferring the value of risk reduction from choices made in actual market transactions, they instead conduct surveys to query people directly. This technique, referred to as *stated* or *expressed* preference,[14] avoids the pitfalls of *revealed* preference techniques, although it introduces other challenges. For one, when asked about spending hypothetical money, survey respondents often seem willing to pay unrealistically large sums for health improvements.[15] They also often seem insensitive to the magnitude of the relevant benefit. For example, when surveys ask people what they would pay to save migrating birds (an ecological "good" that, like health, cannot be readily valued from market data), the responses seem to depend little on the number of hypothetical birds saved, whether 50 or 5,000. Respondents instead seem to express a general preference for rescuing birds, rather than valuing the quantity of birds saved.[16] That result is inconsistent with the idea that when it comes to a positive outcome (saving birds, reducing risk, etc.), a rational individual should be willing to pay more for greater quantities.

Another problem is that responses to surveys can depend on how questions are framed.[17,18] For example, physicians view therapy as more effective when shown data on the treatment's *relative* risks of achieving an outcome (e.g., a 20% reduction) and less effective when shown *absolute* risk data (e.g., a fatality reduction from, say, 1% to 0.8%).[19] Respondents are willing to pay more for a surgery if informed there is a 10% chance they would otherwise die from a disease rather than a 90% chance that they would not. They may be willing to pay more for treatments to reduce a small fatality risk when a survey scenario *labels* the disease (e.g., cancer), as opposed to providing a generic disease description, presumably because explicitly naming the disease provokes a more emotional response (although the evidence on this point seems mixed).[20,21]

Despite these challenges, the stated preference literature can help us think about the value of nonmarketed goods and services. Studies judged to have used the best methods have yielded a reasonably consistent set of estimates for the value of a statistical life, ranging from $4.2 million to $13.7 million.[22] Although using such information has been controversial,[23] parts of the US federal government—including the US Environmental Protection Agency[24] and the US Department of Transportation[25]—regularly employ values in this range to estimate the value of health benefits for new regulations (and then compare those benefits to the regulations' costs). The approach that William Petty developed more than 300 years ago in his attempt to apportion the tax burden in England has evolved into a sophisticated set of methods to compare the costs and health benefits of life-saving regulations so that policymakers can judge which ones are worthwhile.

Cost-Effectiveness Analysis

Money Isn't Everything (and Everything Isn't Money)

In November 1962, *Life Magazine* described a novel treatment for patients whose kidneys had ceased to function.[26] The new procedure, called dialysis, required patients to sleep at a medical center two nights every week so they could be connected to a machine that cleaned their blood of toxins and excess fluid that had accumulated during the preceding days. Without treatment, patients would die within a week or two. But dialysis machines were scarce: only a tiny fraction of the 100,000 Americans who died of chronic kidney disease each year in the early 1960s could be treated. As described in the *Life* story entitled, "They decide who lives, who dies," an anonymous committee of seven community members selected which patients would receive treatment.

Dialysis was also expensive. To be eligible, patients had to demonstrate that they could pay for at least three years of treatment at its annual cost of $10,000—around $80,000 in inflation-adjusted 2020 dollars.[27] Given the life-and-death implications, pressure grew for the federal government to foot the bill for all patients in need. That prospect concerned the Federal Bureau of the Budget (later renamed the Office of Management and Budget), which responded in 1966 by convening its own committee of experts.[28]

At first, the committee's charge seemed unclear. Some members wanted to use cost–benefit analysis to assess and prioritize dialysis compared to competing health concerns.[28p8] Others, noting that the government had already designated chronic kidney disease of high importance, wanted the committee to prioritize alternative ways of addressing the condition. On top of that, the committee's two economists, Herbert Klarman and Jerry Rosenthal, had given up on conducting a cost–benefit analysis,[28p8] believing they could not place a monetary value on human life. Klarman later recalled that while he was dissatisfied with the human capital approach because it failed to recognize value beyond a person's income earning capacity,[29] he did not believe that people could meaningfully place a more holistic value on extending life.[30p589]

Consequently, instead of expressing health impacts in pecuniary terms, Klarman and Rosenthal expressed them as "life years gained" (or lost), thus avoiding the need to monetize human life. However, because the costs and health effects were now expressed in different units (dollars and life years), the economists could not sum them to compute an intervention's net benefit (and determine whether it was "worthwhile"). Still, they could describe the value of each intervention as the ratio of its incremental costs to its incremental benefits. Using this *cost-effectiveness analysis*, they estimated that over the remaining life of a chronic kidney disease patient, dialysis in a medical center would cost $104,000 and extend life by nine years (roughly $11,600 per life year gained); dialysis at home would cost $38,000 over a lifetime and also extend life for nine years (around $4,200 per life year gained). Finally, transplantation of a donor kidney would cost $44,500 and add 17 years of life (around $2,600 per life year gained).[31]

These results can be thought of as "prices." Smaller ratios, like lower prices, are more favorable because they indicate that an intervention produces health at a lower cost. In the case of kidney disease treatment, transplantation seemed the most efficient way to gain life years (assuming there are enough donor kidneys for everyone in need); at-home dialysis was the second most efficient approach; and in-center dialysis, the least efficient.

By expressing health benefits in terms of life-years gained, cost-effectiveness analysis avoids the nettlesome step of explicitly valuing human lives in monetary terms. However, Klarman and Rosenthal also recognized that transplantation not only extends life but—by obviating twice-weekly dialysis sessions—also improves quality of life. Transplant recipients, they noted, "have greater vitality, escape restrictive regimens, can continue to live in the same community, yet are free to travel without encumbrance or special arrangements."[31p50] To maintain the cost-effectiveness analysis framework, in which all benefits are expressed with a common benchmark, Klarman and Rosenthal added "quality adjustments" to the life years gained for dialysis patients and transplant recipients. They assumed that if each added year of life for dialysis patients has a value of 1.0 life year "adjusted for quality," then a year of life for transplant recipients would be worth 1.25 life years "adjusted for quality." Hence, the nine life years added by dialysis (at-home or in-center) would be worth 9.0 life years adjusted for quality, but the 17 adjusted life years added by transplant would be worth 20.6 life years after the quality adjustment. (The 17 years represents 13.3 years on transplant, which is scaled up by 25% for a contribution of 16.6 life years adjusted for quality; added to that is the remaining four years on dialysis.) Rather than gaining 1 life year *unadjusted* for quality for every $2,600 in costs, the cost-effectiveness ratio for transplant would then be even more favorable at $2,200 per life year *adjusted* for quality.

Common Ground: The Quality-Adjusted Life Year

The Klarman and Rosenthal assessment was one of several cost-effectiveness analyses in the 1960s conducted to help the federal government address a fundamental health policy question: "If additional money were to be allocated to disease control programs, which programs would show the highest payoff in terms of lives saved and disability prevented per dollar spent?"[32p1209] Ranking programs depended on having a common health yardstick so that cost-effectiveness ratios could be properly compared. Klarman and Rosenthal had expressed the benefits of both dialysis and transplant in terms of" "life years adjusted for quality," but they offered no empirical basis or rationale for their quality adjustments, noting only, "In this paper the differential [between dialysis and transplant] is set at one-quarter of a life year."[31p50] As a result, others could not readily apply the Klarman and Rosenthal approach to a wider range of health conditions and programs. For example, what quality adjustment is appropriate for a moderate stroke or for late-stage breast cancer?

Other researchers in the 1960s labored to develop a common benchmark for different health outcomes. Their proposed solutions had limitations. For example, Sanders measured population health in terms of "productive man-years," which downplayed illnesses affecting people outside the workforce, including children and retirees (not to mention using the now wince-inducing gender-specific terminology).[33] Katz measured health in terms of lost "activities of daily living (ADLs)" (e.g., one's ability to bathe, dress, use the toilet).[34] However, the index did not specify weights for each level of dependence. Thus, one could not say how much worse it was to lose three ADLs compared to losing two. Chiang measured health in terms of time not in full health.[35] However, because that approach did not distinguish levels of illness severity, a day with *any* condition other than perfect health—including being dead—had the same value. At around the same time, researchers in the United Kingdom began their own efforts to address these issues.[36,37]

The field required a conceptually-grounded, replicable procedure, rather than ad hoc judgments, for assigning values to a wide range of health conditions. Two groups of researchers would independently develop approaches that would come to dominate the field.

Time Trade-Off

In the late 1960s, James W. Bush, a physician with an interest in public policy, worked for the New York State Planning Commission helping to implement universal health insurance.[38] The program's budgetary demands made Bush keenly aware of the need to assess, compare, and prioritize varied health services. Working with an engineer named Sol Fanshel, Bush suggested a "health status index"[39] based on the amount of time people might spend in each of eleven generic states, arranged from most to least favorable: A—well-being, B—dissatisfaction, C—discomfort, D—minor disability, E—major disability, F—disabled, G—confined, H—bedridden and confined, I—isolated, J—coma, and K—death. Bush assigned each state a "functional value" between zero and 1, with State A (well-being) anchored at 1 and State K (death) anchored at zero. Other states were assigned values between zero and 1, with more desirable states closer to 1. Any health scenario's value would be expressed in terms of years of life, with each year scaled by the *functional value* of the health state experienced that year. For example, spending 90 years in State A (well-being) with a functional value of 1) would yield 90 "well years." Spending 80 years in State A and then 10 years with a health condition with a functional value of 0.5 would yield $(80 \times 1.0) + (10 \times 0.5) = 85$ well years.

Crucial to this approach was the estimation of meaningful health state functional values. Bush and Fanshel realized that to place a value on something amounts to declaring what one would be willing to *trade* for it. That tradability implies that one can value the cure of a major disability (State E) by asking, for example, how many days living with a minor disability (State D) one would tolerate to avoid one day with the major disability. If we would accept two days with the minor disability to avoid a single day with the major disability, then curing the major disability is worth twice what curing a minor disability is worth.

The problem with this thought experiment, though, is that it tells us only the *relative* value of a cure for each health state and not an actual useable value that informs the impact between zero (dead) and 1 (full health). So Bush and Fanshel concocted an extension of this thought experiment in which people would essentially trade off time in State A (functional value of 1) in exchange for curing a health condition that diminished quality of life.[39] As described in Box 4.1 using a closely related approach, the more life expectancy a respondent is willing to forego for a cure, the less desirable the health state must be and, hence, the lower its functional value. This approach, the *time trade-off method*, remains in use today.

Standard Gamble

Recalling his time in graduate school in industrial engineering at the State University of New York at Buffalo in the 1960s, George Torrance explained that he had come close to writing his doctoral thesis on a problem pertaining to production planning and inventory control.[40] His advisor, however, suggested that Torrance talk to David Sackett, a physician-researcher who had just landed a faculty position at McMaster University in Toronto. McMaster was an hour and a half drive from Buffalo, but Torrance had a teaching job there, so he decided to stop by to see Sackett.

Sackett was interested in improving decision-making in healthcare. Torrance, drawing upon his own training, considered the problem as one of optimizing health system effectiveness. Like Bush and Fanshel, he realized that any health system's output could be conceived in terms of the value-weighted sum of time spent in each of multiple health states, with each state having value ranging from zero to 1. Because of his roots in operations research, Torrance was familiar with an approach—called the "standard gamble"—to estimate these kinds of values. Like the time trade-off method, it asked respondents what they would forego in exchange for curing a health condition. Specifically, respondents are asked to imagine that they could be cured of some condition (let us suppose again, a major disability), but that in exchange, they would incur a risk of immediate, painless death. The question posed was: how large a risk of death would make the respondent indifferent

Box 4.1 Eliciting Functional Values for Health States: An Example

An approach closely related to that outlined by Fanshel and Bush suggests eliciting functional values for each health state by asking respondents how much life expectancy they would forego in exchange for curing a health condition that diminishes quality of life. For example, for State E (major disability), Fanshel and Bush imagine people who, without treatment, will live with a major disability (with its unknown functional value of V_E) for 90 years (a "standard lifetime"). Now imagine that the condition can be cured, resulting in a transition to State A (well-being, with its functional weight of 1.0), but with a shorter life expectancy. The question is, *How much loss of life expectancy makes the respondent indifferent between a longer life at diminished quality and a shorter life in ideal health?*

Suppose that a respondent is willing to give up 10% of their 90-year life expectancy (i.e., nine years) to achieve ideal health. Because Fanshel and Bush measure health impact in terms of functional value summed over time, the "cured scenario," with its ideal health and shorter life expectancy, has a value of $81 \times 1.0 = 81$ "well years." The "untreated scenario," with its full life expectancy but diminished quality of life, has a value of $90 \times V_E = 90V_E$ well years. Because the respondent judges these two scenarios as having the same value, 81 well years $= 90V_E$ well years, implying that $V_E = 0.9$. More generally, indifference between ideal health for a lifetime shortened from its standard value by X% and a full lifetime at a diminished quality of life implies that the functional value for the diminished quality of life state is $1 - X$%.

While the algebra outlined here shows how health state functional values can be estimated from trade-offs between length and quality of life, it is fair to ask whether people can meaningfully answer questions about how much life expectancy they would sacrifice for improved quality of life. Although people arguably do make such trade-offs in real life (e.g., many of us accept the small increased risk of a fatal heart attack that attends habitual consumption of desserts), few people think about *how much* life expectancy they are sacrificing. Nonetheless, health economists frequently use the "time trade-off" elicitation method to estimate health state "preference weights" that range from zero to 1. The algebra described and a well-developed branch of mathematics called "utility theory"[1] provides a reasonable foundation for this approach. Despite its abstract nature, in the absence of other information, it is better to use people's expressed preferences for alternative health states than to make arbitrary judgments or ignore quality of life altogether.

[1] Fishburn, P.C. 1968. "Utility theory." *Management Science* 14 (5): 335–378.

between the disability on one hand and the cure and its potentially lethal side effect on the other? Willingness to accept a larger probability of death suggested that the condition to be cured was more severe (less favorable). In general, willingness to accept a fatality risk of probability "p" implied the health state's value is 1 − p. In the ensuing years, the standard gamble, like the time trade-off, has become a common approach for eliciting health state preference weights. It is somewhat less popular than the time trade-off, likely because it is more difficult to explain to respondents and because people have a harder time thinking about probabilities (and the risk of immediate death) than they do about trading off life expectancy.

With the introduction of the time trade-off and standard gamble methods, the concept used by Klarman and Rosenthal to put dialysis and transplant on a comparable footing could now be systematically extended to a wide range of health technology assessment problems. Klarman and Rosenthal had referred to "life years adjusted for quality." In 1976, Harvard University's Richard Zeckhauser and Donald Shephard employed the term "quality-adjusted life year" (QALY),[41] which may be the first formal usage of that term (the actual provenance is somewhat murky and debated).[36] Since that time, researchers have published about 9,000 cost-effectiveness analysis that collectively report more than 20,000 cost-per-QALY ratios;[42] those studies document some 30,000 "utility weights" (i.e., preference weights or, as Fanshel and Bush referred to them, "functional values") that quantify the desirability of many health states.[42]

Drawing Boundaries—How Much Is a Quality-Adjusted Life Year Worth?

With methods to assign preference weights to different health conditions, it was now possible to compute cost-effectiveness ratios for many different interventions. By comparing cost-effectiveness ratios, decision makers could identify health interventions (including prescription drugs) with the lowest cost per QALY gained. However, arraying interventions from most to least efficient did not indicate which gained QALYs at a sufficiently low enough cost to warrant spending money on them.

The well-known (at least in health economics circles) "shopping spree problem" is instructive. As explained in a popular textbook by Myriam Hunink and colleagues, imagine having a fixed budget and many health interventions from which to select.[43] Suppose further that decisions about each intervention can be made independently—that is, spending on one intervention does not preclude spending on the others and does not affect their cost-effectiveness. In this situation (with some additional plausible assumptions), we can maximize population health gains by spending first on the intervention with the most favorable cost-effectiveness ratio, and then, when there are no additional patients who can benefit from that first intervention, spending on the intervention with the *second* most favorable ratio, and so on, until we run out of money, patients, or health-improving interventions.

There are objections to this approach. For one, prioritizing the most efficient programs can omit programs for people with conditions that are expensive and difficult to treat, which seems unjust. For another, it may prioritize "minor" conditions that can be inexpensively treated over severe conditions that cost a lot to treat. These objections center on prioritization of efficiency over other criteria (e.g., helping those suffering the most). Indeed, critics raised these sorts of objections when, in the early 1990s, Oregon famously used an approach resembling the "shopping spree" to select the interventions for which its Medicaid program would pay (see Chapter 5, this volume).

Setting aside these concerns, the shopping spree approach is also impractical because it depends on knowing cost-effectiveness ratio values for all interventions under consideration so that they can be ranked. Even with the thousands of cost-effectiveness studies conducted over the last half century, the cost-effectiveness of most interventions remains uncertain and, in many cases, unknown.[44] We could instead compare each intervention's cost-effectiveness to a benchmark representing a QALY's value. For example, if a QALY is worth $50,000, then interventions costing less than $50,000 per QALY gained would be deemed "cost-effective" and approved, while interventions costing more than $50,000 per QALY gained would be deemed "not cost-effective" and rejected.

But how to determine a QALY's value? No marketplace openly prices QALYs. For many years, most cost-effectiveness analyses in the United States referred to a benchmark of $50,000 per QALY, despite its lack of any clear conceptual or empirical basis.[45] One rationale sometimes advanced was that it corresponded to the cost-effectiveness of dialysis, which Medicare had decided to fund, hence in the early 1970s signifying that "purchasing" QALYs at this price must reflect societal preferences.[46] But observers have argued that the $50,000 per QALY benchmark first came into use in the 1990s, and the studies that first cited it did not mention dialysis as a basis.[45,47] Moreover, use of the $50,000 benchmark persisted even as Medicare paid for dialysis at a cost of as much as $95,000 per QALY towards the end of the 1990s.[46] In any case, Medicare's decision to pay for dialysis at $50,000 per QALY suggested that Medicare (and society) placed a value of $50,000 *or more* on each QALY.

To estimate a QALY's value, researchers from the University of Michigan in 2000 reviewed the existing literature, including six human capital assessments, which examined individual economic output; eight expressed preference studies, which asked people to put a value on health and longevity; and 27 revealed preference assessments, 19 of which relied on worker pay premiums for additional occupational risk and 8 of which were premised on the amount people pay for consumer product safety features.[46] These studies generally did not directly measure the value of a QALY or a life year, however. Instead, they measured the value of avoiding *fatalities*, which the Michigan group then converted to life years by making assumptions about the average age at which people in different groups died and hence about how many life years each avoided fatality represented. Other assumptions also entered into their calculations.

The results hardly seemed to clarify matters. The median value of a QALY from the human capital studies was $25,000, but among the expressed preference studies, the median value was $160,000, and for revealed preference studies based on occupational wage and risk trade-offs, the median value was $430,000. In somewhat of an understatement, the authors characterized these findings as a "failure to find a strong central tendency in the values per QALY."[46] The human capital study results could be set aside, however, because, as previously explained, productive output represents only *a portion* of a life's value.

Subsequent studies also reported wide variation in estimates. A review of 24 expressed and revealed preference studies published from 1998 to 2014 found willingness to pay values for a QALY (or life-year) ranging from €1000 ($1,130 in 2020) to €4,800,000 ($5.4 million).[48] The authors concluded that the wide variation may be explained by differences in methodology, preference elicitation methods, the perspective taken (whether individual or societal—see discussion below), and the sample population (what country and whether from the general population or specific patient groups).

Other researchers have attempted to estimate the value of a QALY from actual spending decisions made by individuals or government authorities. One study examined the incremental costs and health effects of individual health insurance purchasing decisions in the United States and inferred a lower bound of $183,000 per life-year gained.[49] Another examined Medicare officials' reimbursement decisions for new technologies but "found no clear evidence of an implicit threshold" (i.e., benchmark) for the value of a QALY above which the US Medicare program would not pay for health interventions.[50] Researchers in the United Kingdom found that NICE decisions reflected a "broad notion of a threshold"[51] in that as a technology's cost per QALY increased, the probability that authorities would issue a rejection increased (e.g., a 2015 study found that technologies costing £40 000 per QALY had a 50% chance of NICE rejection, while those costing £52,000/QALY had a 75% chance of rejection).[52]

The American health economist Chuck Phelps (updating his own work with Alan Garber from 1997)[53] in 2019 developed a theoretical model to explore how people might balance purchases of healthcare against other goods and services.[54] Given a series of plausible assumptions, he found that people would be willing to pay about twice their annual incomes (or about $110,000) for a QALY—and that as incomes increase, so does a QALY's value.

Still others addressed the problem of estimating the value of a QALY from a different angle, producing very different results. Karl Claxton is a brilliant, motorcycle-riding, e-cigarette smoking, jazz-loving professor of health economics at the University of York in the United Kingdom. In 2015, Andrew Ward opined in the *Financial Times* that "for pharmaceuticals companies and their investors, Karl Claxton might be the most dangerous man in economics."[55] Claxton and his York colleagues were skeptical of thinking about a QALY's value in terms of expressed or revealed willingness to pay to improve health. The problem with willingness to pay valuations was that they might be inconsistent with the amount of money available to spend on healthcare.

Suppose, for example, that willingness to pay valuations indicate that a QALY is worth $100,000. Then it makes sense to fund all interventions that improve health at a cost of less than $100,000 per QALY and defund those that cost more. But what if the healthcare budget is not big enough to fund all the programs that gain QALYs at less than $100,000 per QALY? A new intervention that gains eight QALYs at a cost of $400,000 ($50,000 per QALY gained) seems like a "good buy" and should be funded. Budget limitations might mean, however, that another program must be cut to produce that funding. If the displaced program has a cost of $400,000 but gains 10 QALYs, its elimination saves the money needed for the new program but also results in a net loss of two QALYs (i.e., the gain of eight QALYs from the funding of the new program minus the 10 QALY loss from the defunding of the displaced program).

To avoid this unintended outcome (i.e., funding a new, ostensibly attractive program by cutting an even more efficient program), the York group called for a focus on the "marginal cost of health production."[56,57] The idea is to estimate the cost per QALY gained for programs "at the margin" and hence likely to be cut when funding is needed to support new healthcare initiatives. The QALY production cost for those programs that will be cut represent the QALY's de facto value. A program that improves health at a cost below the marginal cost of health production is worthwhile, whereas one that produces health more expensively is not. In the example in the preceding paragraph, a QALY is worth $40,000 because new programs that produce health at a cost below this level are worthwhile.

The York group argued that the marginal cost of health production implied a much lower QALY value than willingness to pay approaches suggested. Looking at the average marginal cost of health production for the UK National Health Service's four largest program budget categories (cancer, circulatory problems, respiratory problems, and gastrointestinal problems), they estimated a QALY's value to be approximately £10,600,[57] or approximately $14,000 at an exchange rate of $1.30 per UK pound.

The York group's QALY value of roughly $14,000 falls considerably below the $100,000 to $200,000 per QALY (and higher) benchmarks from the revealed and expressed preference literature described earlier. Researchers using similar methods have estimated QALY value benchmarks in a number of other countries and have found it is generally less than each country's GDP per capita.[58–62] Studies can sometimes arrive at different estimates because of "noisy data." But other factors may be involved here. For example, occupational revealed preference studies can *overstate* QALY values by incorrectly attributing too much of the variation in pay across jobs to differences in risk, rather than to other job characteristics, such as physical comfort. Alternatively, the York group's approach may *understate* a QALY's value by overstating the QALY reduction associated with lower healthcare spending. Depending on the statistical methods used, that could happen if lower spending on health (say, in less wealthy health districts) is associated with other factors (e.g., inferior nutrition or more smoking) that also harm health.

With such a wide range of QALY values—from $14,000 based on the York group's analysis in the United Kingdom to as much as $200,000 based on revealed and expressed preference studies—what should the QALY benchmark be? As we will see in Chapters 5 and 6, to the extent that health programs in the United States use cost-effectiveness assessments for decision-making, the QALY value benchmarks used to characterize program value seem to be much higher (more generous or lenient) than in the United Kingdom. Differences in per capita income between the two countries (which is roughly 30% higher in the United States) explain only a fraction of the difference.

The larger issue relates to philosophical approaches in terms of whether to base estimates of the QALY's value on consumer preferences (sometimes called "demand-side" approaches) or on the opportunity costs of healthcare services implicit in fixed budgets ("supply side").[54,63] Examining willingness to pay estimates directly through surveys, or exploring how hypothetical individuals might trade off health against other purchases given their incomes and risk attitudes, tends to yield higher estimates for the QALY's value. Still, even if a policymaker favors one of these methods, how should they aggregate them for policy decisions, which involve society's collective views on how the healthcare sector should be financed, organized, and delivered?[54] A key question is whether the benchmark should be the same for all citizens (or different, say, for individuals willing to pay more for health insurance beyond a "basic package" of services).[54] In theory, voters can help decide such matters, but in practice, opinions vary, debates are contentious, and consensus elusive.

Moreover, the York group's QALY value may be more pertinent to settings like the United Kingdom if, like in that country, it is delivered by a central authority (e.g., the United Kingdom's National Health Service) with a fixed annual budget—set in advance and approved by Parliament—for all healthcare, implying that new spending must indeed be paid for by cutting existing measures—just as the scenario contemplated by the York analysis assumes.[63] In contrast, decision-making in the United States is distributed across multiple government programs (e.g., Medicare, state Medicaid programs, the Veterans Administration) and private insurance companies. Budgets are *not* as explicit. The link between new spending and cuts to existing health measures is less definitive. For that reason, in the United States, there may be less need to examine what existing health measures would be cut to pay for a new intervention—because in the United States, perhaps new funding can instead be raised from outside the healthcare sector to pay for new interventions. If that is the case, US decision makers can think more about how much people are willing to pay for a QALY, rather than thinking about what other healthcare spending must be cut to raise new funds and how those reductions affect health.

While the budgets of US payers may be more malleable than those in the United Kingdom, they are not unconstrained. Most states have restrictions on how much private health insurer premiums may increase annually. The introduction of a costly new drug can mean displacing other needed services or passing costs on to patients in the form of higher deductibles or coinsurance.[64] For states, the trade-offs might come in the form of spending cuts to nonhealth programs and services, such as education or infrastructure.

Debates about appropriate value benchmarks will undoubtedly continue. The World Health Organization's (WHO) experience with cost-effectiveness benchmarks is instructive in this regard. In the early 2000s, the WHO suggested that an appropriate benchmark for the value of a disability-adjusted life year (DALY), which is similar to a QALY but measured on an inverse scale so that improving population health means averting DALYs rather than gaining QALYs. WHO stated that in most countries the benchmark should lie somewhere between one to three times gross domestic product (GDP) per capita—that is, that

> interventions that avert one DALY . . . for less than average per capita income for a given country or region are considered very cost-effective; interventions that cost less than three times average per capita income per DALY averted are still considered cost-effective; and those that exceed this level are considered not cost-effective"[65,66]

But economists from the WHO later backed away from this finding, arguing in 2016:

> The use of cost-effectiveness ratios in decision-making remains an area without consensus. Our view is that a fixed cost-effectiveness threshold should never be used as a stand-alone criterion for decision-making. Above all, the indiscriminate sole use of the most common threshold—of three times the per-capita GDP per DALY averted—in national funding decisions or for setting the price or reimbursement value of a new drug or other intervention must be avoided.[67]

Instead, the WHO recommended that

> cost–effectiveness information should be used alongside other considerations— e.g. budget impact and feasibility considerations—in a transparent decision-making process, rather than in isolation based on a single threshold value.[67]

Neumann, Cohen, and Weinstein cautioned in 2014 against trying to find a single threshold or benchmark to represent society's willingness to pay for QALYs gained in the United States, noting that "in the United States, no single decision maker knows the opportunity costs of alternative health investments and issues healthcare decisions under a single budget."[45p797] They suggested that a QALY could be valued at $100,000 to $150,000 or even higher and that $50,000 might be considered a reasonable lower bound in the United States. But they added that "searching for a single benchmark is at best a quixotic exercise because there is no threshold that is appropriate in all decision contexts."[45p797]

Do We Need QALYs at All?

Although QALYs provide an approach for assessing value for a wide range of health interventions, it is fair to ask whether value can be measured without going to the trouble—and as described in later chapters, the controversy—of expressing health in those terms. Some countries make healthcare decisions without using QALYs. For example, Germany's Institute for Quality and Efficiency in Healthcare evaluates the clinical evidence for newly approved pharmaceuticals. If it finds that a new drug provides no better clinical benefit than drugs already available, Germany pays the same price for the new drug as other countries pay. If the Institute for Quality and Efficiency in Healthcare finds that a new drug *does* confer added benefit, the national association of insurers negotiates a price with the manufacturer. Germany's QALY-free pricing procedure reflects deep suspicion within government that QALYs are flawed, and even an "industry trick" to generate opaque measures of health gain that can be used to justify higher prices.

France's approach is somewhat similar. For new therapies, the French National Authority for Health determines added benefit relative to existing drugs, designating this benefit categorically from 1 (major improvement) to 5 (no improvement).[68] If the new drug represents a major improvement (level 1), it is priced between the highest and lowest prices charged for this drug in four "reference" countries. A drug that represents only a minor improvement (level 4) must be priced on par with what France pays for one of the existing alternatives. A drug that does not improve health at all compared to alternatives (level 5) must be priced at a discount to these alternatives.[68]

Although Germany and France can boast drug prices substantially below those in the United States, their systems have limitations.[69] First, while the relative prices for drugs treating the *same* condition may seem sensible (e.g., drugs with no added benefits have the same price as existing drugs), the German and French systems cannot readily compare the reasonableness of spending *across* diseases. That is because the system lacks a common metric—like the QALY—to compare treatment health benefits across disparate conditions. Second, the German system relies on negotiations to arrive at a price for new drugs with added benefits. However, the trade-offs and values that drive those negotiations are opaque, and there is no way to assess their consistency across decisions. Finally, in some cases, Germany and France rely on "reference pricing" (i.e., drug prices set by other countries). This "outsourcing" means that they import the decision-making criteria from those countries. For example, France uses reference prices from the United Kingdom, Germany, Italy, and Spain.[68] The United Kingdom prominently uses cost-per-QALY ratios to help establish its prices. Hence, although France rejects *explicit* use of the QALY, it ends up relying on QALYs *implicitly*.

The bottom line is that it is difficult to assess a treatment's value without a standard benefit measure. Without the QALY (or something like it), decision makers have a harder time comparing therapies—and hence setting priorities—across diseases. Because of these challenges, health systems that have tried to sidestep the QALY have ended up importing decisions from other countries that continue to use it.

A Matter of Time—Making Sense of "Discounting"

Some drug therapies (e.g., new treatments for hepatitis C) have high one-time costs but benefits that continue for long periods of time. Others (e.g., statins or antiretroviral therapies for HIV) have costs that are spread more evenly over a patient's lifetime. How to consider the differential timing of costs and benefits?

Everyone knows that borrowing money typically involves paying back interest, in addition to paying back the original principal. The interest payment compensates the lender for the risk that the borrower may default. Moreover, the dollars paid back have historically been worth less than the dollars advanced because of inflation. For example, a dollar today (early 2020) buys what 85 cents would have purchased in 2010.

But even if there were no default risk and no inflation, many creditors would still agree to lend money only if they could collect interest with the return of the principle, and many borrowers would be willing to pay that interest in exchange for immediate access to money—to pay for tuition, automobiles, a home, or even daily expenses. The fact that people willingly pay interest on loans implies that *a sum of money today must be worth more than the same amount of money at a point of time in the future*. For example, if a lender and borrower agree on a loan of $1,000, with the original principle to be paid back plus $250 interest in five years, then $1,000 today must have the same value as $1,250 five years from now. That is, one dollar today has the same value as $1.25 five years from now. Equivalently, a dollar *five years from now* is worth only 80 cents *today*.

The (generally) declining value of money over time means that a proper economic analysis cannot simply add costs incurred and savings accrued over an extended period. Instead, quantities must be placed on an equal footing by first converting them to their "present value." For example, in the preceding paragraph, the "present value" of one dollar five years from now is 80 cents.

So if we could purchase a medication today for $100 that would avert a $100 hospitalization in five years, the *present value* of the savings from the averted hospitalization would be $80, making the present value of the medication's *net cost* $100 − $80, or $20. Box 4.2 details the arithmetic for computing the present value of a stream of costs and savings.

Although the discounting of monetary costs and savings over time has been well-accepted for centuries, the proper treatment of *nonmonetized* health benefits has been more controversial. Should analyses also discount health consequences (e.g., lives, life years, or QALYs gained)? And, if so, should the evaluation discount them in the same way that we discount money?

The conventional view in health economics is that both monetary impacts and health outcomes should be discounted. As explained in Box 4.3, if we do *not* discount health impacts, then it seems as though we should indefinitely delay health spending—even on efficient interventions. That conclusion makes no sense. Indeed, a review of the health economics literature suggests that health economists consider the discounting of health benefits to be a settled matter. Although there is variation across countries and time, the vast majority of published papers discount monetary costs, monetary savings, and QALYs; moreover, they often use the same discount rate—3% per year— to discount both monetary quantities and health benefits, consistent with recommendations promulgated by the Original Panel on Cost-Effectiveness in Health and Medicine and the Second Panel's revision.[44,70]

Although most health economists are comfortable with discounting health benefits, the practice remains controversial. One set of objections stems from the use of discounting in evaluating environmental protection programs. In this context, benefits accrue over a far longer time horizon than is typical for health interventions. That has two important implications. First, it raises the thorny issue of *intergenerational* trade-offs. It is one thing for individuals to contemplate the merits of health benefits they themselves might gain now or in the future and conclude that near-term health benefits are more important than comparable benefits in the distant future. It is another to declare health benefits to be gained by future generations to be worth less than the same benefits accrued by people who are alive today. As this judgment does not reflect the preferences of all affected parties, its legitimacy is challenged. Second, for some environmental issues—particularly those involving climate change—health impacts can occur hundreds (or thousands) of years in the future. As one observer noted, using a plausible discount rate, "the death of a billion people 500 years from now becomes less serious than the death of one person today."[23p1571]

Box 4.2 Computing the Present Value of a Stream of Costs and Savings

Because the value of a cost or benefit depends on both its magnitude and how far in the future it occurs, costs and savings that occur at different times cannot simply be summed to arrive at an aggregate value. Before they are summed, costs and benefits must instead be discounted to their "present value equivalent."

The present value equivalent of a cost incurred at some point in the future is the cost that if incurred immediately has an equivalent value. To compute the present value equivalent for a cost incurred 1 year in the future, that "nominal" cost (the cost expressed before discounting) must be divided by the annual discount factor, which is $1 + r$, where r is the annual discount rate. For example, if the annual discount rate is 3% (a commonly used value), and the annual discount factor is hence 1.03, a nominal cost of $100 incurred one year in the future has a present value of $\frac{\$100}{1.03} = \$97.09$.

We can apply the same conversion rule repeatedly to compute the present value equivalent for costs incurred at more distant points in the future. Consider a nominal cost of $100 incurred two years in the future. One year from now, it will have a present value of $\frac{\$100}{1.03}$. That quantity, in turn, has a present value right now of $\frac{\$100}{1.03}$ divided once again by 1.03. That is, it has a present value of $\frac{\$100}{1.03 \times 1.03} = \frac{\$100}{1.03^2} = \$94.26$. In general, a nominal cost of X incurred n years in the future has a present value of $\frac{\$X}{(1+r)^n}$. Once costs and savings occurring at different times have been converted to their present value equivalents, they can be summed because the impact of time on their value has been "removed." When summing positive and negative elements—like costs and savings or costs and benefits—the result is sometimes referred to as the "net present value."

For example, consider the net present value of the monetary costs and savings for a drug that costs $1,000 now ("time zero") and $500 at Year 1 and which averts a hospitalization at Year 10 that would have cost $1,600. If costs are, by convention, expressed as positive values and savings as negative values, then the incremental net present value of this drug (compared to doing nothing right now and undergoing hospitalization in 10 years) would be $\$1,000 + \frac{\$500}{1.03} - \frac{\$1,600}{1.03^{10}} = \$1,000 + \$485.44 - \$1,190.55 = \$294.89$. Without taking into account discounting, the drug achieves a net savings of $100 (i.e., $1,000 + $500 − $1,600 = *savings of* $100. But with discounting, the drug has a net cost of nearly $295.

Box 4.3 Why Health Outcomes Should Be Discounted

One argument in favor of discounting health benefits starts by claiming that an intervention's cost-effectiveness should be the same—and hence receive the same priority—whether we adopt it now or at some point in the future. For example, consider a health program that costs $100,000 and saves one QALY (i.e., has a cost-effectiveness of $100,000 per QALY). Suppose we could instead adopt this program in five years for $100,000 and that $100,000 in five years has a present value of $80,000 because of discounting. If we do not discount the QALYs accrued in five years, then the cost-effectiveness ratio for the same program adopted in five years is $80,000 per QALY saved. If the cost-effectiveness benchmark is $90,000 per QALY, the same program might look like a poor investment if implemented now, but a good investment if implemented in five years. If we believe that the advisability of investing in an intervention should remain the same if the costs and benefits remain unchanged, then this result makes no sense.

This argument can be reframed in the form of a paradox.[1] Suppose that we discount monetized costs each year but leave health benefits undiscounted. In that case, each year we delay adopting the health program reduces the present value of its costs but leaves its health benefits unchanged. As a result, the cost-effectiveness ratio's numerator (the cost) declines each year we delay, thus making the cost-effectiveness ratio smaller (i.e., *more favorable*). The longer we delay implementation, the more favorable the cost-effectiveness ratio becomes. Indeed, this formulation suggests that delaying a program's implementation by another year always improves the cost-effectiveness ratio. Because delaying is always advantageous, *it never makes sense to adopt the intervention*; hence the paradox.

At the root of this reasoning is an assumption that the same health benefits can always be bought with money. Because money declines in value over time and because health benefits and money are interchangeable, health benefits must *also* decline in value over time (and *at the same rate*). Proponents of this argument add that discounting health benefits also makes sense because people tend to favor the immediate gratification of receiving benefits sooner rather than later[43p275]; that is, health benefits received earlier are worth more than benefits received later (in the same way that money received sooner is worth more than an identical sum received later).

[1] Keeler, E.B., and Cretin, S. 1983. "Discounting of life-saving and other nonmonetary effects." *Management Science* 29 (3): 300–306. https://doi.org/10.1287/mnsc.29.3.300.

Where does this theorizing leave us? Most everyone agrees that monetary costs and savings should be discounted. Leaving health benefits undiscounted makes them appear especially large as we project an intervention's consequences into the future, giving rise to the "indefinite delay" paradox described in Box 4.3. On the other hand, discounting health benefits makes long-term investments in population health (e.g., to prevent climate change) seem especially unfavorable.

As a practical matter, health economists seem to have largely settled on discounting both monetary impacts and health benefits and to discount them at the same rate. For programs with a long-term horizon, it makes sense for investigators to consider how changing assumptions about discounting affects estimated cost-effectiveness, as in some cases, discounting monetary and health impacts differently can substantially influence results.

A Matter of Perspective—Whose Benefits and Costs?

A joke in academia is about how a paper's lead author should acknowledge the contributions of colleagues: "I would like to thank my co-authors, without whose help this paper would have been finished six months earlier." A version of this story transpired for a particular section of the 500-page volume produced by the Second Panel on Cost-Effectiveness in Health and Medicine (disclosure: one of this book's authors, PJN, was a member).[71] Chapter 3 of the panel's report (pp. 67–73) is entitled "Recommendations on Perspectives for the Reference Case." (The term "reference case" refers to the primary cost-effectiveness analysis used to inform a policy or decision.) In that chapter's second paragraph, the authors hint at the group's backroom discord, noting that the panel "debated at length the issue of what perspective the Reference Case should take."[71]

"Perspective" reflects what costs and benefits an analysis should include. At first glance, the question may seem relatively unimportant. But the perspectives of different decision makers can diverge substantially. Consider the patient versus the health plan. Once a patient becomes ill, they may desire all potentially beneficial healthcare regardless of cost, whereas the health plan, which must consider the impact on its own net costs[72] (which can affect premiums paid by all members), will presumably be more judicious about its healthcare resources.

The patient and health plan perspectives can be reconciled to some degree by considering only decisions made before the onset of illness (in economic terms, the ex ante view). Acting as the agents of potential patients, health plans select the package of services (e.g., hospital care, physician visits, and prescription drugs) available to health plan enrollees. Though their choices are often limited, people reveal their preferences to some extent indirectly through their selection of a health plan. For example, they might choose a more expensive option (i.e., with higher premiums) that covers, say, a wider network of physicians or better access to novel and expensive medications. Even then there are important differences. For example, the patient (and their family) may have a much stronger interest than the health plan in preventing and treating conditions (e.g., dementia) that impose a substantial burden on informal caregivers. The regular transition of enrollees from one plan to another (e.g., with a job change) could mean that US plans may place less value on interventions (e.g., preventive care) with benefits that accrue well into the future.[73]

Treatments can affect others beyond the patient (and his or her family) and the health plan. For example, treatment of attention deficit/hyperactivity disorder can affect education costs. Treatment of opioid use disorder affects both the criminal justice system and employers. A "societal perspective" incorporates these broader considerations, in addition to impacts affecting patients and health plans.

All of which returns us to the debate of the Second Panel on Cost-Effectiveness. The Second Panel explained that the original Panel on Cost-Effectiveness, which published its findings in 1996, had defined its "Reference Case" to reflect a societal perspective.[74] The Second Panel explained, "The societal perspective has the advantages of capturing the full consequences of investments in interventions designed to improve health and of reflecting the broad public interest."[71p68] Limiting attention to "the healthcare payer or health system perspective . . . would potentially ignore many important consequences of healthcare investment decisions."[71p69] The Second Panel noted that, consistent with the government's overall responsibilities, administrators of public health programs (including Medicare, Medicaid, and the Veterans Administration, which together cover tens of millions of people), "should consider the full consequences of their choices and recommendations"[71p69] and hence should take a societal perspective.

However, the Second Panel also supported use of a healthcare perspective. They noted that despite the original panel's recommendation in favor of a societal perspective, "many, if not most [of the thousands of cost-effectiveness analyses published since that time] have *not* used the societal perspective (emphasis in original)."[71pp67–68] Indeed, the Second Panel noted that many of the studies that claimed to use a societal perspective omitted many of that perspective's elements. The Second Panel speculated that some authors had ignored societal perspective elements because they believed the omission would not materially influence their analysis. But they also noted that "in practice . . . it seems that analysts have seldom given [societal perspective] elements serious consideration" and that "decision-making bodies— primarily in Europe, Australia, and Canada— . . . generally have not adopted a societal perspective."[71p68] The problem with a societal perspective, it seems, is that it provides "advice that is not closely tied to any particular decision maker or budget holder."[71p68] (Another problem is that data gaps may preclude the quantification of certain societal perspective elements.) In short, though, while it might be useful if decision makers considered a broad range of impacts spanning multiple sectors, in practice, they often do not.[75] Hence, even if the Second Panel were to convince health economists to use a societal perspective, the ultimate impact might be to (figuratively) relegate cost-effectiveness analyses to dusty, unvisited shelves in the recesses of university health economics departments.

Faced with this dilemma, and following lengthy debate, the Second Panel recommended that the Reference Case include *both* societal and healthcare perspective analyses. In part, this outcome reflected the kind of workable compromise produced by a committee. But it also reflected an acknowledgment by the Second Panel that cost-effectiveness analysis is never used as a single input in a formulaic manner. Instead, decisions about (sometimes expensive) drugs and other health interventions involve complex factors involving many parties and interests (see Chapters 5, 6, and 10 of this volume). Cost-effectiveness analysis helps these parties consider how much health can be acquired given finite resources, but because different parties have different preferences and care about different resource pools, different populations, and other factors, a single analysis will never suffice.

References

1. Nichol, G., Hallstrom, A.P., Ornato, J.P., Riegel, B., Stiell, I.G., Valenzuela, T., Wells, G.A., White, R.D., and Weisfeldt, M.L. 1998. "Potential cost-effectiveness of public access defibrillation in the United States." *Circulation* 97 (13): 1315–1320. https://doi.org/doi:10.1161/01.CIR.97.13.1315.
2. Groeneveld, P.W., Kwong, J.L., Liu, Y., Rodriguez, A.J., Jones, M.P., Sanders, G.D., and Garber, A.M. 2001. "Cost-effectiveness of automated external defibrillators on airlines." *JAMA* 286 (12): 1482–1489. https://doi.org/10.1001/jama.286.12.1482.
3. Cram, P., Vijan, S., and Fendrick, A.M. 2003. "Cost-effectiveness of automated external defibrillator deployment in selected public locations." *Journal of General Internal Medicine* 18 (9): 745–754. https://doi.org/10.1046/j.1525-1497.2003.21139.x.
4. Andersen, L.W., Holmberg, M.J., Granfeldt, A., James, L.P., and Caulley, L. 2019. "Cost-effectiveness of public automated external defibrillators." *Resuscitation* 138: 250–258. https://doi.org/10.1016/j.resuscitation.2019.03.029.

5. "Free exchange: Petty impressive." 2013, December 21. *The Economist*. https://www.econo-mist.com/finance-and-economics/2013/12/21/petty-impressive.

6. Kiker, B.F. 1966. "The historical roots of the concept of human capital." *Journal of Political Economy* 74 (5): 481–499.

7. Warner, K.E., and Luce, B.R. 1982. *Cost–benefit and cost-effectiveness analysis in health care: Principles, practice, and potential.* Ann Arbor, MI: Health Administration Press.

8. Fisk, E.L. 1921. "Health of industrial workers." In *Waste in industry*, edited by Committee on Elimination of Waste in Industry of the Federated American Engineering Societies, 342–373. New York, NY: McGraw-Hill. https://archive.org/stream/wasteinindustry00ameriala/wasteinindustry00ameriala_djvu.txt.

9. Mishan, E.J. 1971. "Evaluation of life and limb: A theoretical approach." *Journal of Political Economy* 79 (4).

10. Schelling, T.C. 1968. "The life you save may be your own." In *Problems in public expenditure analysis: Studies of government finance*, edited by S.B. Chase, 687–705. Washington, DC: The Brookings Institution.

11. Jennings, W.P., and Jennings, P.R. 2000. "Risk, the willingness-to-pay, and the value of a human life." *Journal of Insurance Issues* 23 (2): 180–184. www.jstor.org/stable/41946188.

12. Johannesson, M. 1996. "The revealed preference approach." In *Theory and methods of economic evaluation of health care*, 65–74. New York: Springer-Verlag US.

13. Ashenfelter, O. 2005. "Measuring the value of a statistical life: Problems and prospects." *Industrial Section, Princeton University* (Working paper #505). https://citeseerx.ist.psu.edu/viewdoc/download?doi=10.1.1.536.6890&rep=rep1&type=pdf.

14. Johannesson, M. 1996. "The expressed preference approach." In *Theory and methods of economic evaluation of health care*, 75–100. New York: Springer.

15. Johannesson, M., Liljas, B., and Johansson, P. 1998. "An experimental comparison of dichotomous choice contingent valuation questions and real purchase decisions." *Applied Economics* 30: 643–647. https://www.tandfonline.com/doi/abs/10.1080/000368498325633.

16. Diamond, P.A., and Hausman, J.A. 1994. "Contingent valuation: Is some number better than no number?" *Journal of Economic Perspectives* 8 (4): 45–64. https://doi.org/10.1257/jep.8.4.45.

17. Tversky, A., and Kahneman, D. 1981. "The framing of decisions and the psychology of choice." *Science* 211 (4481): 453. https://doi.org/10.1126/science.7455683.

18. McNeil, B.J., Pauker, S.G., Sox, H.C., and Tversky, A. 1982. "On the elicitation of preferences for alternative therapies." *New England Journal of Medicine* 306 (21): 1259–1262. https://doi.org/10.1056/nejm198205273062103.

19. Naylor, C.D., Chen, P.E., and Strauss, B. 1992. "Measured enthusiasm: Does the method of reporting trial results alter perceptions of therapeutic effectiveness?" *Annals of Internal Medicine* 117 (11): 916–921. https://doi.org/10.7326/0003-4819-117-11-916.

20. Viscusi, W.K., Huber, J., and Bell, J. 2013. "Assessing whether there is a cancer premium for the value of a statistical life." *Health Economics* 23 (4): 384–396. https://doi.org/10.1002/hec.2919.

21. Morrell, L., Wordsworth, S., Rees, S., and Barker, R. 2017. "Does the public prefer health gain for cancer patients? A systematic review of public views on cancer and its characteristics." *PharmacoEconomics* 35 (8): 793–804. https://doi.org/10.1007/s40273-017-0511-7.

22. Robinson, L.A., and Hammitt, J.K. 2016. "Valuing reductions in fatal illness risks: Implications of recent research." *Health Economics* 25 (8): 1039–1052. https://doi.org/10.1002/hec.3214.

23. Ackerman, F., and Heinzerling, L. 2002. "Pricing the priceless: Cost–benefit analysis of environmental protection." *University of Pennsylvania Law Review* 150: 1553–1584. https://doi.org/10.2307/3312947.

24. "Mortality risk valuation." *US Environmental Protection Agency*. Accessed November 15, 2020. https://www.epa.gov/environmental-economics/mortality-risk-valuation.
25. Moran, M.J., and Monje, C. 2016. *Guidance on treatment of the economic value of a statistical life (VSL) in U.S. Department of Transportation Analyses—2016 adjustment*. Washington, DC: U.S. Department of Transportation, Office of the Secretary of Transportation.
26. Alexander, S. 1962. "They decide who lives, who dies." *Life Magazine*. Accessed November 30, 2020. http://www.nephjc.com/news/godpanel.
27. "Who shall live?" 1965. *NBC News*.
28. Hogness, J.R. 1981. *The implications of cost-effectiveness analysis of medical technology: Background paper #2: Case studies of medical technologies: Case study #1: Formal analysis, policy formulation, and endstage renal disease*. Washington, DC: OTA.
29. Klarman, H. 1998. *History of health services research project interview with Herbert Klarman*, edited by E. Berkowitz. Baltimore, MD: National Information Center on Health Services Research and Health Care Technology.
30. Klarman, H.E. 1982. "The road to cost-effectiveness analysis." *The Milbank Memorial Fund Quarterly. Health and Society* 60 (4): 585–603. https://doi.org/10.2307/3349692. www.jstor.org/stable/3349692.
31. Klarman, H.E., Francis, J.O.S., and Rosenthal, G.D. 1968. "Cost effectiveness analysis applied to the treatment of chronic renal disease." *Medical Care* 6 (1).
32. Grosse, R.N. 1969. "Problem of resource allocation in health." In *The analysis and evaluation of public expenditures: The PPB system, a compendium of papers submitted to the subcommittee on economy in government of the joint economic committee*, edited by Joint Economic Committee, vol. 3, 1197. Washington, DC: US Government Printing Office.
33. Sanders, B.S. 1964. "Measuring community health levels." *American Journal of Public Health and the Nation's Health* 54 (7): 1063–1070. https://doi.org/10.2105/ajph.54.7.1063.
34. Katz, S., Ford, A.B., Moskowitz, R.W., Jackson, B.A., and Jaffe, M.W. 1963. "Studies of illness in the aged: The index of ADL: A standardized measure of biological and psychosocial function." *JAMA* 185 (12): 914–919. https://doi.org/10.1001/jama.1963.03060120024016.
35. Chiang, C.L. 1965. "An index of health: Mathematical models." *National Center for Health Statistics*. Originally accessed December 17, 2019. Accessed again on January 21, 2021. https://www.cdc.gov/nchs/data/series/sr_02/sr02_005acc.pdf.
36. MacKillop, E., and Sheard, S. 2018. "Quantifying life: Understanding the history of quality-adjusted life-years (QALYs)." *Social Science & Medicine* 211: 359–366. https://doi.org/10.1016/j.socscimed.2018.07.004.
37. Williams, A. 2005. "Discovering the QALY, or how Rachel Rosser changed my life." In *Personal Histories in Health Research*, edited by A. Oliver, 191–206. London: The Nuffield Trust.
38. Kaplan, R.M. 2005. "Measuring quality of life for policy analysis: Past, present, and future." In *Advancing health outcomes research methods and clinical applications*, edited by W.R. Lenderking and D.A. Revicki, 1–35. Milwaukee, WI: International Society for Quality of Life Research.
39. Fanshel, S., and Bush, J.W. 1970. "A health-status index and its application to health-services outcomes." *Operations Research* 18 (6): 1021–1066. https://doi.org/10.1287/opre.18.6.1021.
40. Torrance, G.W. 2002. "Looking back and looking forward: Viewed through the eyes of George Torrance." *Medical Decision Making* 22 (2): 178–181. https://doi.org/10.1177/0272989x0202200215.
41. Zeckhauser, R., and Shepard, D. 1976. "Where now for saving lives?" *Law and Contemporary Problems* 40 (4).

42. Center for the Evaluation of Value and Risk in Health. *The Cost-Effectiveness Analysis Registry*. Boston: Institute for Clinical Research and Health Policy Studies (Tufts Medical Center).

43. Hunink, M., Glasziou, P., Siegel, J., Weeks, J., Pliskin, J., Elstein, A., and Weinstein, M. 2001. *Decision making in health and medicine.* Cambridge, UK: Cambridge University Press.

44. Neumann, P.J., Thorat, T., Shi, J., Saret, C.J., and Cohen, J.T. 2015. "The changing face of the cost-utility literature, 1990–2012." *Value in Health* 18 (2): 271–277. https://doi.org/10.1016/j.jval.2014.12.002.

45. Neumann, P.J., Cohen, J.T., and Weinstein, M.C. 2014. "Updating cost-effectiveness—the curious resilience of the $50,000-per-QALY threshold." *New England Journal of Medicine* 371 (9): 796–797. https://doi.org/10.1056/NEJMp1405158.

46. Hirth, R.A., Chernew, M.A., Miller, E., Fendrick, A.M., and Weissert, W.G. 2000. "Willingness to pay for a quality-adjusted life year: In search of a standard." *Medical Decision Making* 20 (3): 332–342. https://doi.org/10.1177/0272989X0002000310.

47. Grosse, S.D. 2008. "Assessing cost-effectiveness in healthcare: History of the $50,000 per QALY threshold." *Expert Review of Pharmacoeconomics & Outcomes Research* 8 (2): 165–178. https://doi.org/10.1586/14737167.8.2.165.

48. Ryen, L., and Svensson, M. 2015. "The willingness to pay for a quality adjusted life year: A review of the empirical literature." *Health Economics* 24 (10): 1289–1301. https://doi.org/10.1002/hec.3085.

49. Braithwaite, R.S., Meltzer, D.O., King, J.T., Leslie, D., and Roberts, M.S. 2008. "What does the value of modern medicine say about the $50,000 per quality-adjusted life-year decision rule?" *Medical Care* 46 (4): 349–356. www.jstor.org/stable/40221668.

50. Chambers, J.D., Neumann, P.J., and Buxton, M.N. 2010. "Does Medicare have an implicit cost-effectiveness threshold?" *Medical Decision Making* 30 (4): E14–E27. https://doi.org/10.1177/0272989X10371134.

51. Devlin, N., and Parkin, D. 2004. "Does NICE have a cost-effectiveness threshold and what other factors influence its decisions? A binary choice analysis." *Health Economics,* 13 (5): 437–452.

52. Dakin, H., Devlin, N., Feng, Y., Rice, N., O'Neill, P., and Parkin, D. 2015. "The influence of cost-effectiveness and other factors on NICE decisions." *Health Economics* 24 (10): 1256–1271. https://doi.org/10.1002/hec.3086.

53. Garber, A.M., and Phelps, C.E. 1997. "Economic foundations of cost-effectiveness analysis." *Journal of Health Economics* 16 (1): 1–31. https://doi.org/10.1016/S0167-6296(96)00506-1.

54. Phelps, C.E. 2019. "A new method to determine the optimal willingness to pay in cost-effectiveness analysis." *Value in Health* 22 (7): 785–791. https://doi.org/10.1016/j.jval.2019.03.003.

55. Ward, A. 2015, February 18. "Expensive drugs cost lives, claims report." *Financial Times.* Accessed September 13, 2020. https://www.ft.com/content/d00c4a02-b784-11e4-981d-00144feab7de.

56. Kohli-Lynch, C.N. 2019. "Beyond ten-year risk: Novel approaches to the primary prevention of cardiovascular disease." *Institute of Health and Wellbeing, University of Glasgow.* http://theses.gla.ac.uk/74296/1/2019Kohli-LynchPhD.pdf.

57. Claxton, K., Martin, S., Soares, M., Rice, N., Spackman, E., Hinde, S., Devlin, N., Smith, P., and Sculpher, M. 2015. "Methods for the estimation of the National Institute for Health and Care Excellence cost-effectiveness threshold." *Health Technology Assessment* 19 (14). https://doi.org/10.3310/hta19140.

58. Vallejo Torres, L., Garcia, B., Castilla Rodríguez, I., Valcarcel-Nazco, C., García-Pérez, L., Linertová, R., Polentinos, E., and Serrano-Aguilar, P. 2016. "On the estimation of the cost-effectiveness threshold: Why, what, how?" *Value in Health* 19 (5): 558–566. https://doi.org/10.1016/j.jval.2016.02.020.

59. Woods, B., Revill, P., Sculpher, M., and Claxton, K. 2016. "Country-level cost-effectiveness thresholds: Initial estimates and the need for further research." *Value in Health* 19 (8): 929–935. https://doi.org/10.1016/j.jval.2016.02.017.

60. Edney, L.C., Haji Ali Afzali, H., Cheng, T.C., and Karnon, J. 2018. "Estimating the reference incremental cost-effectiveness ratio for the Australian health system." *PharmacoEconomics* 36 (2): 239–252. https://doi.org/10.1007/s40273-017-0585-2.

61. Siverskog, J., and Henriksson, M. 2019. "Estimating the marginal cost of a life year in Sweden's public healthcare sector." *The European Journal of Health Economics* 20 (5): 751–762. https://doi.org/10.1007/s10198-019-01039-0.

62. van Baal, P., Perry-Duxbury, M., Bakx, P., Versteegh, M., van Doorslaer, E., and Brouwer, W. 2019. "A cost-effectiveness threshold based on the marginal returns of cardiovascular hospital spending." *Health Economics* 28 (1): 87–100. https://doi.org/10.1002/hec.3831.

63. Hernandez-Villafuerte, K., Zamora, B., and Towse, A. 2018. "Issues surrounding the estimation of the opportunity cost of adopting a new health care technology." *Office of Health Economics.* https://www.ohe.org/news/opportunity-costs-new-health-care-technologies-research-agenda.

64. Norman, R., Augustine, G.M., and Sharyl, J. 2018. *Making medicines affordable: A national imperative.* Washington, DC: National Academies Press.

65. World Health Organization. 2001. *Macroeconomics and health: Investing in health for economic development.* https://www.who.int/pmnch/topics/economics/2001_who_cmh/en/.

66. Hutubessy, R., Chisholm, D., Edejer, T.T.-T., and Who, C. 2003. "Generalized cost-effectiveness analysis for national-level priority-setting in the health sector." *Cost Effectiveness and Resource Allocation* 1 (1): 8. https://doi.org/10.1186/1478-7547-1-8.

67. Bertram, M.Y., Lauer, J.A., De Joncheere, K., Edejer, T., Hutubessy, R., Kieny, M.-P., and Hill, S.R. 2016. "Cost-effectiveness thresholds: Pros and cons." *Bulletin of the World Health Organization* 94 (12): 925–930. https://doi.org/10.2471/BLT.15.164418.

68. Rodwin, M.A. 2019. "What can the United States learn from pharmaceutical spending controls in France?" *The Commonwealth Fund.* Accessed July 10, 2020. https://www.commonwealthfund.org/publications/issue-briefs/2019/nov/what-can-united-states-learn-drug-spending-controls-france.

69. Sarnak, D.O., Squires, D., and Bishop, S. 2017. "Paying for prescription drugs around the world: Why is the U.S. an outlier?" *The Commonwealth Fund.* Accessed August 4, 2020. https://www.commonwealthfund.org/publications/issue-briefs/2017/oct/paying-prescription-drugs-around-world-why-us-outlier.

70. Kwok, M.Q.T., Kareem, M.A., Cash, M.J., Lafferty, F., Tobin, K., and O'Mahony, J.F. 2020. "Adherence to discounting guidelines: Evidence from over 2000 published cost-effectiveness analyses." *PharmacoEconomics* 38 (8): 809–818. https://doi.org/10.1007/s40273-020-00916-4.

71. Neumann, P.J., Sanders, G.D., Russell, L.B., Siegel, J.E., and Ganiats, T.G. 2017. *Cost-effectiveness in health and medicine* (2nd ed.). New York: Oxford University Press.

72. Garrison, L.P., Pauly, M.V., Willke, R.J., and Neumann, P.J. 2018. "An overview of value, perspective, and decision context—a health economics approach: An ISPOR special task force report." *Value in Health* 21 (2): 124–130. https://doi.org/10.1016/j.jval.2017.12.006.

73. Kim, D., Wilkinson, C., Pope, E., Chambers, J., Cohen, J., and Neumann, P. 2017. "The influence of time horizon on results of cost-effectiveness analyses." *Expert Review of Pharmacoeconomics & Outcomes Research* 17 (6): 615–623.

74. Gold, M.E., Siegel, J.E., Russell, L.B., and Weinstein, M.C. 1996. *Cost-effectiveness in health and medicine* (1st ed.). New York: Oxford University Press.

75. Kim, D.D., Silver, M.C., Kunst, N., Cohen, J.T., Ollendorf, D.A., and Neumann, P.J. 2020. "Perspective and costing in cost-effectiveness analysis, 1974–2018." *PharmacoEconomics* 38: 1135–1145. https://doi.org/10.1007/s40273-020-00942-2.

PART II

EXPERIENCES MEASURING A DRUG'S VALUE IN THE US AND ABROAD

5

Measuring Drug Value

Whose Job Is It Anyway?

NICE: A "Terrible Beauty" or Just a Beast?

In 1995, Gerry Malone, a Minister of State at the Department of Health in the United Kingdom, wrestled with a dilemma: Should the country's National Health Service pay for beta-interferon, an expensive new treatment for multiple sclerosis? While the therapy showed promise for reducing the frequency and severity of "flares" in the disease's neurologic, cognitive, and other major symptoms, the drug's effects and how long it would continue to work were highly uncertain. The cost to the country could run as high as £380 million, equivalent to 10% of the nation's total drug budget.[1] Malone, a lawyer and journalist by background, was flummoxed. "How the hell am *I* meant to make that decision?" he wondered.[2p32]

The choice highlighted a recurring problem for Malone and the United Kingdom's health system, namely the absence of a central authority to assess whether therapies like beta-interferon were worth the expense, and for which patients and under what circumstances. To be sure, the country had clinical guidelines (sometimes multiple conflicting ones) and no shortage of opinions about such questions. What it lacked was a systematic, independent, science-based review of the clinical and economic evidence. The consequence was sometimes wide geographic variation across Britain in patients' access to specific treatments, a phenomenon known as the "postcode lottery," reflecting the dependence of the availability of therapies on the resources available and idiosyncratic decisions made in a particular town or health district.[2p24]

In the late 1990s, Tony Blair's Labour Government adopted the cause and launched the National Institute for Health and Care Excellence (NICE), a special health authority for the "speedy uptake of cost-effective innovations."[2p34] NICE drew upon the United Kingdom's rich intellectual foundation for understanding the evidence underpinning medical practice. The physician Archie Cochrane (1909–1988) had pioneered the concept of "evidence-based medicine," the idea that rather than relying on their intuition, clinicians should

The Right Price. Peter J. Neumann, Joshua T. Cohen, and Daniel A. Ollendorf, Oxford University Press (2021).
© Peter J. Neumann, Joshua T. Cohen, and Daniel A. Ollendorf. DOI: 10.1093/oso/9780197512883.003.0005

deliver care with solid empirical foundations, preferably substantiated by data from randomized controlled trials.[3] Around the same time, British health economists, including Alan Williams (1927–2005) of the University of York, helped develop and refine the field of cost-effectiveness analysis, including efforts to advance the quality-adjusted life year (QALY).[4] The mid-1980s saw important economic evaluations for heart transplantation and breast cancer screening that informed decisions by the National Health Service.[5]

If you want to learn about how an organization can measure the value of prescription drugs (and other technologies) and use the results to inform decision-making, you would be hard pressed to find a better starting place than NICE. While not the world's oldest body conducting such evaluations, it is likely the most renowned, recognized widely as an international leader in the methods and process for conducting clinical and economic reviews. One observer has called it "one of Britain's greatest cultural exports along with Shakespeare, Newtonian physics, the Beatles, Harry Potter, and the Teletubbies."[6]

As of September 2020, NICE has evaluated over 600 technologies in partnership with a network of academic research collaborators.[7] The agency, with a remit that includes the issuance of clinical guidelines and that has expanded to encompass reports about public health and social services, is now called the National Institute for Health and Care Excellence, although the acronym "NICE" endures, and continues to inspire a thousand puns (e.g., "Is the latest decision NICE or nasty?").[2p113]

NICE's 20-year history reveals the benefits and pitfalls inherent in assessing a drug's value. A charitable view would depict an organization that has provided health authorities with a structured, rational, consistent approach to value measurement, bringing evidence and scientific reasoning to an unruly and inequitable healthcare system.[8] Its reports have demonstrated the merits of using cost-effectiveness analysis, not only as a means to benchmark a therapy's relative costs and benefits, but also as a framework for comparing alternatives, exploring scenarios, testing the strength of underlying assumptions, and considering tradeoffs, all in an explicit, quantitative, and systematic way.[8]

At the same time, controversy has followed NICE at many turns. In the fall of 1999, the agency's very first evaluation, of zanamivir (Relenza®, GlaxoSmithKline), an antiviral for influenza, caused a stir. NICE recommended against routine prescribing of the drug based on the lack of evidence of the treatment's benefit in older and sicker populations and a finding that, at its proposed price, the therapy was not cost-effective.[2p9,9] A public outcry ensued, as well as threats from GlaxoSmithKline, the product's

UK-based manufacturer, to move its operation elsewhere.[10] NICE held firm and weathered the storm. The case set an important precedent and signaled that the upstart agency would adhere to its interpretation of the evidence and not easily bow to external pressure.

Other disputes followed. "Cancer Patients Denied Better, Cheaper Care" and "Sentenced to Death by NICE" are just two examples of newspaper headlines that appeared after unfavorable NICE reviews.[2pp81-82] Patient advocates, the drug industry, medical societies, and others have criticized particular decisions and protested generally about "NICE blight," the delays in access that patients experience while the organization undertakes its sometimes-lengthy review process.

Still, the agency has endured and mostly earned the respect, if not love, of external groups for the rigor, transparency, and fairness of its process. Evoking a poem by W. B. Yeats, authors of a 2016 history of NICE called the agency a "terrible beauty"—terrible because of treatments denied that offered hope to patients and profits to companies, but a beauty in the way NICE has sought to improve population health given resource constraints.[2p135] Indeed, over the years, NICE has received political support from parties on opposite sides of the ideological spectrum—in no small measure by taking sensitive decisions out of politicians' hands. The organization and its academic partners are generally admired for the thoroughness of their reviews and critiques of drug company-submitted economic models, the openness of the process, and the nuances considered in its deliberations on the evidence. In most cases, NICE issues a "yes, but" recommendation regarding the value of a new drug, meaning the treatment is cost-effective in certain circumstances or patient subgroups but not others.

Critically, the organization has proven flexible at key junctures. It has shortened review times with a fast-track appraisal option for lone technologies applying for a single indication. It has amended (i.e., made more generous) its usual cost-effectiveness benchmark of £20,000 ($28,000) per QALY gained to £30,000 ($42,000) per QALY gained for certain situations, such as "end-of-life" care and ultra-rare diseases (see Chapter 8 of this volume). It has established and refined a Cancer Drugs Fund to provide faster access to cancer therapies, even those that did not meet standard cost-effectiveness benchmarks (Chapter 8 of this volume). These exceptions and the creation of the Cancer Drugs Fund have been controversial in their own rights, but they have also provided an escape valve for political pressures and helped NICE endure. As close observers of the process have noted, one of the principal takeaways from NICE's history has been "don't let perfect be the enemy of good."[2p169]

The agency has also developed "managed entry agreements," which provide drug companies an avenue for confidential discounts and flexible coverage arrangements under which additional evidence on a drug is gathered while offering patients some access to products. For example, in 2002 NICE concluded that beta-interferon and glatiramer acetate—by then established treatments for multiple sclerosis—were not cost-effective at their prevailing prices.[11] The resulting backlash—from patient groups, medical societies, and the drug industry—led to a compromise in which NICE allowed access to the medications in exchange for a confidential price discount and additional concessions if the drugs did not work as advertised.[12] As of September 2020, there were over 250 instances of managed entry agreements across a range of products, and NICE had established a special office to facilitate them.[13]

Valuing Drugs Across the Globe

Efforts to assess a drug's value have also proliferated elsewhere. Canada and Australia, for example, have long-standing health technology assessment (HTA) programs to assess the value of drugs and other technologies.[14] A 2017 report found that of the 20 western/southern European or Scandinavian members of the European Union or European Economic Area, 17 have at least one HTA organization with a national mandate to inform drug coverage, pricing, and/or reimbursement.[15] Although at earlier stages of implementation, HTA in eastern Europe has accelerated (a 2019 survey found that 9 of 13 countries in the region consider economic evaluation explicitly in drug coverage or pricing decisions).[16]

The idea has also spread to Latin America and Asia, although lack of expertise and training opportunities, as well as insufficient public investment, remain challenges.[17,18] Brazil and Colombia have relatively established HTA organizations and efforts have grown elsewhere in the region.[19] Thailand's Health Intervention and Technology Assessment Program has one of the world's most productive and visible HTA bodies and has advised other countries including Singapore and Malaysia.[20] South Korea's National Evidence-based Healthcare Collaborating Agency is also well established, contributing to regional and global HTA policy discussions.[21] China has seen fledgling efforts to adopt value-driven approaches to drug price negotiations, although HTA remains largely fragmented and decentralized, mirroring the country's health system.[22]

A growing trend is cross-national collaborative HTA initiatives to foster efficiencies and bargaining power for drug price negotiations. The European

Network for Health Technology Assessment, for example, includes 80 HTA bodies from 30 countries, with European Union backing and funding to conduct assessments.[23] On a smaller scale, the BeNeLuxA pilot initiative combines HTA organizations of Belgium, Ireland, the Netherlands, Luxembourg, and Austria to improve the consistency of assessments across jurisdictions and leverage the countries' ability to negotiate prices.[24]

In all settings, policymakers have grappled with methodological challenges and often faced determined opposition from the drug industry, patient advocates, and other groups.[25] Health officials have navigated the political terrain with different approaches, varying in whether they consider economic evaluations explicitly, whether they use QALYs, whether analyses assume a health payer or societal perspective, and in terms of the processes undertaken.

As noted in Chapter 4 of this volume, authorities in Germany and France have chosen not to use cost-per-QALY analyses as the basis for determining a drug's value. Instead, they judge value by considering the magnitude and nature of a medicine's clinical benefit (i.e., whether the effects are viewed as major or minor), and while economic evaluations are permitted, they are rarely performed.[15] In contrast, neighboring countries, including the Netherlands, Sweden, and others, conduct economic evaluations explicitly using cost-per-QALY analyses, in a manner similar to NICE. We return to the pros and cons of cost-per-QALY analyses later in the book. But as Chapter 4 of this volume observed, comparing treatment health benefits across disparate conditions or interventions depends on having a common metric. As a result, those systems that have rejected the QALY tend to instead rely on opaque negotiations to arrive at drug prices and on "reference pricing," which often means "importing" assessments from countries that *do* use cost-per-QALY analyses. Countries also use different benchmarks to identify ranges of acceptable cost-effectiveness values. Finally, they differ in their consideration of affordability and budget impact concerns.[26]

Worldwide, most HTA bodies are government organizations or receive direct appropriations from government. Still, they vary widely in terms of their reporting structures, whether they conduct analyses for regional or national authorities, whether their recommendations are binding or advisory, and whether and how value their assessments influence a drug's price. For example, the Canadian Agency for Drugs and Technologies in Health issues national reports, but implementation of recommendations varies across provinces, depending on available budgets, priorities, and political considerations.[27] In theory, interprovincial transfer payments address inequities in access, although generally these efforts have disappointed.[28] Australia's Pharmaceutical Benefits Scheme cannot list a medication unless it has been recommended by the Pharmaceutical Benefits Advisory Committee, the national HTA body. Positive recommendations may also be reviewed by the cabinet if the potential budget impact exceeds AU$20 million annually.[29,30]

HTA bodies also vary in terms of whether they conduct their own assessments or simply review dossiers submitted by drug companies. Other differences across HTA bodies include the duration of their assessments, the transparency of their reviews, opportunities for stakeholder input, and the ability of external parties to appeal decisions.[15,31-33]

There are also subtle but important differences in how organizations reach conclusions. Nearly all HTA bodies relegate deliberations on clinical and economic evidence to committees of experts and stakeholders appointed by, but independent from, the organization. Stakeholder representation on these committees varies; for example, drug industry and payer representatives participate fully on some committees, while other HTA organizations restrict or prohibit such participation.[34,35] Some committees vote on their conclusions, while others attempt to forge consensus, making the chair's role in managing the process critical.[36 37] The setting for deliberation also varies. Committees convened by the Institute for Clinical and Economic Review (see Chapter 6 of this volume) conduct their proceedings in public, while NICE committees deliberate partially in the open, and committees in Canada and France review and discuss evidence privately.[36,38]

A takeaway is that while HTA organizations may draw from the same methodological toolbox, the manner in which they consider the techniques and integrate them into deliberations varies. Each application is influenced by the politics, culture, and values of the society in which it operates.

American Exceptionalism?

Green Shoots for Value Assessment in the United States

The health cost pressures that have pushed other countries toward formal value assessment have also, of course, existed in the United States. Concerns about the cost of dialysis for patients with end-stage renal disease motivated the federally sponsored assessment of that technology, as described in Chapter 4 of this volume.

The US government has long been involved in value assessment, particularly for preventative care and screening. The Office of Technology Assessment conducted congressionally requested cost-effectiveness analyses between the late 1970s and early 1990s to inform Medicare's adoption of pneumococcal vaccination, screening for breast cancer, cervical cancer, and colorectal cancer.[39–42] The Centers for Medicare and Medicaid Services reviewed cost-effectiveness evidence in considering coverage for human immunodeficiency virus (HIV) screening in 2010 and lung cancer screening in 2015 and for screening and behavioral counseling for alcohol misuse in 2011.[43,44] The Advisory Committee for Immunization Practices, which makes immunization recommendations for the Centers for Disease Control and Prevention, uses cost-effectiveness analysis.[45,46]

Other government agencies, such as the Agency for Healthcare Research and Quality, the Centers for Disease Control and Prevention and National Institutes of Health, have funded or conducted cost-effectiveness analyses in selected areas.[47] The Department of Veterans Affairs and the Department of Defense's health authority review the cost-effectiveness of pharmaceuticals in their reimbursement policies.[48p84]

A few private health plans have adopted economic evaluation explicitly in drug formulary policies. For example, Premera Blue Cross, a large regional health plan primarily serving Washington State and Alaska, offers its employees lower co-payments on favorably cost-effective drugs and imposes higher co-payments on drugs with less favorable cost-effectiveness (see Chapter 10 of this volume).[49] The Academy of Managed Care Pharmacy has promoted guidelines encouraging health plans to request cost-effectiveness information from drug companies.[50,51]

These "green shoots" suggest a demand in certain quarters for value assessment to help guide drug policy decisions. Overall receptiveness to these approaches has remained limited in the United States, however. The experience in Oregon offers a cautionary example.

Lessons From Oregon

In the late 1980s and early 1990s, John Kitzhaber seemed the perfect champion for a bold new health policy experiment. An emergency room physician and Oregon's Senate president (he would later serve three terms as the state's governor), the iconoclastic Kitzhaber, who wore jeans to the office and disdained neckties before such sartorial choices became *de rigueur*, was a determined advocate for a better health system.

Kitzhaber was the chief architect of the Oregon Health Plan, an audacious experiment in policymaking. The impetus had been the experiences of a seven-year-old Oregon resident, Coby Howard, a boy with leukemia in need of a bone marrow transplant. The state would not pay because of budget shortfalls and other pressing health priorities. Coby's family had privately managed to raise $70,000 of the $100,000 needed when Coby died in December 1987.[52] To Kitzhaber, the case, agonizing as it was, revealed a larger truth about the unfairness and inefficiency of the system and spurred a call to action. "What we can do with our limited money is to reduce the number of deaths to the maximum," Kitzhaber said. "Save as many people as we can, because we can't save them all."[52]

The Oregon plan that followed sought to ensure coverage for a greater proportion of state residents through a mix of employer-funded plans and public health insurance. Importantly, coverage of additional residents by public insurance would be funded in part by restricting the range of services covered in the standard public benefit package. In particular, the Oregon plan would (a) develop a prioritized list of paired medical conditions and treatments that ranked the value of services from most important to least important *according to information on their costs and effects* and (b) cover only those services that fell above a line reflecting the state's budgetary resources. Notably, Oregon's priority list would use a formula to estimate the cost-effectiveness of treatments.[8pp58-70]

The plan seemed to herald a new era in health policymaking, one grounded in a more honest, rational, empirically driven approach to prioritizing care and apportioning resources based on formal cost-effectiveness analysis. Indeed, cost-effectiveness analysis would take center stage as a tool to help the state obtain better value for its spending. It would enable Oregon to provide health insurance to many more low-income residents. Advocates of the plan also lauded the public and participatory nature of the process, a "classic exercise of American democracy in the sunlight."[52p7,53] It involved elected officials, community leaders, and health professionals who assembled to define an adequate minimum standard of healthcare in a manner that was seen as politically accountable, reflecting community values, and subject to a vote of the legislature.[52] Newspaper stories and journal articles followed. Policymakers from around the country and the world watched closely and in some cases visited Salem, the state capitol, to learn about what would surely be the future of health policy.

Except that it wasn't. The plan was controversial from the start. Critics— including US Senator Albert Gore, US Representative Henry Waxman, and groups ranging from the Children's Defense Fund and the American Academy of Pediatrics to the National Association of Community Health Centers, US Catholic Conference, and the National Association of Children's Hospitals[54]—attacked the plan for unfairly singling out the state's poorest citizens (who also happened to be disproportionately young, nonwhite, and female) for the "rationing" scheme (Medicaid recipients would be denied medically necessary services that fell "below the line"). One pair of critics called it "politically convenient and ethically execrable."[55p395] The Children's Defense Fund contended that the process amounted to 1,000 healthy, upper-middle-class people making decisions for poor children on what services to take away.[54]

The cost-effectiveness methodology was also criticized. Senator and future Vice President Al Gore said the plan amounted to "playing God by playing with spreadsheets."[54p39] Bruce Vladeck, who would later head the Health Care Financing Administration (now the Centers for Medicare and Medicaid Services), called it a "misbegotten mishmash of second-rate policy analysis and cynical budgetary politics."[54p39] "The methodological basis for this is insane," complained one vocal opponent.[56p2135]

In the end, cost-effectiveness analysis played little role in Oregon's plan. It proved so contentious and difficult to implement that it was largely abandoned even as a priority list was salvaged. To obtain a federal waiver for the plan (required for Medicaid experiments of this kind) and to comply with the Americans with Disabilities Act, Oregon amended its priority list, basing it more on the judgments of an external commission comprised of health professionals and consumer representatives. Moreover, the plan seemed to *increase* overall healthcare costs: Medicaid expenditures rose 39% in Oregon in the three years following enactment as opposed to 30% nationally. Even after the plan's implementation, few services were denied. The main exclusions seemed to be for clinically marginal or ineffective therapies or for self-limiting conditions.[53,57]

Most important, no other state—or public or private health plan—ever emulated the model. Instead, they dealt with the same problems without the explosive priority list, in part by eliminating certain benefits, but mostly by redefining eligibility, reducing reimbursement to providers, and rapidly expanding managed care options.[52,58,59] The idea was never transportable across state lines.[60] The plan's proponents assumed that rising spending and the public's insatiable appetite for medical technology would force Americans to recognize limits more directly—and, inevitably, employ cost-effectiveness analysis as the best solution to its dilemma. However, there was no such groundswell among policymakers or politicians. In retrospect, the application of cost-effectiveness analysis in Oregon as a means to valuing care seemed in fundamental ways to cut against the grain of American values.

Lessons From Elsewhere

Oregon was not an anomaly. A National Center for Health Care Technology existed for a short time in the late 1970s and early 1980s but was eliminated by the Reagan administration amid criticisms by the Health Industry Manufacturers Association (now the Advanced Medical Technology Association), the American Medical Association, and others who argued that the agency impeded the judgment of physician and focused more on cost control than on technology assessment.[61–63] Congress created an Office of Technology Assessment in 1972 to inform that body about technologies, including healthcare technologies. The office conducted numerous well-regarded assessments before being abolished in 1995 as part of the Republican-controlled Congress's elimination of what it described as wasteful spending (in particular redundancies in assessment activities across other government agencies) and its concerns about politically biased evaluations and a strong and independent advisory board that could usurp Congress's own authority. The Agency for Healthcare Research and Quality faced threats of extinction in the 1990s because of fears about overly prescriptive clinical practice guidelines.[64]

The government-funded technology assessment functions that have endured have generally focused on clinical (not economic) evidence and on preventive services, as opposed to treatments. Some state efforts to assess the value of drugs, such as those conducted by the Drug Effectiveness Review Project, a collaborative of state Medicaid and public pharmacy programs, have considered the strength of clinical evidence but shied away from using cost-effectiveness analysis.[65] The US Preventive Services Task Force, which makes evidence-based recommendations about clinical preventive services, has considered using cost-effectiveness analysis[66] but in practice has chosen not to do so. The Medicare program for years attempted to incorporate cost-effectiveness analysis into its decision-making processes for new drugs and other technologies but has been thwarted by legal and political hurdles.[67] The 2010 Patient Protection and Affordable Care Act (commonly known as the ACA) created a Patient-Centered Outcomes Research Institute to conduct comparative clinical effectiveness research but prohibited the institute from developing or employing cost-per-QALY benchmarks or "thresholds" (see Box 9.4 in Chapter 9 of this volume).[68]

Most commercial plans have been reluctant to use economic evaluations too openly when pricing or covering drugs. Plans have adopted ever more aggressive policies that aim to constrain cost growth by discouraging use (e.g., increasing copayments for expensive medications drugs), but historically they have avoided explicit consideration of cost-effectiveness.[8,pp23-25,69]

Americans' Distaste for Rationing

The pushback against government-led efforts to value drugs seems particularly acute in the United States, although to be sure, concerns are not unique to Americans. Many scholars have written about the roots of American attitudes and its enduring influence on public policy, including health policy.[70] The term "American exceptionalism," coined by the French historian Alexis de Tocqueville during a trip to the still young United States in 1835, refers to the idea that the United States is different than other developed nations because of its unique origins, evolution, and institutions.[70] Briefly stated and somewhat oversimplified, the idea is that Americans are characterized by their optimism, their religiosity, and, above all, their predilection for personal and economic freedom.[70,71] The concept of American exceptionalism has been debated extensively in the academic literature—what it means, whether there indeed even exists such a thing and, if so, whether it is good or bad for the United States and the world.[72-74]

The Hollywood image and caricature of the American cowboy—freedom-loving, individualistic, mistrustful of authority—animates themes de Tocqueville identified in the 1830s. In *Democracy in America* he noted the country's strong commitment to liberty and egalitarianism, a streak of anti-authoritarianism and a laissez faire attitude about private enterprise. He also observed a fundamental optimism and patriotism among the people.

Even today, observers point to exceptionalism in various aspects of American life. For consumers it has translated into low savings rates, big cars, high rates of obesity, and a self-reliant—but also more litigious—people. In business, the term conveys a commitment to competition ("cowboy capitalism"), free markets, a tolerance for seemingly outrageous executive pay and income inequality, longer work hours and less vacation time, low union membership, and less regulation. In politics, it has meant more culturally conservative voters and domestic policies, ranging from the right to bear arms to low income taxes. Of course, making general statements about the preferences of Americans is a fraught exercise. Still, policies in the United States stand in contrast to the relatively more regulated and taxed social-democratic models of western Europe.

"American exceptionalism in health care is notable in several respects, particularly the US's high spending on health services relative to its GDP, its lack of universal health care, its poor health outcomes compared to other high income nations" and "faster and more flexible access to new drugs, though with significantly more cost sharing than elsewhere."[70p4,75,76] It has also meant mistrust of centralized value assessment activities.[70,77]

The ferocious backlash to the US Preventive Services Task Force's advice to raise the age limit for breast cancer screening based in part on misconceptions that costs were being used to deny needed services serves as an example.[78] The statutory language prohibiting the Patient-Centered Outcomes Research Institute to use cost-effectiveness analysis is another example of an aversion towards "big government" healthcare and "death panels."[68]

Of course, the United States "rations" in healthcare in other, less visible ways. Despite expansions of coverage in recent years, some 28 million Americans still lack health insurance. Millions more are underinsured with inadequate benefits (e.g., in terms of high deductibles and co-payments), resulting in excessive medical debt or bankruptcy and the postponement of needed care because of costs.[79] The question is not whether America rations but whether payers use tools such as cost-effectiveness analysis to help determine which services to pay for.

The answer to this question seemed to be no, America would not consider cost-effectiveness openly in healthcare decisions. With a deep-rooted antipathy to top–down decision-making stretching back to the early days of the republic, and a decades-long track record of resisting the prominent use of cost-effectiveness methods so popular elsewhere, it seemed that the situation would never change.

And then it did.

References

1. Walley, T., and Barton S. (cited in Timmins 2016). 1995. "A purchaser perspective of managing new drugs: Interferon beta as a case study." *BMJ* 311 (7008): 796–799. https://doi.org/10.1136/bmj.311.7008.796.
2. Timmins, N., Rawlins, M., and Appleby, J. 2016. *A terrible beauty: A short history of NICE.* London: Health Intervention and Technology Assessment Program.
3. Stavrou, A., Challoumas, D., and Dimitrakakis, G. 2014. "Archibald Cochrane (1909–1988): The father of evidence-based medicine." *Interactive Cardiovascular and Thoracic Surgery* 18 (1): 121–124. https://doi.org/10.1093/icvts/ivt451.
4. Williams, A. 2005. "Discovering the QALY, or how Rachel Rosser changed my life." In *Personal Histories in Health Research*, edited by A. Oliver, 191–206. London: The Nuffield Trust.
5. Buxton, M.N. 1987. "The economic evaluation of high technology medicine: The case of heart transplants." In *Health and Economics*, edited by A. Williams, 162–172. London, UK: Palgrave Macmillan.

6. "The triumph of NICE." 2004. *British Medical Journal* 329: 0-g

7. National Institute for Health and Care Excellence. 2020. "Technology appraisal data: Appraisal recommendations." https://www.nice.org.uk/about/what-we-do/our-programmes/nice-guidance/nice-technology-appraisal-guidance/data/appraisal-recommendations.

8. Neumann, P.J. 2005. *Using cost-effectiveness analysis to improve health care: Opportunities and barriers.* New York: Oxford University Press.

9. National Institute for Health and Care Excellence. 2009. "Amantadine, oseltamivir and zanamivir for the treatment of influenza: Technology appraisal guidance [TA168]." Accessed January 25, 2021. https://www.nice.org.uk/guidance/ta168.

10. Mitchell, P. 1999. "Glaxo Wellcome disputes NICEs recommendation against zanamivir." *The Lancet* 354 (9186): 1275. https://doi.org/10.1016/S0140-6736(05)76055-4.

11. National Institute for Health and Care Excellence. 2002. "Beta interferon and glatiramer acetate for the treatment of multiple sclerosis: Technology appraisal guidance [TA32]." Last modified June 27, 2018. Accessed January 25, 2021. https://www.nice.org.uk/guidance/ta32.

12. Multiple Sclerosis Trust. "The Department of Health risk-sharing scheme." Accessed January 25, 2021. https://www.mstrust.org.uk/department-health-risk-sharing-scheme.

13. National Institute for Health and Care Excellence. 2020. "Technologies recommended by NICE that include a commercial arrangement." https://www.nice.org.uk/about/what-we-do/patient-access-schemes-liaison-unit.

14. International Network of Agencies for Health Technology Assessment. "INAHTA members list." Accessed January 25, 2021. https://www.inahta.org/members/members_list/.

15. Chamova, J. 2017. "Mapping of HTA national organisations, programmes and processes in EU and Norway." *European Union.* https://op.europa.eu/en/publication-detail/-/publication/971cf96d-0aef-11e8-966a-01aa75ed71a1.

16. García-Mochón, L., Espín Balbino, J., Olry de Labry Lima, A., Caro Martinez, A., Martin Ruiz, E., and Pérez Velasco, R. 2019. "HTA and decision-making processes in Central, Eastern and South Eastern Europe: Results from a survey." *Health Policy* 123 (2): 182–190. https://doi.org/10.1016/j.healthpol.2017.03.010.

17. Simoens, S. 2010. "Health technology assessment and economic evaluation across jurisdictions." *Value in Health* 13 (6): 857–859. https://doi.org/10.1111/j.1524-4733.2010.00756.x.

18. Rosselli, D., Quirland-Lazo, C., Csánadi, M., Ruiz de Castilla, E.M., Cisneros González, N., Valdés, J., Abicalaffe, C., Garzón, W., and Kaló, Z. 2017. "HTA implementation in Latin American countries: Comparison of current and preferred status." *Value Health Reg Issues* 14: 20–27. https://doi.org/10.1016/j.vhri.2017.02.004.

19. Castro, H.E. 2017. "Advancing HTA in Latin America: The policy process of setting up an HTA agency in Colombia." *Global Policy* 8 (S2): 97–102. https://doi.org/10.1111/1758-5899.12333.

20. "Policy brief: Conducive factors to HTA development in Asia." *HITAP International Unit.* Accessed January 25, 2021. http://www.globalhitap.net/projects/policy-brief-conducive-factors-to-hta-development-in-asia-2/.

21. "NECA—National Evidence-Based Healthcare Collaborating Agency." *International Network of Agencies for Health Technology Assessment.* Accessed January 25, 2021. https://www.inahta.org/members/neca/.

22. Chen, Y., He, Y., Chi, X., Wei, Y., and Shi, L. 2018. "Development of health technology assessment in China: New challenges." *BioScience Trends* 12 (2): 102–108. https://doi.org/10.5582/bst.2018.01038.

23. "EUnetHTA Network: EUnetHTA partner organisations and institutions." *European Network for Health Technology Assessment.* Accessed January 25, 2021. https://eunethta. eu/about-eunethta/eunethtanetwork/.

24. O'Mahony, J.F. 2019. "Beneluxa: What are the prospects for collective bargaining on pharmaceutical prices given diverse health technology assessment processes?" *PharmacoEconomics* 37 (5): 627–630. https://doi.org/10.1007/s40273-019-00781-w.

25. Wong, J. 2014. "The history of technology assessment and comparative effectiveness research for drugs and medical devices and the role of the federal government." *Biotechnology Law Report* 33 (6): 221–248. https://doi.org/10.1089/blr.2014.9967.

26. Schwarzer, R., Rochau, U., Saverno, K., Jahn, B., Bornschein, B., Muehlberger, N., Flatscher-Thoeni, M., Schnell-Inderst, P., Sroczynski, G., Lackner, M., Schall, I., Hebborn, A., Pugner, K., Fehervary, A., Brixner, D., and Siebert, U. 2015. "Systematic overview of cost-effectiveness thresholds in ten countries across four continents." *Journal of Comparative Effectiveness Research* 4 (5): 485–504. https://doi.org/10.2217/cer.15.38.

27. Rocchi, A., Chabot, I., and Glennie, J. 2015. "Evolution of health technology assessment: Best practices of the pan-Canadian oncology drug review." *ClinicoEconomics and Outcomes Research* 7: 287–298. https://doi.org/10.2147/CEOR.S82549.

28. Di Matteo, L. n.d. Federal transfer payments and how they affect healthcare funding in Canada. *Making Evidence Matter.* http://evidencenetwork.ca/federal-transfer-payments-and-how-they-affect-healthcare-funding-in-canada/.

29. Grove, A. 2016. "The pharmaceutical benefits scheme: A quick guide." *Parliament of Australia.* https://www.aph.gov.au/About_Parliament/Parliamentary_Departments/ Parliamentary_Library/pubs/rp/rp1516/Quick_Guides/PBS.

30. Pearce, A. 2012, November 21. "Why medicines take so much time to get listed on the PBS." *The Conversation.* https://theconversation.com/why-medicines-take-so-much-time-to-get-listed-on-the-pbs-10902.

31. Akehurst, R.L., Abadie, E., Renaudin, N., and Sarkozy, F. 2017. "Variation in health technology assessment and reimbursement processes in Europe." *Value in Health* 20 (1): 67–76. https://doi.org/10.1016/j.jval.2016.08.725.

32. International Society for Pharmacoeconomics and Outcomes Research. n.d. "Pharmacoeconomic guidelines around the world." Accessed January 25, 2021. https:// tools.ispor.org/peguidelines/.

33. Barnieh, L., Manns, B., Harris, A., Blom, M., Donaldson, C., Klarenbach, S., Husereau, D., Lorenzetti, D., and Clement, F. 2014. "A synthesis of drug reimbursement decision-making processes in Organisation for Economic Co-operation and Development countries." *Value in Health* 17 (1): 98–108. https://doi.org/10.1016/j.jval.2013.10.008.

34. Bond, K. 2020. "2020 HTAi Global Policy Forum." *HTAi.* https://htai.org/wp-content/ uploads/2020/02/HTAi_GPF-newOrleans_program_background-paper.pdf.

35. Ollendorf, D.A., and Krubiner, C. 2019, November 5. "The dynamics of health technology assessment: Is it just about the evidence?" *Center for Global Development.* https://www. cgdev.org/blog/dynamics-health-technology-assessment-it-just-about-evidence.

36. Bond, K. 2020. "Deliberative processes in health technology assessment: Prospects, problems, and policy proposals." *Health Technology Assessment International.* https://htai. org/wp-content/uploads/2020/02/HTAi_GPF-newOrleans_program_background-paper. pdf.

37. Ollendorf, D.A., and Krubiner, C. 2019. "The dynamics of health technology assessment: Is it just about the evidence?" *Center for Global Development.* https://www.cgdev.org/blog/ dynamics-health-technology-assessment-it-just-about-evidence.

38. National Institute for Health and Care Excellence. 2014. "Developing NICE guidelines: The manual." Last modified October 15, 2020. Accessed January 25, 2021. https://www.nice.org.uk/process/pmg20/resources/developing-nice-guidelines-the-

manual-appendices-ag-i-2549710189/chapter/appendix-d-guideline-committee-terms-of-reference-and-standing-orders.

39. Office of Technology Assessment, Congress of the United States. 1979. *A review of selected federal vaccine and immunization policies: Based on case studies of pneumococcal vaccine.* https://catalog.hathitrust.org/Record/000758700.

40. Office of Technology Assessment, Congress of the United States. 1987. *Breast cancer screening for Medicare beneficiaries: Effectiveness, costs to Medicare and medical resources required.* https://catalog.hathitrust.org/Record/002976847.

41. Office of Technology Assessment, Congress of the United States. 1990. *The costs and effectiveness of cervical cancer screening in elderly women.* http://www.princeton.edu/~ota/disk2/1990/9012_n.html.

42. Office of Technology Assessment, Congress of the United States. 1990. *Costs and effectiveness of colorectal cancer screening in the elderly.* http://www.princeton.edu/~ota/disk2/1990/9013_n.html.

43. Chambers, J.D., Cangelosi, M.J., and Neumann, P.J. 2015. "Medicare's use of cost-effectiveness analysis for prevention (but not for treatment)." *Health Policy* 119 (2): 156–163. https://doi.org/10.1016/j.healthpol.2014.11.012.

44. Centers for Medicare & Medicaid Services. 2015. *Decision memo for screening for lung cancer with low dose computed tomography (LDCT).* https://www.cms.gov/medicare-coverage-database/details/nca-decision-memo.aspx?NCAId=274.

45. Smith, J.C. 2010. "The structure, role, and procedures of the U.S. Advisory Committee on Immunization Practices (ACIP)." *Vaccine* 28: A68–A75. https://doi.org/10.1016/j.vaccine.2010.02.037.

46. Ahmed, F. 2013. "U.S. Advisory Committee on Immunization Practices (ACIP) handbook for developing evidence-based recommendations." *Centers for Disease Control and Prevention.* https://www.cdc.gov/vaccines/acip/recs/grade/downloads/handbook.pdf.

47. Siegel, J.E., Byron, S.C., and Lawrence, W.F. 2005. "Federal sponsorship of cost-effectiveness and related research in health care: 1997–2001." *Value in Health* 8 (3): 223–236. https://doi.org/10.1111/j.1524-4733.2005.04037.x.

48. Neumann, P.J., Sanders, G.D., Russell, L.B., Siegel, J.E., and Ganiats, T.G. 2017. *Cost-effectiveness in health and medicine* (2nd ed.). New York: Oxford University Press.

49. Sullivan, S.D., Yeung, K., Vogeler, C., Ramsey, S.D., Wong, E., Murphy, C.O., Danielson, D., Veenstra, D.L., Garrison, L.P., Burke, W., and Watkins, J.B. 2015. "Design, implementation, and first-year outcomes of a value-based drug formulary." *Journal of Managed Care & Specialty Pharmacy* 21 (4): 269–275. https://doi.org/10.18553/jmcp.2015.21.4.269.

50. Fry, R.N., Avey, S.G., and Sullivan, S.D. 2003. "The Academy of Managed Care Pharmacy format for formulary submissions: An evolving standard—a foundation for managed care pharmacy task force report." *Value in Health* 6 (5): 505–521. https://doi.org/10.1046/j.1524-4733.2003.65327.x.

51. Academy of Managed Care Pharmacy. 2016. "A format for submission of clinical and economic evidence in support of formulary considerations." http://www.amcp.org/sites/default/files/2019-03/AMCP-Format-V4.pdf.

52. Fox, D.M., and Leichter, H.M. 1991. "Rationing care in Oregon: The new accountability." *Health Affairs* 10 (2): 7–27. https://doi.org/10.1377/hlthaff.10.2.7.

53. Leichter, H.M. 1999. "Oregon's bold experiment: Whatever happened to rationing?" *Journal of Health Politics, Policy and Law* 24 (1): 147–160. https://doi.org/10.1215/03616878-24-1-147.

54. Brown, L.D. 1991. "The national politics of Oregon's rationing plan." *Health Affairs* 10 (2): 28–51. https://doi.org/10.1377/hlthaff.10.2.28.

55. Himmelstein, D.U., and Woolhandler, S. 1998. "The Oregon health plan." *New England Journal of Medicine* 338 (6): 395–396. https://doi.org/10.1056/NEJM199802053380615.

56. Eddy, D.M. 1991. "Oregon's methods. Did cost-effectiveness analysis fail?" *JAMA* 266 (15): 2135–2141. https://pubmed.ncbi.nlm.nih.gov/1920704/.

57. Ham, C. 1998. "Retracing the Oregon trail: The experience of rationing and the Oregon health plan." *BMJ* 316 (7149): 1965–1969. https://doi.org/10.1136/bmj.316.7149.1965.

58. Bodenheimer, T. 1997. "The Oregon health plan—lessons for the nation." *New England Journal of Medicine* 337 (9): 651–656. https://doi.org/10.1056/NEJM199708283370923.

59. Gold, M. 1997. "Markets and public programs: Insights from Oregon and Tennessee." *Journal of Health Politics, Policy and Law* 22 (2): 633–666. https://doi.org/10.1215/03616878-22-2-633.

60. Jacobs, L., Marmor, T., and Oberlander, J. 1999. "The Oregon health plan and the political paradox of rationing: What advocates and critics have claimed and what Oregon did." *Journal of Health Politics, Policy and Law* 24 (1): 161–180. https://doi.org/10.1215/03616878-24-1-161.

61. Perry, S. 1982. "The brief life of the National Center for Health Care Technology." *New England Journal of Medicine* 307 (17): 1095–1100. https://doi.org/10.1056/NEJM198210213071738.

62. Blumenthal, D. 1983. "Federal policy toward health care technology: The case of the national center." *The Milbank Memorial Fund Quarterly. Health and Society* 61 (4): 584–613. https://doi.org/10.2307/3349874.

63. Cotter, D. 2009, January 22. "The national center for health care technology: Lessons learned." *Health Affairs*. https://www.healthaffairs.org/do/10.1377/hblog20090122.000490/full/.

64. Deyo, R.A., Psaty, B.M., Simon, G., Wagner, E.H., and Omenn, G.S. 1997. "The messenger under attack—intimidation of researchers by special-interest groups." *New England Journal of Medicine* 336 (16): 1176–1180. https://doi.org/10.1056/NEJM199704173361611.

65. Neumann, P.J. 2006. "Emerging lessons from the drug effectiveness review project." *Health Affairs (Millwood)* 25 (4): W262–W271. https://doi.org/10.1377/hlthaff.25.w262.

66. Saha, S., Hoerger, T.J., Pignone, M.P., Teutsch, S.M., Helfand, M., and Mandelblatt, J.S. 2001. "The art and science of incorporating cost effectiveness into evidence-based recommendations for clinical preventive services." *American Journal of Preventive Medicine* 20 (3): 36–43. https://doi.org/10.1016/S0749-3797(01)00260-4.

67. Neumann, P.J., and Chambers, J.D. 2012. "Medicare's enduring struggle to define "reasonable and necessary" care." *New England Journal of Medicine* 367 (19): 1775–1777. https://doi.org/10.1056/NEJMp1208386.

68. Neumann, P.J., and Weinstein, M.C. 2010. "Legislating against use of cost-effectiveness information." *New England Journal of Medicine* 363 (16): 1495–1497. https://doi.org/10.1056/NEJMp1007168.

69. Chambers, J.D., Kim, D.D., Pope, E.F., Graff, J.S., Wilkinson, C.L., and Neumann, P.J. 2018. "Specialty drug coverage varies across commercial health plans in the US." *Health Affairs* 37 (7): 1041–1047. https://doi.org/10.1377/hlthaff.2017.1553.

70. Neumann, P.J. 2009, March. "American exceptionalism and American health care: Implications for the US debate on cost-effectiveness analysis." *Office of Health Economics*. https://www.ohe.org/publications/american-exceptionalism-and-american-health-care-implications-us-debate-cost.

71. Wilson, J.Q. 2006. "American exceptionalism." *American Enterprise Institute*. https://www.aei.org/articles/american-exceptionalism-3/.

72. Lipset, S.M. 1996. *American exceptionalism.* New York: W. W. Norton.

73. Madsen, D.L. 1998. *American exceptionalism.* Jackson: University Press of Mississippi.

74. Kohut, A., and Stokes, B. 2006. *America against the world: How we are different and why we are disliked.* New York: Times Books.

75. Cohen, J., Cairns, C., Paquette, C., and Faden, L. 2006. "Comparing patient access to pharmaceuticals in the UK and US." *Applied Health Economic Health Policy* 5 (3): 177–187. https://doi.org/10.2165/00148365-200605030-00004.

76. Cohen, J., Faden, L., Predaris, S., and Young, B. 2007. "Patient access to pharmaceuticals: An international comparison." *The European Journal of Health Economics* 8: 253–266. https://doi.org/10.1007/s10198-006-0028-z.

77. Blendon, R.J., Brodie, M., Benson, J.M., Altman, D.E., Levitt, L., Hoff, T., and Hugick, L. 1998. "Understanding the managed care backlash." *Health Affairs* 17 (4): 80–94. https://doi.org/10.1377/hlthaff.17.4.80.

78. Partridge, A.H., and Winer, E.P. 2009. "On mammography—more agreement than disagreement." *New England Journal of Medicine* 361 (26): 2499–2501. https://doi.org/10.1056/NEJMp0911288.

79. Collins, S.R., Rasmussen, P.W., Beutel, S., and Doty, M.M. 2015, May 20. The problem of underinsurance and how rising deductibles will make it worse. *The Commonwealth Fund.* Accessed August 6, 2020. https://www.commonwealthfund.org/publications/issue-briefs/2015/may/problem-underinsurance-and-how-rising-deductibles-will-make-it.

6
Institute for Clinical and Economic Review

Origins

To a drug company representative, Steven Pearson may at first blush seem to have the demeanor of an accountant who has just inspected your company's books. Well-mannered and spectacled with a slender build and thinning brown hair, he speaks with precision, but also a trace of bemusement. He may have unpleasant news to share, but he recognizes the cleverness that landed you in your predicament.

In fact, Pearson is a physician-bioethicist-researcher, trained in internal medicine. He might appear an unlikely threat to the $500 billion US prescription drug industry. However, his private, nonprofit organization, the Institute for Clinical and Economic Review (ICER), has emerged as a singular concern for pharmaceutical companies. While there are other individuals and organizations that oppose and sometimes pressure Big Pharma, they do so with conventional tactics—by lobbying Congress in support of federal price controls, for example. In contrast, ICER has two features these other groups lack: a compelling methodology for calculating the value of prescription drugs and the keen attention of health insurers, the public, and some state and federal lawmakers.

How did ICER come to play this role? The short version is that Pearson, who had a long-standing interest in health policy, spent a year at the United Kingdom's National Institute for Health and Care Excellence's office in London in 2004 to learn how the British used cost-effectiveness analysis to price medical technologies for their National Health Service. Pearson found the approach appealing. "It didn't provide the answers but it provided the context for a conversation around value that I found very powerful," he would later recall.[*] In 2006, Pearson, back in the United States, founded ICER. For much of the next decade, ICER operated mostly under the radar, until early 2015, when its analysis of a new, highly effective but expensive hepatitis C

---

[*] Interview with the authors, February 12, 2020.

The Right Price. Peter J. Neumann, Joshua T. Cohen, and Daniel A. Ollendorf, Oxford University Press (2021).
© Peter J. Neumann, Joshua T. Cohen, and Daniel A. Ollendorf. DOI: 10.1093/oso/9780197512883.003.0006

treatment resonated powerfully with those seeking to rein in rapidly rising prescription drug costs.

In truth, the real story did not unfold quite so linearly. Pearson indeed founded ICER with cost-effectiveness analysis in mind—its acronym is a tease on the term "incremental cost-effectiveness ratio." In early 2020, reflecting on ICER's origins, Pearson would remember,

> I realized there was a way to use a very technical method such as cost effectiveness . . . in a way that would feel more transparent, explicit, and ultimately fair, because it forced you out of hierarchal goal or categorical thinking like, "cancer drugs are more expensive," or "orphan drugs were more expensive," and made you think broadly around what fairness really means.[†]

But pharmaceuticals did not figure prominently in ICER's assessment portfolio during much of its first decade. Instead, the organization focused on evaluating technologies and services, such as community health workers, obesity management, and palliative care,[1] reflecting issues of interest to its regional advisory councils and national health plans.

Events changed following the US Food and Drug Administration's approval of sofosbuvir (Sovaldi®; Gilead Sciences, Inc.) in December 2013 to treat hepatitis C.[2] With a cure rate above 90% and a favorable side-effect profile compared to standard therapies, expectations rose that sales could easily surpass the previous drug launch record of $5 billion in Sovaldi's first year (see Box 6.1).[3]

The prospect of spending tens of billions of dollars for a single new drug caught the attention of one of ICER's advisory councils. In response, ICER evaluated Sovaldi, concluding in April 2014 that, compared to an older, less effective treatment with more side effects (interferon), the medication's added cost—at $300,000 per additional patient cured (i.e., per patient achieving a *sustained virologic response*)—exceeded the corresponding added cost for another hepatitis C therapy called telaprevir ($189,000 per additional patient cured).[4] By that metric, Sovaldi could seem *overpriced*. Indeed, 11 of the 14 members of the expert panel ICER had convened concluded that at its then current price, compared to telaprevir, Sovaldi conferred "low value."[4] Yet the response to ICER's finding was muted. While several news stories quoted Steve Pearson warning that "this is the tip of the iceberg," and "we have about a year or two as a country to sort this out,"[5] the report generated relatively little attention.

[†] Interview with the authors, February 12, 2020.

Box 6.1 Cost-Effective but Unaffordable: Sovaldi Challenges the System

Sofosbuvir (Sovaldi®; Gilead Sciences, Inc.) was not the most expensive drug ever to enter the US market. But at $84,000 per 12-week treatment course, the $1,000-per-day drug breakthrough galvanized public attention and ignited debate about how to value curative treatments. The US Food and Drug Administration approved sofosbuvir in late 2013 for use in combination with other medications for certain hepatitis C genotypes. Compared to existing interferon-based regimens, Sovaldi decreased treatment duration from 24 to 48 weeks to 12 weeks, while nearly doubling cure rates from 46% to 90% for people with the most prevalent genotype.[1-3] Moreover, the new treatment was more tolerable than prevailing interferon-based regimens, whose side effects—fever, muscle aches, and nausea—were often described as worse than the disease. And the drug arrived just in time. Most of the approximately 4 million Americans with chronic hepatitis C were born between 1945 and 1965, before the US blood supply was routinely screened for such pathogens.[4]

Despite Sovaldi's clinical superiority, its manufacturer, Gilead, was vilified for its pricing because hepatitis disproportionately affects low-income and uninsured Americans. The company argued that Sovaldi would offset other health costs in the long run by reducing or eliminating spending for liver cancer, liver failure, and cirrhosis.[5]

Still, the main issue was not price, per se (in the sense that other drugs for cancer and rare diseases cost several times more) or even cost-effectiveness (published studies estimated that Sovaldi and its successor products had cost/QALY ratios in the range of $2,000 to $70,000).[6] At issue was the size of the hepatitis C population. Providing the new drug to just half of the 4 million people in the United States with hepatitis C could cost in excess of $200 billion. To put that figure into perspective, in 2018, the United States spent $500 billion on *all* prescription drugs (see Box 1.1). Sovaldi seemed cost-effective but unaffordable (see following paragraphs for a discussion of the conundrum).

Meanwhile, many hepatitis C patients, after considering the side effects of existing therapies, the slow progression of disease, and the potential for a shorter and more effective drug regimen on the horizon, had deferred treatment in anticipation of Sovaldi's approval. Payers scrambled to squeeze these "warehoused" patients into their budgets, in many cases by restricting treatment with Sovaldi to the sickest individuals whose disease had already progressed to liver damage. Most state Medicaid programs required patients wishing to use Sovaldi to undergo examination to establish disease severity, and testing for drug and alcohol use.[7] Patients eager to begin treatment were returned to the warehouse list.[8]

Nonetheless, Sovaldi and follow-on hepatitis C therapies became blockbuster products for Gilead, although prices and sales eventually declined. In its first year, Sovaldi's sales exceeded $10 billion.[9] The following year, Gilead launched the first all-oral hepatitis C drug, Harvoni®, at $94,500 per 12-week treatment.[10] Harvoni's revenue soared before falling 34% in 2016 and 52% the following year.[11] The decline resulted from increased competition, as other companies, including AbbVie and Merck, introduced competing products at substantially lower prices. Gilead responded by offering discounts of up to 46%.[12] As less expensive, more convenient treatments entered the market, manufacturers became more willing to offer price concessions and engage in innovative contracting arrangements.

Five years after Sovaldi's approval, 85% of hepatitis C-infected Americans still awaited treatment. In Louisiana in 2017, only 384 of the estimated 35,000 afflicted individuals on Medicaid or in prison had received treatment. According to the state's Secretary of Health, treating the entire state population would cost $760 million, or "more than the state spends on K–12 education, Veteran's Affairs, and Corrections combined."[13] In response, the state negotiated an arrangement under which it could treat an unlimited number of hepatitis C patients with another Gilead hepatitis C therapy, Epclusa® (a combination of sofosbuvir and velpatasvir), for a set payment of roughly $290 million spread over five years. This fixed-price subscription (the "Netflix" model) provided revenue certainty for the manufacturer (see Chapter 10 of the volume). For the state, which aimed to treat 31,000 individuals by the end of the contract period, the arrangement provided treatment access at a much lower per-patient cost (under $10,000 per individual) and offered budget predictability. Australia also reached a similar arrangement with the manufacturer in 2015.[14]

[1] Fried, M.W., Shiffman, M.L., Reddy, K.R., Smith, C., Marinos, G., Gonçales, F.L., Häussinger, D., Diago, M., Carosi, G., Dhumeaux, D., Craxi, A., Lin, A., Hoffman, J., and Yu, J. 2002. "Peginterferon alfa-2a plus ribavirin for chronic hepatitis C virus infection." *New England Journal of Medicine* 347 (13): 975–982. https://doi.org/10.1056/NEJMoa020047.

[2] Lawitz, E., Mangia, A., Wyles, D., Rodriguez-Torres, M., Hassanein, T., Gordon, S.C., Schultz, M., Davis, M.N., Kayali, Z., Reddy, K.R., Jacobson, I.M., Kowdley, K.V., Nyberg, L., Subramanian, G.M., Hyland, R.H., Arterburn, S., Jiang, D., McNally, J., Brainard, D., Symonds, W.T., McHutchison, J.G., Sheikh, A.M., Younossi, Z., and Gane, E.J. 2013. "Sofosbuvir for previously untreated chronic hepatitis C infection." *New England Journal of Medicine* 368 (20): 1878–1887. https://doi.org/10.1056/NEJMoa1214853.

[3] Messina, J.P., Humphreys, I., Flaxman, A., Brown, A., Cooke, G.S., Pybus, O.G., and Barnes, E. 2015. "Global distribution and prevalence of hepatitis C virus genotypes." *Hepatology* 61 (1): 77–87. https://doi.org/10.1002/hep.27259.

[4] Spach, D. 2020. "HCV epidemiology in the United States: Screening and diagnosis of hepatitis C infection." *University of Washington.* Accessed July 9, 2020. https://www.hepatitisc.uw.edu/go/screening-diagnosis/epidemiology-us/core-concept/all.

⁵ Pagliarulu, N. 2016. "Gilead: 'We stand behind the pricing of our therapies.'" https://www.biopharmadive.com/news/gilead-we-stand-behind-the-pricing-of-our-therapies/423859/.

⁶ Luhnen, M., Waffenschmidt, S., Gerber-Grote, A., and Hanke, G. 2016. "Health economic evaluations of sofosbuvir for treatment of chronic hepatitis C: A systematic review." *Applied Health Economic Health Policy* 14 (5): 527–543. https://doi.org/10.1007/s40258-016-0253-2.

⁷ Barua, S., Greenwald, R., Grebely, J., Dore, G.J., Swan, T., and Taylor, L.E. 2015. "Restrictions for Medicaid reimbursement of sofosbuvir for the treatment of hepatitis C virus infection in the United States." *Annals of Internal Medicine* 163 (3): 215–223. https://doi.org/10.7326/M15-0406.

⁸ Rice, J.P. 2015. "Hepatitis C treatment: Back to the warehouse." *Clinical Liver Disease (Hoboken)* 6 (2): 27–29. https://doi.org/10.1002/cld.490.

⁹ Pollack, A. 2015, February 3. "Sales of Sovaldi, New Gilead hepatitis C drug, soar to $10.3 billion." *New York Times.* https://www.nytimes.com/2015/02/04/business/sales-of-sovaldi-new-gilead-hepatitis-c-drug-soar-to-10-3-billion.html.

¹⁰ Pollack, A. 2014, October 10. "Harvoni, a hepatitis C drug from Gilead, winds F.D.A. approval." *New York Times.* https://www.nytimes.com/2014/10/11/business/harvoni-a-hepatitis-c-drug-from-gilead-wins-fda-approval.html.

¹¹ Middleton, J. 2018. "2017 sales review: Big names soldier on as Harvoni sinks." *Thepharmaletter.* https://www.thepharmaletter.com/article/2017-sales-review-big-names-soldier-on-as-harvoni-sinks#:~:text=Sales%20fell%20to%20%249.08%20billion,most%20businesses%20across%20the%20world.

¹² Britt, R. 2015, February 4. "Gilead to discount its pricey Sovaldi drug." *Market Watch.* Accessed July 7, 2019. https://www.marketwatch.com/story/gilead-to-discount-its-pricey-sovaldi-drug-2015-02-04.

¹³ Simmons-Duffin, S., and Kodjak, A. 2019, June 26. "Louisiana's novel 'subscription' model for pricey hepatitis C drugs gains approval." *NPR.* Accessed July 9, 2020. https://www.npr.org.

¹⁴ Moon, S., and Erickson, E. 2019. "Universal medicine access through lump-sum remuneration: Australia's approach to hepatitis C." *New England Journal of Medicine* 380 (7): 607–610. https://doi.org/10.1056/NEJMp1813728.

However, ICER was not finished analyzing hepatitis C drugs. Because ICER's analysis characterized health using a disease-specific measure (i.e., the cost per case of hepatitis C cured), it could only compare the value of hepatitis C treatments to each other. Its subsequent January 2015 analysis instead used the more general measure of value—cost per quality-adjusted life year (QALY) gained. That measure, which incorporates the prevention of liver-related complications caused by hepatitis C—including liver cancer, cirrhosis, and liver failure, as well as premature death from any or all of these—suggested that Sovaldi's benefits were so substantial, that despite its cost, Sovaldi was *reasonably cost-effective.*[6]

On the other hand, ICER also observed that because so many people might need treatment, total population costs—and hence insurance premiums—could increase substantially. To limit Sovaldi's contribution to insurance cost growth to no more than 0.5 to 1.0%, ICER concluded that *Sovaldi's price would nonetheless have to be reduced by at least half.* That finding struck a chord with payers. It would also put ICER on a new path.[6]

Philanthropists John Arnold, a former whiz-kid Enron energy trader in the early 2000s, and wife Laura Arnold, a mergers-and-acquisitions lawyer, had established the Laura and John Arnold Foundation (now Arnold Ventures) in 2008. Their goal, powered by a net worth of approximately $3 billion,[7] was to promote transparent science and evidence generation to address a range of societal issues in criminal justice, education, public finance (pension systems, in particular), and healthcare.[8] Sovaldi's $1,000 per day price—which John Arnold had called arbitrary—drew the foundation's attention.[9] To the analytically inclined Arnolds, ICER's systematic, evidence-based approach for developing a value-based price was appealing.

The result was a $5.2 million grant from the Arnold Foundation to ICER in 2015, enabling the organization to double its staff and begin issuing regular reports assessing the value of drugs.[10] While ICER continued to review diagnostics and medical procedures, it would concentrate most of its fire on new and emerging prescription medications. With the prospect of ramping up production, ICER announced its Emerging Therapy Assessment and Pricing program in July 2015.[11] The program's foundation was ICER's newly formulated *value assessment framework*—a uniform approach for evaluating drugs.[12]

The new framework made assumptions about how to quantify health benefits, how much weight to give to a drug's effect on population costs—the "budget impact"—and how broadly to project costs and savings. While other issues and controversies arose, the value-based pricing framework remains the centerpiece of ICER's efforts and has drawn the lion's share of public attention. Thus, scrutinizing the framework and how it has evolved is instructive. Because of the stakes, the potential for disagreements was substantial, and ICER has refined its approach partly in response to criticisms. After releasing its first framework in 2015, ICER issued a second, revised framework in mid-2017 and a third in early 2020.

The QALY as Lightning Rod

Although Steve Pearson returned from the United Kingdom in 2004 well versed in QALY methodology, ICER's use of this metric was uneven during the decade that followed ICER's founding in 2006. Pearson worried that QALYs would not appeal to his advisory councils, which comprised clinicians and others generally unfamiliar with cost-effectiveness analyses. He would later explain, "We had to work with Medicaid medical directors who never learned any decision science, and health care people who if they heard of the QALY it was, 'Oh, that's what we don't do. That's some international thing. I don't know why, but we don't do that.'"[‡] Nor were QALYs popular at the US federal grant agencies that had historically funded some of ICER's work (see Chapter 5 of this volume). Instead, during its first decade, ICER often reported economic findings in terms of "natural units" (e.g., cost per case of disease averted or cured).

ICER's initial assessment of Sovaldi, published in April 2014, continued this trend. But in light of its experience using QALYs to reevaluate hepatitis C drugs in January of 2015 (see previous discussion), ICER's decision to make QALYs a permanent feature of its framework was understandable. Most assessments would resemble the hepatitis C drug evaluation in requiring a combination of disparate health impacts. Moreover, ICER's mission was not simply to estimate a drug's costs and benefits, but rather to assess whether a therapy's benefits *justified* its costs. ICER required a common benchmark applicable across assessments, no matter the disease. The cost-per-QALY ratio—which Pearson had witnessed being used as the basis of England's health technology assessment (HTA) process during his UK sojourn a decade earlier—would be a centerpiece to ICER's "care value" criterion (later renamed "long-term value for money" (Figure 6.1), although clinical findings and "contextual elements" outside the cost-effectiveness calculation play important roles (see Box 8.3 in Chapter 8 of this volume) According to the group, *an appropriately priced drug would have a cost-effectiveness ratio no less favorable than $100,000 to $150,000 per QALY*[12] (see Chapter 4 of this volume for a discussion of the value of a QALY).

ICER's use of QALYs raised familiar concerns. In December 2015, the National Pharmaceutical Council (NPC), for example, highlighted the challenge of placing meaningful, reproducible numbers between zero (dead) and 1 ("perfect health") on different health conditions to represent patient preferences for avoiding them. NPC catalogued other known complaints, including inconsistent results depending on how survey questions were framed. They noted systematic differences between weights assigned by people who have experienced a disease and those who have not. In addition to technical issues that, at least in theory, could be addressed by developing better tools and more extensive health preference datasets, NPC also suggested that cost-effectiveness was inherently limited because it is "unlikely to fully capture all

---

[‡] Interview with the authors, February 12, 2020.

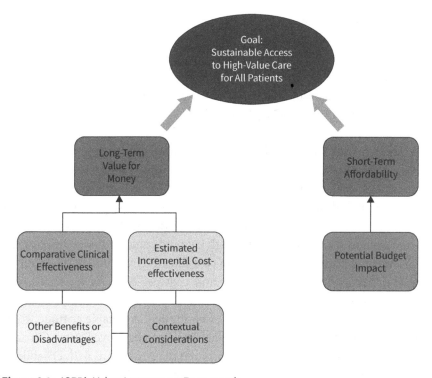

Figure 6.1: ICER's Value Assessment Framework

Source: "ICER value assessment framework." Institute for Clinical and Economic Review. Accessed August 12. https://icer.org/methodology/icers-methods/icer-value-assessment-framework-2/.

of the benefits important to patients"—such as long-term survival potential, ease of therapy use, and other attributes.[13]

In 2016, ICER released a proposed draft of a revised framework for analyses conducted from 2017 through 2019. It received more than 50 sets of comments totaling more than 300 pages of feedback. About two dozen submissions called ICER's use of QALYs problematic. Many complained that QALYs failed to capture relevant attributes of value. As an example, representatives from Celgene argued,

Cost effectiveness (cost per QALY) analyses . . . are not appropriate for assessing either value or price of innovative medicines. Value is a multi-dimensional concept and, therefore, a flexible, multi-criteria method for value assessment is required. . . . A cost-effectiveness analysis . . . is rigid and applies a narrow understanding of value."[14p93]

Eli Lilly officials wrote,

Given that the QALY is often not a good fit for some evaluations, it should be replaced with the most suitable alternative . . . rather than relying on a metric that tries to force comparison between disease states that may be at very different stages in scientific understanding."[15pp110-111]

Astellas contended that QALYs do not capture differences in preferences across individuals.[16p35] Others questioned the validity of theoretical assumptions underlying QALYs—and hence the idea that health benefits can be quantified by scaling life-years by preference weights and summing the results.[17pp98-100,18p161] ICER attempted to address these complaints in its second framework, saying that although it would continue using the cost-per-QALY ratio as its primary measure of cost-effectiveness, it would also report results in terms of cost-per-*life-year* and cost-per-*consequence* ratios (e.g., cost-per-case of disease cured).[19]

Still, attacks on ICER's use of QALYs continued. A notable critique would come from Tony Coelho, chair of the Partnership to Improve Patient Care and a former congressman who had co-authored the Americans with Disabilities Act and chaired President Clinton's Committee on Employment of People with Disabilities. Coelho, who has often spoken of his own experiences with epilepsy, argued in 2018 that the QALY "discriminates against people with disabilities and other vulnerable groups like the elderly because it assigns higher value to people in 'perfect health' than people in less-than-perfect health."[20] The scenario Coelho envisioned was a treatment that extends the lives of people with a disabling disease without improving their quality of life. Coelho noted that each added life year would be "worth less" than a life year for a nondisabled individual, and as a result, the cost-effectiveness ratio would be less favorable. Put another way, if two therapies each extend life by the same amount, one for people with disabilities and one for persons without, cost-effectiveness analysis will prioritize the therapy for those without disabilities.

While defending its use of QALYs, ICER further responded, "ICER's future reports will incorporate more prominently a calculation of the Equal Value of Life Years Gained (evLYG) [see Box 6.2], which evenly measures any gains in length of life, regardless of the treatment's ability to improve patients' quality of life."[21] By comparing the cost-per-evLYG results and the cost-per-QALY results, ICER would identify cases where use of QALYs might indeed make a therapy look less favorably cost-effective. ICER pledged that if their "analysis

Box 6.2 The Equal Value Life Year Gained

Consider an assessment of two medications to treat a cancer that without treatment diminishes quality of life to 0.2 QALYs per year and causes imminent death. Suppose that both treatments extend life by two years. However, the first treatment extends length of life without improving symptoms (quality of life continues at 0.2 QALYs per year), while the second improves quality of life to 0.8 QALYs per year. Compared to the alternative of no treatment and imminent death (approximately 0 QALYs), the QALY assessment credits the first treatment with a gain of $2 \times 0.2\ QALYs = 0.4\ QALYs$, and the second treatment with a gain of $2 \times 0.8\ QALYs = 1.6\ QALYs$. The difference between the two treatments of $1.6\ QALYs - 0.4\ QALYs = 1.2\ QALYs$ represents the incremental clinical value of treatment 2 (compared to treatment 1) recognized by the QALY measure.

In contrast, the evLYG measure credits both treatments in this example with the same gain—for simplicity, let's say the equal value is 0.9 evLYGs per year, resulting in 1.8 evLYGs for each treatment. Although the evLYG measure does not "discriminate" against cancer patients by designating a year of life with their condition as "worth less" than a year of life for an individual in typical health, it can fail to recognize the value of medications that improve symptoms for these patients (in addition to extending their lives). In the context of a decision, the evLYG can harm cancer patients by failing to warrant even a small additional expenditure for the second treatment (which improves quality of life), compared to the first (which does not).

finds a major difference in these two measures, we will include specific language in our report describing the underlying characteristics of the treatment and the condition that led to the difference."[21]

Despite introduction of the evLYG, ICER was unequivocal in its support of QALYs, stating, "The QALY remains the gold standard in cost-effectiveness analyses for many reasons, and a systematic departure from using the QALY would risk undervaluing treatments that improve the quality of life more than other alternatives for that condition."[21] ICER saw the evLYG as a way to address apprehensions. It continued,

By drawing greater attention to the analysis of a treatment's evLYG . . . ICER hopes to provide peace of mind to concerned patients and policymakers, while furthering the ability of cost-effectiveness analysis to support explicit, transparent discussions in the U.S. on how best to align a drug's price with its benefits for patients.[21]

Indeed, QALYs can *advantage* people with disabilities by valuing improvements to their quality of life. As the authors of this book pointed out in a 2018 blog post in response to Partnership to Improve Patient Care's criticisms, "the diminished weight QALYs assign to life with disability does not represent discrimination. Instead, diminished weight represents recognition that treatments mitigating disability confer value by restoring quality of life to levels typical among most of the population."[22] In short, to recognize gains from improving quality of life, we must acknowledge that a year lived with these negative factors is valued less than a life year without them. For the QALY, placing a smaller value on life years in a diminished state of health is the flip side of awarding value for improving quality of life. For example, suppose an analyst planned to attach a utility weight of 0.5 to a neurodegenerative disease, but because doing so was deemed discriminatory, the weight was raised to 0.85, the average in the general population. The consequence is to reduce the headroom for improvement in quality of life that a new treatment for the condition might provide by 70% (because perfect health has a utility weight of 1.0, and 1.0 – 0.85 is 70% less than 1.0 – 0.5).

ICER's third value framework, released in early 2020, consolidated its position on QALYs. It stated that henceforth ICER would express health gains in terms of QALYs, life years, evLYGs, and condition-specific outcomes ("e.g., treatment response, [or] event[s] avoided"[23p22]). Nonetheless, the QALY remained ICER's "gold standard" for its value-based price calculation for drugs. ICER directly addressed the discrimination argument, noting,

> Economic analyses using the QALY make treatments that alleviate serious illness look especially valuable. Because the QALY records the degree to which a treatment improves patients' lives, treatments for people with serious disability or illness have the greatest opportunity to demonstrate more QALYs gained and justify a higher price.[23p22]

Finally, ICER again explained the need for a common metric, stating, "a common measure of improved outcomes for patients is needed for cost-effectiveness analyses to support broader efforts to make more transparent, evidence-based coverage policies and pricing decisions."[23p23] At least for now at ICER, the QALY is here to stay.

Budget Impact Hullabaloo

In its 2015 framework, ICER's calculation of a drug's value-based price depended not only on its cost-per-QALY ratio (which ICER at that time termed its "care value criterion") but also on the drug's budget impact—that is, the medication's cost, summed over the population—which ICER called its "health system value" criterion (later changed to "short-term affordability") (see Figure 6.1).[12] The framework sounded "an 'alarm bell'" if short-term costs might increase overall health spending significantly faster than the US national economy is growing."[24] In concrete terms, the alarm sounded when a drug might increase annual national healthcare spending by around $900 million or more. ICER developed that limit by determining that if all new drugs adhered to it, resulting healthcare cost growth would be consistent with the national economy's growth rate, plus 1%.[25] To meet criteria for a value-based price, a drug had to satisfy both the *care value* (i.e., cost-effectiveness) and *health system value* (i.e., budget impact) constraints. For example, if ICER projected that a new drug would cost the United States. $1.8 billion per year, it would recommend making adjustments (e.g., seeking other budget savings or prioritizing subpopulations at greatest need) or cutting the price until the annual budget impact dropped to $900 million. The bottom line was that the drug had to satisfy both the cost-effectiveness criterion and the budget criterion.[26–28]

ICER's framework included "health system value" because of the critical role that budget impact had played in some of its assessments. Recall that without this criterion, ICER would have found the price of new hepatitis C drugs to reflect reasonable value because of their favorable cost-effectiveness profiles (roughly $20,000 per QALY gained). Budget impact would prove a major concern for other drugs evaluated through ICER's freshly minted value framework. With the potential to reduce cholesterol levels for the millions of Americans who struggled to do so even when treated with statins, newly approved proprotein convertase subtilisin/kexin type 9 (PCSK9) inhibitors loomed as potential blockbusters for drug companies *and* budget busters for payers (see Box 6.3).

Indeed, ICER's budget impact criterion played a key role in its 2015 PCSK9 inhibitor assessment. On the basis of cost-effectiveness, ICER had recommended that the prices of two new PCSK9 inhibitors should be reduced by 46% to 62% (roughly from $14,000 per year to $5,000–$7,500). However, on the basis of budget impact, ICER instead recommended a reduction of nearly 85% off the $14,000 annual price to roughly $2,200 per year. After several years of often-contentious negotiations with payers, manufacturers of

Box 6.3 Should Budget Impact Affect a Value Assessment? ICER's Review of PCSK9 Inhibitors

In 2014, many predicted blockbuster status for the forthcoming cholesterol-reducing drugs, called proprotein convertase subtilisin/kexin type 9 (PCSK9) inhibitors. Statins had revolutionized the treatment of high cholesterol over the previous decades, but millions of Americans still struggled to control their levels. Adding PCSK9 inhibitors promised to address the problem. Moreover, the new drugs were advanced biologics and could attract premium pricing. Predictions for annual prices ranged from $7,000 to $12,000.[1]

Still, the clinical evidence supporting PCSK9 inhibitors was limited. Clinical trial results did show that the drugs substantially reduced low-density lipoproteins, the so-called bad cholesterol, in different types of patients, including those with an inherited and dangerous form of high cholesterol, as well as individuals who could not tolerate statins.[2] However, the drugs' impact on longer-term outcomes, such as heart attacks and strokes, was unknown, and studies to investigate those endpoints were ongoing.

The approval of the first PCSK9 inhibitor, alirocumab (Praluent®; Sanofi US/ Regeneron Pharmaceuticals, Inc.), in July 2015 came with a surprise. The list price was even higher than predicted, at over $14,000 a year.[3] The second product, evolocumab (Repatha®; Amgen Inc.), followed with nearly identical pricing. Did the clinical benefits of these drugs justify their costs?

ICER had just released its first framework for estimating a drug's "value-based price."[25] PCSK9 inhibitors would serve as the guinea pigs to test the new framework. In its review of the drugs' clinical benefits, ICER confirmed the positive findings from the clinical trials. Moreover, ICER projected that, based on the impressive low-density lipoproteins reductions, the drugs could potentially avert about 7 million heart attacks and strokes in the United States over approximately 20 years (a duration corresponding to the remaining life expectancy for individuals in their early 60s participating in the PCSK9 trials).[26]

But the value calculations proved more challenging. After considerable analysis, ICER estimated that the cost-effectiveness ratio for PCSK9 inhibitors would range from $274,000 to $302,000 per QALY across all major patient subgroups.[26] ICER also projected that the budget impact for these drugs could reach $36 billion per year, even if only half of potentially eligible patients received these therapies. The budget impact would be around $18 billion a year even if the drug's price dropped enough to bring its cost-effectiveness ratio down to the benchmark of $150,000 per QALY.[26] While ICER found that an annual price of $7,735 for PCSK9 inhibitors would bring the drug's cost-effectiveness ratio within the $150,000 per QALY benchmark, that reduction did not satisfy its budget impact criteria. To address that issue, ICER reported a value-based price benchmark for PCSK9 inhibitors of $2,177 per year, an 85% discount on the drug's full annual wholesale acquisition cost of $14,350.[26]

"New Class of Cholesterol Drugs Should Cost Much Less, Report Says," declared the *Wall Street Journal*.[4] In response, the manufacturers of PCSK9 inhibitors aggressively condemned ICER. Amgen stated that ICER had assumed an unrealistically low rate for cardiac events (thus understating its drug's benefit in preventing those events) and severely exaggerated the likely budget impact. The company also decried ICER's use of "arbitrary budget caps."[5]

Rather than becoming billion dollar blockbusters, PCSK9 sales reached only several hundred million dollars by 2017, despite favorable positioning in clinical guidelines, the publication of subsequent trial results showing the drugs produced major reductions in heart attacks and strokes, and increasingly aggressive discounting with payers and pharmacy benefit managers.[6]

Then came another unexpected twist. In late 2017, on the eve of public release of trial data on its drug's (alirocumab's) impact on cardiac events, Regeneron and Sanofi approached ICER with a proposal to submit clinical data to the organization, even before it was presented publicly, to allow ICER to revise its analyses. More surprising still was the companies' commitment to increase the drug's discount to levels falling within ICER's range for a value-based price.[7] In October 2018, Amgen subsequently announced that it was reducing *its* list price by more than 60%, to just under $6,000 per year.[8] Regeneron and Sanofi followed suit a few months later.[9]

[1] Silverman, E. 2015. "How much?! Those New cholesterol drugs could cost $23 billion a year." *Wall Street Journal*. Accessed July 14, 2020. https://www.wsj.com/articles/BL-270B-2050.

[2] Joshi, P.H., Martin, S.S., and Blumenthal, R.S. 2014. "The fascinating story of PCSK9 inhibition: Insights and perspective from ACC." *Cardiology Today* 17 (5): 32.

[3] Pollack, A. 2015. "New drug sharply lowers cholesterol, but it's costly." *The New York Times*. Accessed July 14, 2020. https://www.nytimes.com/2015/08/28/health/fda-approves-another-in-a-new-class-of-cholesterol-drugs.html.

[4] Loftus, P. 2015. New class of cholesterol drugs should cost much less, report says. *The Wall Street Journal*. Accessed July 14, 2020. https://www.wsj.com/articles/new-class-of-cholesterol-drugs-should-cost-much-less-report-says-1441752760.

[5] Ofman, J. 2015. "Amgen response to ICER PCSK9i report." https://www.amgen.com/~/media/amgen/full/www-amgen-com/downloads/perspectives/amgen_response_to_icer_pcsk9i_report.ashx?la=en.

[6] Munjal, R. 2019, May 27. "Are PCSK9 inhibitors about to take off?" *PharmaTimes*. Accessed July 14, 2020. http://www.pharmatimes.com/web_exclusives/are_pcsk9_inhibitors_about_to_take_off_1289184.

[7] "Regeneron CEO puts conditions on lowering his $14,000-per-year cholesterol drug. 2018, March 12." *CNBC*. https://www.cnbc.com/2018/03/12/regeneron-ceo-puts-conditions-on-lowering-his-14000-cholesterol-drug.html.

[8] Dangi-Garimella, S. 2018, October 24. "Amgen announces 60% reduction in list price of PCSK9 inhibitor evolocumab." *AJMC*. Accessed July 14, 2020. https://www.ajmc.com/view/amgen-announces-60-reduction-in-list-price-of-pcsk9-inhibitor-evolocumab.

[9] Terry, M. 2019, February 11. "Sanofi and Regeneron cut price of cholesterol med Praluent by about 60%." *STAT*. Accessed July 14, 2020. https://www.statnews.com/2019/02/11/regeneron-sanofi-praluent-price-cholesterol/.

the PCSK9 inhibitors agreed to lower their prices to about $5,900 annually, roughly mirroring ICER's pricing guidance based on cost-effectiveness.[29] To be sure, other factors (e.g., the ability of payers to restrict patient access to these drugs, lackluster sales, and questions about the impact of these drugs on long-term clinical outcomes) apart from ICER's assessment played a role in drug company actions. Still, concessions by companies signaled ICER's growing influence.

The idea of including budget impact as a component of a drug's value-based price remained compelling to many audiences. After all, an expensive purchase, no matter how "great a deal" (i.e., no matter how cost-effective), forces difficult trade-offs and can perhaps make the buyer worse off. For example, acquiring a pair of Manolo Blahnik shoes for $500 is a marvelous bargain (or so this book's authors have been told), but purchasing half a dozen pairs at that price is problematic because it would leave the daughter of one of the authors unable to pay her rent, and housing is even more important than footwear. (Her father, sensing her disappointment and feeling guilty about spending too much time at the office during her childhood, could "subsidize" the shoe purchase, although this happens only in an alternate universe. But we digress.)

Economists love to remind us that "value" is what you receive in exchange for what you give up. A cost-effectiveness ratio represents value because it compares spending (the incremental dollars in its numerator) to the acquired benefit (the incremental QALYs in its denominator). Because a budget impact calculation refers to dollars expended but ignores benefits received (excepting any cost savings from reduced use of health services such as hospital or emergency room admissions), it does not, strictly speaking, represent *value*.

But shouldn't budget impact figure someplace in value considerations? If total spending cannot increase beyond a "cap," any spending above this level means that some other spending must be foregone. The budget serves as a tool to force consideration of the tradeoffs involved in purchasing decisions. A new drug might seem cost-effective, but if it replaces other essential spending, it could decrease overall welfare. Put another way, a sufficiently expensive purchase of a valuable commodity can seem "cost-effective but unaffordable."

New hepatitis C drugs presented a real-world example. Individuals with the condition often depend on government programs like Medicaid or the Veterans Administration for their medications. Because these programs cannot always easily increase their budgets, it follows that a large, new expense like Sovaldi and other antiviral drugs can lead to cuts elsewhere. As one Medicaid plan chief executive explained, "for the price of Sovaldi for one patient, we could provide health insurance through Medicaid for [up to] 26 people for an entire year."[30] Although the novel antiviral drugs seemed to have favorable cost-effectiveness ratios (see Chapter 4 of this volume), limiting spending on them could help preserve overall healthcare coverage, which could be even more important.

Still, reducing a new drug's price to meet a predetermined budget target, as in ICER's framework, presented problems. While a budget limit may make sense to protect essential spending (e.g., basic health coverage), it can be unreasonable when new spending addresses a sufficiently important problem. Would we reject a cure for cancer or Alzheimer's disease if its cost would exceed ICER's $900 million annual budget benchmark? ICER's budget ceiling would have designated statin drugs, which reduce heart disease risk by lowering cholesterol levels, as too expensive. These drugs cost over $300 billion during their first 20 years of use but, according to some estimates, have returned health benefits worth over $1.2 trillion.[31]

Another concern was that ICER's short-term budget impact would send inappropriate signals to innovators. In public comments submitted to ICER, Sanofi argued, "Imposing a uniform threshold for all new products can stifle innovation for high-value treatments that affect diseases with the highest prevalence."[32p6] In response to ICER's assessment of treatments for nonsmall cell lung cancer, Bristol Myers Squibb noted, "Patients subjected to a cancer of high incidence or prevalence are worth 'less' than patients who have a more rare form of cancer, creating disincentives for innovation and healthcare investment."[33]

In mid-2017, ICER released its second framework, defending the importance of a drug's budget impact in determining "affordability." ICER explained,

> A rapid increase in costs resulting from the significant budget impact of a new drug might lead to decisions to forgo hiring of needed new staff, or delay of introduction of other new services. Quite simply: budget impact, and not long-term cost-effectiveness, determines how affordable health care insurance will be in coming years and shapes what health care can be provided with the resources available.[19p9]

Nonetheless, ICER amended its framework, making cost-effectiveness (which it now called "long-term value for money") the sole determinant of the value price. In an important symbolic change, ICER changed how it characterized its budget impact criterion, replacing the phrase "health system *value*" with "short-term affordability." In addition, the Institute's independent voting panels had already stopped voting on health system value by mid-2016.

While ICER's first framework (covering 2015–2017) had assumed that all patients who could benefit from a drug would use it and then calculated the price that kept total annual spending below $900 million, the new framework (2017–2019) declared that "ICER will no longer attempt to estimate the uptake of a new intervention."[19p25] Instead, ICER would estimate "potential budget impact" for different combinations of prices and population "uptake" rates. Finally, while ICER's new framework would issue an "affordability and access alert" if its projected budget impact exceeded its $900 million benchmark, it did not explicitly say it would recommend a lower price.[19pp25-26]

Perspective Revisited: Healthcare or Societal?

As discussed in Chapter 4, the "perspective" of an economic analysis determines whether the study considers only consequences to the health system (or, similarly, the "healthcare payer"), or also broader "societal" effects, such as those influencing unpaid family caregivers and worker productivity. Although ICER's initial framework (2015–2017) contained little about perspective,[11] the organization's assessments during that period assumed a "payer perspective." For example, ICER's assessments of Sovaldi and PCSK9s assumed a health system perspective. At the time, the decision seemed to generate little debate. Only one set of public comments in response to ICER's Sovaldi evaluation recommended inclusion of societal benefits (in particular, the benefit of prevented infections among other members of the community). One responder to ICER's PCSK9 assessment suggested that ICER take a "broad societal perspective related to the costs and benefits of healthcare interventions" but offered no elaboration.[34p8]

ICER's approach stood in contrast to recommendations of the Second Panel on Cost Effectiveness Analysis and Medicine, which, as Chapter 4 noted, called for both a healthcare and societal perspective for cost-effectiveness analyses. ICER partially addressed this difference in its framework 2.0 (covering the period 2017–2019), declaring that it would include a "scenario analysis including work productivity when feasible" in addition to its "base case" analysis, which would continue to reflect a health system perspective.[19p18]

For advocates of a societal perspective, this amendment represented a limited change. Crucially, the societal perspective would appear only as a "scenario analysis" rather than in the base case, which served as the basis for ICER's main findings, including its recommended value-based price. In short, the price recommendations issued from an ICER review would not reflect the elements of a drug's value that accrue to society.

ICER advanced several reasons for its continued emphasis on a health system perspective. The first was pragmatic. The organization explained that societal impacts—including effects on productivity, income taxes, educational outcomes, criminal justice outcomes, and disability and social security benefits—depend on uncertain long-term projections. ICER argued, "Finding reliable estimates for long-term effects of health interventions on these broader outcomes is usually not possible."[19p18] Second, as noted, ICER continued to argue that a health system perspective remained "most relevant for decision-making by public and private insurers, risk-bearing provider groups, and health care policymakers."[19] It added that ICER would present societal impact information not only in scenario analyses but also in qualitative discussions of "other potential benefits and disadvantages."[19] Finally, ICER warned that recognition of societal impacts could disadvantage groups not earning income. ICER stated that it was "also conscious that a full societal analysis has concerning ethical implications (e.g. favoring treatments for younger working adults over treatments for the elderly and disabled)."[19p14]

ICER's second framework provided one further adjustment. For ultra-rare conditions (i.e., those affecting no more than 10,000 individuals in the United States), ICER might include two co-base case scenarios, one from a health system and one from a limited societal perspective, when feasible and when including societal costs substantially influenced the results. Elevating the societal perspective to a co-base case would play an important role in ICER's 2018 evaluation of voretigene neparvovec (Luxturna˚; Spark Therapeutics, Inc.), a gene therapy for a rare congenital vision disorder (see Box 6.4). However, in ICER's 16 drug assessments (published through April 2019) using its second framework from the 2017–2019 period, the institute designated a societal analysis as "co-base case analyses" in only three cases—treatments for amyloidosis, hemophilia A, and Luxturna. In other reports, if ICER included a societal perspective, it appeared as a scenario analysis and hence did not affect ICER's calculation of its value-based prices. Since 2018, ICER has also included an "Impact Inventory," or checklist of all health and nonhealth items included in its cost-effectiveness analyses. ICER has explained that it added the impact inventory to "document specific health care and societal impacts

Box 6.4 Contextual Considerations: ICER's Assessment of Luxturna

Imagine a young child, full of wonder at his emerging world, except he is having trouble seeing it. A rare, genetic retinal disease (biallelic RPE65 mutation-associated retinal dystrophy) is causing his eyes to gradually lose their ability to recognize light and integrate it into their visual field. Untreated, his world goes dark—those with mutations in both copies of the gene experience complete blindness. Now imagine that a single injection of a new therapy could halt the disease's progression. If the child had already lost some vision, it would not worsen; if diagnosed early enough, he might be cured entirely.

The gene therapy, Luxturna® (voretigene neparvovec), is a DNA fragment containing a working copy of the RPE65 gene packaged in an inactivated virus.[1] Injected into each eye, the working gene replaces the mutated one. But how effective is the treatment? Does it work in all patients? And, of course, how much does it cost?

Gene replacement therapies like Luxturna present advances that are challenging health systems. In recent years, the field has progressed considerably, after setbacks with the tragic death in 1999 of Jesse Gelsinger, who suffered a catastrophic immune reaction to an early gene therapy infusion.[2]

The first gene therapy, alipogene tiparvovec (Glybera®; uniQure Inc.) for lipoprotein lipase deficiency, was introduced in Europe in 2012. Hailed as a breakthrough, it proved a commercial failure due to the rarity of the condition (one patient per million) and its high cost ($1.2 million for a single injection).[3] Next came Strimvelis® (Orchard Therapeutics plc) in 2016, to treat severe combined immunodeficiency due to adenosine deaminase deficiency, the so-called bubble boy disease, which makes patients susceptible to life-threatening infections. Priced at $667,000, Strimvelis also struggled to find its commercial footing, with only five patients treated in its first two years on the market.[4] The original manufacturer, GlaxoSmithKline, sold the product to another company that was advancing next-generation gene therapies.[4]

With these inauspicious precedents, Spark Therapeutics proceeded with the development of voretigene neparvovec. The company planned to prioritize approval in the potentially friendlier environment of the United States, but it also faced risks. For one, the disease is very rare, with only 3,000 to 4,000 patients in the United States. For another, for patients who had suffered some sight loss, it did not provide a complete cure. Most important, the supporting data were limited. The pivotal clinical trial had only 31 participants, who were followed for only two years. And its major outcome was performance on a new "mobility test"—essentially an obstacle course with varying levels of light. How should regulators and payers evaluate the meaningful-ness of an improvement in a patient's mobility test score?

Despite the uncertainties, Spark's CEO Jeff Marrazzo was confident that Luxturna would prove a breakthrough and command a premium price. He embarked on a media tour, touting the value of the blindness-saving drug and citing court awards to eye damage sufferers of workplace injury cases and the willingness-to-pay litera-ture (see Chapter 4 of this volume) to support the idea that a "$1 million plus" price was could be justified.[5] Complicating matters was pushback from some in the visually impaired community who did not view sight loss as a disability and rejected the idea that they need some form of intervention to improve their lives.[6] The environment seemed ripe for the disappointments that had greeted gene therapies in Europe.

The therapy was approved in the United States in December 2017 and shortly thereafter Spark announced its price of $425,000 per eye, $850,000 total—high to be sure, but lower than some predictions. But given the product's benefits, did the price reflect reasonable value for money?

Luxturna quickly appeared on ICER's radar. A public meeting was set for the end of January 2018. The drug would serve as a test for ICER's adapted value framework for ultra-rare diseases, conditions affecting fewer than 10,000 people in the United States.[7] The adaptation allowed for the presentation of additional cost-effectiveness benchmarks (up to $500,000 per QALY), and consideration of additional contextual elements for ICER voting panels to consider, including benefits not captured by the QALY; positive impacts outside the family, such as effects on schools and communi-ties; and substantial effects on the care infrastructure, including screening, clinician sensitization, and broader knowledge of the condition (see Box 8.3 in Chapter 8 of this volume). Importantly, the rating of clinical evidence and the all-important value-based price range—corresponding to achievement of health improvements at a cost of $100,000 to $150,000 per QALY—remained unchanged.

ICER's report, released a few weeks after Luxturna's approval in December 2017, estimated that Luxturna's cost-effectiveness would be roughly $650,000 per QALY gained. Even under a societal perspective scenario that incorporated education, transportation, work loss, and other nonhealth costs, cost-effectiveness remained in the range of $500,000 per QALY.[8] The cost-effectiveness estimates fell to $150,000 per QALY only in a single scenario conducted from a societal perspective, with addi-tional assumptions that children would be universally screened for the disease and that treatment would be restricted to younger patients who were more likely to ben-efit. Spark challenged the report, stating that the analysis "still fails to account for any benefit of treatment on quality of life for caregivers/family members."[9]

Given the report's findings, the company's expectations for ICER's impending public assembly were glum. But the meeting produced a surprise. Typically, the independent assessment by ICER's committee members as to whether a drug provides high, medium, or low value align with ICER's conclusions regarding cost-effectiveness.[10] For Luxturna, however, only 3 of 12 members voted that the drug (at the price announced by Spark Therapeutics) represented low value. Despite its high price and unfavorable cost-effectiveness, seven members judged Luxturna to represent intermediate value, and two deemed it to represent high value. In explaining these votes, members noted contextual considerations and benefits not accounted for by the cost-per-QALY framework, including the gene therapy's novel mechanism of action, the severity of the condition, and an expectation that, while unmeasured, the therapy would reduce caregiver and family burden. For ICER's panel members, cost-effectiveness clearly represented only one factor among a number of others that influenced their view of the drug's value.

The first patient received the approved Luxturna in March 2018, and the drug generated nearly $30 million in sales for the remainder of the year; it generated nearly that amount of revenue in the first six months of 2019.[11,12] Despite its high price and unfavorable cost-effectiveness profile, US payers have generally granted unrestricted access to Luxturna; an analysis of coverage policies from 17 of the largest 20 commercial insurers in the United States indicated that they all cover Luxturna, although some cover the treatment only for patients meeting certain criteria, including their level of visual impairment and age and only if the patient receives the treatment at an approved institution.[a]

[1] "How does Luxturna** (voretigene neparvovec) work?" *Novartis.* Accessed July 22, 2020. https://novartis.gcs-web.com/static-files/6db84d3d-2f16-4b15-a91b-591596d14cf8.

[2] Sibbald, B. 2001. "Death but one unintended consequence of gene-therapy trial." *Canadian Medical Association Journal* 164 (11): 1612–1612.

[3] Sagonowsky, E. 2017, April 20. "With its launch fizzling out, UniQure gives up on $1M+ gene therapy Glybera." *Fierce Pharma.* Accessed July 22, 2020. https://www.fiercepharma.com/pharma/uniqure-gives-up-1m-gene-therapy-glybera.

[4] Dolgin, E. 2019. "'Bubble boy' gene therapy reignites commercial interest." Nature Biotechnology 37 (7): 699–701.

[5] Carroll, J. 2017, November 8. "How much is your vision worth? Spark CEO Jeff Marrazzo has a price in mind." *Endpoints News.* https://endpts.com/spark-ceo-jeff-marrazzo-has-done-the-math-on-blindness-and-hes-come-up-with-a-blockbuster-price-for-lead-gene-therapy/.

[6] Bondy, H. 2018, August 8. "Blind YouTube star Molly Burke doesn't want a cure—she wants a voice." *NBC News.* https://www.nbcnews.com/know-your-value/feature/blind-youtube-star-molly-burke-doesn-t-want-cure-she-ncna1040376.

[7] "Voretigene Neparvovec for biallelic RPE65-mediated retinal disease: Effectiveness, value, and value-based price benchmarks." 2017, August 7. *Institute for Clinical and Economic Review.* https://icer.org/wp-content/uploads/2020/10/MWCEPAC_SCOPE_VORETIGENE_08072017.pdf

[8] Banken, R., Rind, D., Cramer, G., Synnott, P.G., Chapman, R., Khan, S., Pearson, S.D., Carlson, J., Zimmerman, M., and Lubinga, S.J. 2018. "Voretigene Neparvovec for Biallelic RPE65—mediated retinal disease: Effectiveness and value." *Institute for Clinical and Economic Review.* https://icer.org/wp-content/uploads/2020/10/MWCEPAC_VORETIGENE_FINAL_EVIDENCE_REPORT_02142018.pdf

[9] Pagliarulo, N. 2018. "Price for spark gene therapy too high, ICER says." *BioPharmaDive.* Accessed July 22, 2020. https://www.biopharmadive.com/news/icer-finds-spark-luxturna-gene-therapy-too-expensive-price/514821/.

[10] Neumann, P.J., Silver, M.C., and Cohen, J.T. 2018, November 6. "Should a drug's value depend on the disease or population it treats? Insights from ICER's value assessments." *Health Affairs.* https://doi.org/10.1377/hblog20181105.38350.

[11] George, J. 2019, February 20. "Sales of Philadelphia-born gene therapy product hit $27M during first year." *Philadelphia Business Journal.* Accessed June 12, 2020. https://www.bizjournals.com/philadelphia/news/2019/02/19/sales-of-philadelphia-born-gene-therapy-product.html.

[12] Dunn, A. 2019. "Novartis' Zolgensma starts strong as about 100 infants are treated with gene therapy." *BioPharmaDive.* Accessed June 12, 2020. https://www.biopharmadive.com/news/novartis-zolgensma-sma-gene-therapy-strong-launch/565546/.

[a]*Authors* analysis of the Tufts Medical Center Specialty Drug and Evidence Coverage (SPEC) database.

included" and to "justify the rationale for not including any intervention effect in the analysis, if applicable."[35]

ICER's third framework, released in January 2020 (covering the period 2020–2023), again raised questions about the appropriateness of the societal perspective. It noted that "ICER uses a health care system perspective as its primary base case for several reasons": (a) its relevance to healthcare payers; (b) the more uncertain assumptions needed to account for impacts on tax revenue, productivity, educational outcomes, and criminal justice outcomes; and (c) ethical concerns attending valuation of productivity and the corresponding devaluation of individuals who will not be in workforce, regardless of treatment.[23p24]

Despite these concerns, ICER's new framework declared that it "presents a modified societal perspective as a co-base case for certain topics," in particular, when including societal impacts substantially influences cost-effectiveness estimates.[23p25] With ICER's position now more aligned with the position promoted by Second Panel on Cost Effectiveness, it seemed the idea of a societal perspective had gained purchase and would share top billing when it is judged to influence cost-effectiveness projections.[36p69] That said, in the spring of 2020, when evaluating remdesivir, the first drug to receive emergency use authorization for COVID-19 and for which societal costs seemed crucial, ICER declined to include them in their analysis (see Chapter 9 of this volume).

Table 6.1 Cost-Effectiveness Findings From ICER Reviews Under Second Value Framework From September 2017 to February 2020

Indication	Intervention	Comparator	Annual WAC ($)	ICER ($/QALY)
Acute migraine				
	CGRP receptor antagonists (2)—triptan-ineligible	Usual care	4,896 (estimated)	40,000
	CGRP receptor antagonists (2)—triptan-eligible	Sumatriptan or eletriptan	4,896 (estimated)	Dominated
	Lasmiditan—triptan-ineligible	Usual care	4,610	152,000
	Lasmiditan—triptan-eligible	Sumatriptan or eletriptan	4,610	Dominated
Rheumatoid arthritis[a]				
	Upadacitinib	Adalimumab	59,860	92,000
	Tofacitinib	Conventional DMARDs	54,552	900,000
	Adalimumab	Conventional DMARDs	67,263	1,586,000
Asthma (severe)				
	Biologic agents (4)	Best supportive care	31,000–39,000	325,000–391,000
ATTR amyloidosis				
	Inotersen	Best supportive care	450,000	1,700,000
	Patisiran	Best supportive care	450,000	850,000
Cardiovascular disease				
	Icosapent ethyl	Medical management	3,699	18,000
	Rivaroxaban	Medical management	5,457	36,000
Cystic fibrosis				
	CFTR modulators (3)	Best supportive care	292,000–312,000	841,000–974,000
Depression				
	Esketamine	Placebo	32,400	198,000

Table 6.1 *Continued*

Indication	Intervention	Comparator	Annual WAC ($)	ICER ($/QALY)
Duchenne muscular dystrophy				
	Deflazacort	Prednisone	117,400	361,000
Endometriosis				
	Elagolix—Short-term	Placebo	10,138	126,800
	Elagolix—Lifetime	Placebo	10,138	81,000
Hemophilia A				
	Emicizumab	Bypassing agent prophylaxis	482,000	Cost-saving
Hereditary angioedema				
	Lanadelumab (prophylaxis)	On-demand treatment	566,000	1,100,000
	C1 inhibitors (2) (prophylaxis)	On-demand treatment	510,000–539,000	328,000–5,600,000
Leukemia and lymphoma				
	CAR-T—Tisagenlecleucel	Chemotherapy	475,000	$46,000
	CAR-T—Axicabtagene ciloleucel	Chemotherapy	373,000	$136,000
Migraine				
	CGRP inhibitors (2)—Chronic	Placebo	6,900	90,000–120,000
	CGRP inhibitors (2)—Episodic	Placebo	6,900	150,000
Multiple sclerosis				
	Siponimod	Best supportive care	88,500	433,000
	Siponimod	Other MS Drugs	88,500	1,150,000
Opioid use disorder				
	Buprenorphine implant	Oral buprenorphine	9,900	265,000
Ovarian cancer				
Maintenance	PARP inhibitors (3)	Observation	178,000–195,000	291,000–369,000

Continued

Table 6.1 *Continued*

Indication	Intervention	Comparator	Annual WAC ($)	ICER ($/QALY)
Recurrent disease	PARP inhibitors (3)	Chemotherapy	178,000–195,000	146,000–295,000
Peanut allergy				
	Viaskin Peanut	Avoidance alone	Not available	216,000
	AR101	Avoidance alone	Not available	88,000
Prostate cancer				
	Early anti-androgen therapy (2)	Later anti-androgen therapy	135,000–142,000	$68,000–$84,000
Psoriasis				
	Biologic agents (10)	Placebo	38,000–79,000	$131,000–$188,000
RPE65-Mediated retinal disease				
	Voretigene neparvovec—Treat at age 15	Best supportive care	$850,000	$643,800
	Voretigene neparvovec—Treat at age 3	Best supportive care	$850,000	$288,000
Spinal muscular atrophy				
	Nusinersen	Best supportive care	$750,000	1,100,000
	Onasemnogene	Best supportive care	$2,000,000	$243,000
Tardive dyskinesia				
	Deutetrabenazine	Placebo	$90,071	$1,100,000
	Valbenazine	Placebo	$75,789	$752,000
Type 2 diabetes				
	Oral semaglutide	Liraglutide	$9,404	Cost-saving
	Oral semaglutide	Empagliflozin	$9,404	480,000
	Oral semaglutide	Sitagliptin	$9,404	140,000
	Oral semaglutide	Background therapy	$9,404	110,000

[a]Analysis reflects a one-year time horizon, in contrast to most other models, which use a longer time horizon (often a lifetime horizon).

Source: Authors' analysis of publicly available ICER evaluations accessible at https://icer.org/.

ICER's Influence

The United States and United Kingdom have vastly different approaches to their healthcare systems. Many Americans are inclined to think of theirs as at its best when privately run and free of excessive government or any other bureaucratic oversight. Although sometimes frustrated by service delivery, the British are so proud of their single-payer, government-run, unified health system that the opening ceremony of the 2012 London Olympics featured a tribute to the UK's National Health Service—with dancers dressed as nurses and sick children, a performance that confused many Americans.[37] Yet both countries now possess prominent groups assessing drug value using cost-per-QALYs as their cornerstone (Table 6.1).

Unlike National Institute for Health and Care Excellence, which was created by legislation and is accountable to the United Kingdom's Department of Health, ICER is a private organization with no government authority. Moreover, ICER does not issue reimbursement decisions; it merely provides information to U.S. payers and others who might use their findings. However, ICER's profile continues to rise. As one sign, external parties submitted hundreds of comments in response to 15 pharmaceutical assessments that ICER conducted between 2017 and April 2019.[38]

ICER's reports seem to be affecting the national conversation in the US on drug prices and affordability. The organization's findings have garnered headlines and stirred debate.[39,40] Still, without the force of law to compel decision makers to follow its recommendations, how influential is ICER?

Respondents to surveys overwhelmingly agree on the need for an objective, independent, non-governmental, third-party HTA body in the US or report that they use third-party assessments.[41-44] They generally concur that ICER is influencing their price negotiations, as well as their choices about preferred products within a therapeutic class and conditions of reimbursement.[41,42,44] More than one in three payer representatives said it was "likely or extremely likely that they would request a rebate to match the net ICER cost-effective price."[41] Some payer respondents said they would use ICER reports to amend the requirements they impose to control access to expensive drugs (19%) or to achieve cost-effective pricing (more than a third).[41]

Notably, some drug companies have even reduced their prices to earn a more favorable designation by ICER. In 2018, Sanofi and Regeneron Pharmaceuticals announced they would "offer [US] payers that agree to reduce burdensome access barriers for high-risk patients a further reduced net price for alirocumab (Praluent') Injection in alignment with a new value assessment for high-risk patients from the Institute for Clinical and Economic Review" (Box 6.3).[46]

Behind the scenes, the same manufacturers also shared confidential data with ICER on the impact of dupilumab (Dupixent®) on the quality of life for patients with atopic dermatitis. More recently, Amgen and Novartis set a relatively low price—at least judged against Wall Street expectations—for Aimovig®, their new biologic for migraine prevention. The list price, $6,900 per year, was well below the $8,000 to $10,000 price that investment analysts were anticipating. The companies informed ICER, as well as pharmacy benefit managers and payers, that they would offer discounts and rebates to further drop the price to $5,000 annually, which factored into a favorable review of cost-effectiveness by ICER.[47,48]

As another example, the New York State Medicaid program has attempted to use ICER's findings to obtain lower prices for cystic fibrosis drugs, priced near $300,000 per year, to bring prices in line with cost-effectiveness benchmarks of $100,000 to $150,000 per QALY.[49] Vertex, the manufacturer, has also faced objections elsewhere. The drugs were initially excluded from the market in England and Australia, for example, because of findings that they were not cost-effective at the offered price and only recently became available after years of protracted negotiations.[50,51] Since 2017, the Veterans Administration has formally collaborated with ICER to integrate ICER reports into its evidence review processes and use ICER's value-based price recommendations in negotiations with the drug industry.[52]

ICER's rapid rise to a position of influence is remarkable given its status as a private organization with private funding. Nor was its role preordained, as other organizations had also recognized the need for value assessment and had offered their own value frameworks. Understanding why those alternatives fell short sheds even more light on why ICER's approach has seen more success. It is to these alternatives that we turn next.

References

1. Butcher, L. 2019. "Can ICER bring cost-effectiveness to drug prices?" *Managed Care* 28 (6): 30–33.
2. FDA approves Sovaldi for chronic hepatitis C. 2013. *U.S. Department of Health & Human Services.* Accessed August 6, 2020. https://www.hhs.gov/hepatitis/blog/2013/12/09/fda-approves-sovaldi-for-chronic-hepatitis-c.html.
3. Herper, M. 2014. "Gilead's hepatitis C pill takes off like a rocket." *Forbes.* Accessed May 10, 2020. https://www.forbes.com/sites/matthewherper/2014/02/21/gileads-hepatitis-c-pill-takes-off-like-a-rocket/#56c8ce354093.
4. Tice, J.A., Ollendorf, D.A., and Pearson, S.D. 2014, April 15, "The comparative clinical effectiveness and value of simeprevir and sofosbuvir in the treatment of chronic hepatitis C infection." *Institute for Clinical and Economic Review.* https://icer.org/wp-content/uploads/2020/10/CTAF_Hep_C_Apr14_final.pdf

5. Appleby, J. 2014, May 1. "New hepatitis C drugs' price prompts an ethical debate: Who deserves to get them?" *The Washington Post*. Accessed May 10, 2020. https://www. washingtonpost.com/business/new-hepatitis-c-drugs-price-prompts-an-ethical-debate-who-deserves-to-get-them/2014/05/01/73582abc-cfac-11e3-937f-d3026234b51c_story. html.

6. Tice, J.A., Ollendorf, D.A., Chahal, H.S., Kahn, J.G., Marseille, E., Weissberg, J., Shore, K.K., and Pearson, S.D. 2015. "The comparative clinical effectiveness and value of novel combination therapies for the treatment of patients with genotype 1 chronic hepatitis C infection." *Institute for Clinical and Economic Review* https://icer.org/wp-content/uploads/2020/10/CTAF_HCV2_Final_Report_013015.pdf.

7. Kroll, l., and Dolan, K.A. 2019. "The Forbes 400: The definitive ranking of the wealthiest Americans." *Forbes*. Accessed August 6, 2020. https://www.forbes.com/forbes-400/.

8. "Laura and John Arnold Foundation." 2018. *Influence Watch*. https://www.influencewatch. org/non-profit/laura-and-john-arnold-foundation/.

9. Loftus, P. 2018, October 21. "A billionaire pledges to fight high drug prices, and the industry is rattled: Ex-energy trader John Arnold has put millions behind efforts to curb prices." *The Wall Street Journal*. https://www.wsj.com/articles/a-billionaire-decided-to-fight-high-drug-prices-and-the-industry-is-rattled-1540145686.

10. Loftus, P. 2015, July 21. "Rising U.S. drug prices are focus of research grant." *The Wall Street Journal*. Accessed July 16, 2020. https://www.wsj.com/articles/rising-u-s-drug-prices-are-focus-of-research-grant-1437433550.

11. "Transforming the market for new drugs: The ICER emerging therapy assessment and pricing (ETAP) program." 2015. *Institute for Clinical and Economic Review*. https://icer.org/wp-content/uploads/2021/01/ICER-2015-July-ETAP-Emerging-Therapy-Assessment-and-Pricing.pdf.

12. Pearson, S.D. 2015. "A US approach to value-based drug assessment." *MedNous*. https://www.mednous.com/us-approach-value-based-drug-assessment.

13. Dubois, R.W. 2015. "Cost–effectiveness thresholds in the USA: Are they coming? Are they already here?" *Journal of Comparative Effectiveness Research* 5 (1): 9–12. https://doi.org/10.2217/cer.15.50.

14. *Comments received on ICER's value assessment framework*. 2016. *Institute for Clinical and Economic Review*. https://icer.org/wp-content/uploads/2020/10/ICER_Comments_on_VAF_100316.pdf.

15. Eli Lilly. 2016. "Comments received on ICER's value assessment framework." *Institute for Clinical and Economic Review*. https://icer.org/wp-content/uploads/2020/10/ICER_Comments_on_VAF_100316.pdf.

16. Astellas. 2016. "Comments received on ICER's value assessment framework." *Institute for Clinical and Economic Review*. https://icer.org/wp-content/uploads/2020/10/ICER_Comments_on_VAF_100316.pdf.

17. Hal Singer, Economists Incorporated. 2016. "Comments received on ICER's value assessment framework." *Institute for Clinical and Economic Review*. https://icer.org/wp-content/uploads/2020/10/ICER_Comments_on_VAF_100316.pdf.

18. Janssen. 2016. "Comments received on ICER's value assessment framework." *Institute for Clinical and Economic Review*. https://icer.org/wp-content/uploads/2020/10/ICER_Comments_on_VAF_100316.pdf.

19. "Overview of the ICER value assessment framework and update for 2017–2019." 2018. *Institute for Clinical and Economic Review*. https://icer.org/wp-content/uploads/2020/10/ICER-value-assessment-framework-Updated-050818.pdf.

20. Coelho, T. 2018, August 30. "Patients harmed by 'cost-effectiveness' measures." *RealClear Health*. Accessed January 26, 2021. https://www.realclearhealth.com/articles/2018/08/30/patients_harmed_by_cost-effectiveness_measures_110821.html.

21. "The QALY: Rewarding the care that most improves patients' lives." 2018. *Institute for Clinical and Economic Review*. https://icer.org/wp-content/uploads/2020/12/QALY_evLYG_FINAL.pdf.

22. Cohen, J.T., Ollendorf, D.A., and Neumann, P.J. 2018. "Will ICER's response to attacks on the QALY quiet the critics?" *Center for the Evaluation of Value and Risk in Health, Tufts Medical Center*. Accessed June 11, 2020. https://cevr.tuftsmedicalcenter.org/news/2018/will-icers-response-to-attacks-on-the-qaly-quiet-the-critics.

23. "2020–2023 value assessment framework." 2020. *Institute for Clinical and Economic Review*. https://icer.org/wp-content/uploads/2020/10/ICER_2020_2023_VAF_102220.pdf.

24. "Addressing the myths about ICER and value assessment." 2016. *Institute for Clinical and Economic Review*. https://icer.org/wp-content/uploads/2021/01/ICER-2016-Myths-and-Facts.pdf.

25. "Evaluating the value of new drugs and devices." 2015. *Institute for Clinical and Economic Review*. https://icer.org/wp-content/uploads/2021/01/ICER-2015b-FW-v1-Evaluating-the-value-of-new-drugs.pdf.

26. "PCSK9 inhibitors for treatment of high cholesterol: Effectiveness, value, and value-based price benchmarks final report." 2015. *Institute for Clinical and Economic Review*. https://icer.org/wp-content/uploads/2020/10/Final-Report-for-Posting-11-24-15-1.pdf.

27. CardioMEMS™ HF System (St. Jude Medical, Inc.) and Sacubitril/Valsartan (Entresto™, Novartis AG) for management of congestive heart failure: Effectiveness, value, and value-based price benchmarks final report. 2015, December 1. *Institute for Clinical and Economic Review*. https://icer.org/wp-content/uploads/2020/10/CHF_Final_Report_120115.pdf.

28. Mepolizumab (Nucala®; GlaxoSmithKline plc.) for the treatment of severe asthma with eosinophilia: Effectiveness, value, and value-based price benchmarks final report. 2016, March 14. *Institute for Clinical and Economic Review*. https://icer.org/wp-content/uploads/2020/10/CTAF_Mepolizumab_Final_Report_031416.pdf.

29. Pagliarulo, N. 2019. "Regeneron, Sanofi cut PCSK9 list price, matching earlier move by rival Amgen." *BioPharmaDive*. https://www.biopharmadive.com/news/regeneron-sanofi-cut-pcsk9-list-price-matching-earlier-move-by-rival-amge/548147/.

30. Appleby, J. 2014. "Who should get pricey hepatitis c drugs?" *Kaiser Health News*. Accessed May 10, 2020. https://khn.org/news/sovaldi-who-should-get-pricey-drug/.

31. Grabowski, D.C., Lakdawalla, D.N., Goldman, D.P., Eber, M., Liu, L.Z., Abdelgawad, T., Kuznik, A., Chernew, M.E., and Philipson, T. 2012. "The large social value resulting from use of statins warrants steps to improve adherence and broaden treatment." *Health Affairs* 31 (10): 2276–2285. https://doi.org/10.1377/hlthaff.2011.1120.

32. Greissing, E. 2016. "Public comment letter to the Institute for Clinical and Economic Review on their assessment of "Insulin Degludec (Tresiba®; Novo Nordisk) for the Treatment of Diabetes." *Institute for Clinical and Economic Review*. https://icer.org/wp-content/uploads/2020/10/CTAF_Degludec_Public_Comments_012516.pdf

33. Bristol-Myers Squibb. 2016. "Response to ICER's draft report on non-small cell lung cancer." *Institute for Clinical and Economic Review*. https://icer.org/wp-content/uploads/2020/10/Bristol-Myers-Squibb-2016-Response-to-ICER-Small-Lung-Cancer.pdf.

34. Ofman, J. 2015. "Response to ICER assessment of PCSK9 inhibitors." *Institute for Clinical and Economic Review*. https://icer.org/wp-content/uploads/2020/10/Public-Comments-PCSK9.pdf.

35. "ICER's reference case for economic evaluations: Principles and rationale." 2018. *Institute for Clinical and Economic Review*. http://icer.org/wp-content/uploads/2020/10/ICER_Reference_Case_July-2018.pdf.

36. Neumann, P.J., Sanders, G.D., Russell, L.B., Siegel, J.E., and Ganiats, T.G. 2017. *Cost-effectiveness in health and medicine* (2nd ed.). New York: Oxford University Press.

37. Harris, P. 2012, July 28. "Olympics opening ceremony: US media reacts to 'peculiar' British festival." *The Guardian*. Accessed May 10, 2020. https://www.theguardian.com/media/2012/jul/28/us-media-reacts-olmpics-opening-ceremony.
38. Cohen, J.T., Silver, M.C., Ollendorf, D.A., and Neumann, P.J. 2019. "Does the Institute for Clinical and Economic Review revise its findings in response to industry comments?" *Value in Health* 22 (12): 1396–1401. https://doi.org/10.1016/j.jval.2019.08.003.
39. Pollack, A. 2015, September 9. "New cholesterol drugs are vastly overpriced, analysis says." *The New York Times*. Accessed August 11, 2020. https://www.nytimes.com/2015/09/09/business/new-cholesterol-drugs-are-vastly-overpriced-analysis-says.html.
40. Berkrot, B. 2018, January 12. "Spark's price for Luxturna blindness gene therapy too high: ICER." *Reuters*. Accessed August 11, 2020. https://www.reuters.com/article/us-spark-icer/sparks-price-for-luxturna-blindness-gene-therapy-too-high-icer-idUSKBN1F1298.
41. White, N., Johns, A., and Latch, E. 2019. "Industry perceptions and expectations: The role of ICER as an independent HTA organisation." *ICON*. https://iconplc.com/insights/value-based-healthcare/the-role-of-icer-as-an-independent-hta-organisation/.
42. Sampsel, E., Watkins, J., and Kenney, J. 2019, February 28. "ICER: Payer perspectives on the use and usage of ICER reports." *Dymaxium*. https://www.amcp.org/sites/default/files/2019-03/AMCP%20webinar%20-%20ICER%202-28-19%20FINAL.pdf
43. Schafer, J., Galante, D., and Shafrin, J. 2017. "Value tools in managed care decision making: Current hurdles and future opportunities." *Journal of Managed Care & Specialty Pharmacy* 23 (6-a Suppl): S21–S27. https://doi.org/10.18553/jmcp.2017.23.6-a.s21.
44. Lising, A., Drummond, M.F., Barry, M., and Augustovski, F. 2017, May. "Payers' use of independent reports in decision making—Will there be an ICER effect?" *International Society for Pharmacoeconomics and Outcomes Research: Value & Outcomes Spotlight*. https://www.ispor.org/publications/newsletters/newsletter/newsletter-detail/ebulletin-may-2017/value-outcomes-spotlight.
45. Cohen, J. 2019, April 17. "ICER's growing impact on drug pricing and reimbursement." *Forbes*. Accessed August 11, 2020. https://www.forbes.com/sites/joshuacohen/2019/04/17/icers-growing-impact-on-drug-pricing-and-reimbursement/?sh=1ed316456b53.
46. "Regeneron and Sanofi announce plans to make Praluent® (Alirocumab) more accessible and affordable for patients with the greatest health risk and unmet need." 2018. *Regeneron*. Accessed June 13, 2020. https://investor.regeneron.com/news-releases/news-release-details/regeneron-and-sanofi-announce-plans-make-praluentr-alirocumab.
47. Ellis, A.G., Otuonye, I., Kumar, V., Chapman, R., Seidner, M., Rind, D., Pearson, S.D., Walton, S.M., Lee, T.A., and Quach, D. 2018. "Calcitonin gene-related peptide (CGRP) inhibitors as preventative treatments for patients with episodic or chronic migraine: Effectiveness and value." *Institute for Clinical and Economic Review*. https://icer.org/wp-content/uploads/2020/10/ICER_Migraine_Final_Evidence_Report_070318.pdf /.
48. Taylor, P. 2018. "Novartis, Amgen set low price for first CGRP migraine drug." *PMLive*. http://www.pmlive.com/pharma_news/novartis,_amgen_set_low_price_for_first_cgrp_migraine_drug_1235956.
49. Thomas, K. 2018, June 24. "A drug costs $272,000 a year. Not so fast, says New York state." *The New York Times*. Accessed July 21, 2020. https://www.nytimes.com/2018/06/24/health/drug-prices-orkambi-new-york.html.
50. "Vertex cystic fibrosis drug to be available in England after pricing deal." 2019. *Physicians Weekly*. https://www.physiciansweekly.com/vertex-cystic-fibrosis-drug-2/.
51. Staines, R. 2018. "Vertex's Orkambi CF drug okayed for funding in Australia." *Pharmaphorum*. https://pharmaphorum.com/news/vertexs-orkambi-cf-drug-okayed-for-funding-in-australia/.
52. Glassman, P., Pearson, S.D., Zacher, J., Rind, D., and Valentino, M. 2020, June 15. "VA and ICER at three years: Critics' concerns answered." *Health Affairs*. https://doi.org/10.1377/hblog20200611.662048.

7
Other US Value Assessment Frameworks

The Road to ICER

A traditional view of human evolution imagined our species as progressing in a more-or-less linear fashion. That vision, well represented by the 1965 illustration known as "The March of Progress" (more formally, "The Road to Homo Sapiens") had its allure. The depiction starts at the left with a monkey-like animal, to the right of which is a somewhat more upright ape-like creature, and so on, until the sequence concludes with modern man at the head of the line at the far right of the frame.[1] More recent science suggests a much messier (and more interesting!) history. In the distant past, *Homo sapiens'* ancestors were just one of many coexisting prehistoric human species. For better or worse, modern humans outcompeted those species or at least outlasted them.

With a bit of license, there is an analogy between humanity's evolution and the development of drug value assessment frameworks in the United States. Considering the landscape in the early 2020s, it can seem that the Institute for Clinical and Economic Review (ICER) has always dominated the scene. In reality, not long ago, there were numerous other value assessment frameworks that seemed to coexist along with ICER and seemed poised to compete with the organization. Those alternatives have not exactly vanished, but while they once seemed to garner attention rivaling the focus on ICER, they no longer play as active a role. For now, at least, ICER is the "dominant species." Understanding the alternative frameworks and how they differ from ICER's sheds light on which attributes make a framework well-adapted to the current environment.

The Roads Less Traveled

Before examining how US value assessment frameworks vary, it is worth revisiting the stark differences between drug value assessment in the United States and abroad (see Chapters 4 and 5 of this volume). Elsewhere, the government (or a government-appointed body) drives the assessments, which in

The Right Price. Peter J. Neumann, Joshua T. Cohen, and Daniel A. Ollendorf, Oxford University Press (2021).
© Peter J. Neumann, Joshua T. Cohen, and Daniel A. Ollendorf. DOI: 10.1093/oso/9780197512883.003.0007

turn drives a drug's price and ultimate adoption. Examples include agencies in the United Kingdom, France, Germany, Canada, and Australia. With few exceptions, the US government has assiduously avoided this role (see Chapter 5 of this volume). Even initiatives for the federal government to fund *research* that compares the value of therapies—which does not direct the allocation of health care resources—has elicited congressional language to sideline cost-per-QALY analyses.[2]

The government's reluctance to assess value, however, has not removed the need for this type of information. In the absence of government involvement, other groups sensed a vacuum and an opportunity. Several were privately run nonprofit medical societies with a history of issuing clinical guidelines; now their membership was seeking guidance on whether a drug's price was justified given the medication's clinical evidence. Examples included the American College of Cardiology (ACC)/American Heart Association (AHA), the American Society of Clinical Oncology (ASCO), and the National Comprehensive Cancer Network (NCCN). At New York City's Memorial Sloan Kettering Cancer Center, a group led by Peter Bach, a physician, health policy researcher, and well-known critic of high pharmaceutical prices, also weighed in. Reviews and critiques of drug value frameworks over the past few years have generally highlighted most or all of these frameworks, along with ICER's methodologies.[3,4]

American Society of Clinical Oncology

ASCO has explained that its drug value framework is intended to "enable a physician and patient to assess the value of a particular cancer treatment regimen given the patient's individual preferences and circumstance"[5p1,6] To this end, the framework computes for cancer drugs a "net health benefit score" to be compared to a medication's cost. As described in Box 7.1, the score reflects a drug's clinical benefit (changes in survival or cancer progression rates), toxicity, and a series of "bonus" benefit categories, including reduced pain and discomfort, improved quality of life, reduced treatment frequency, and so on.

Because oncologists comprise its key target audience, ASCO's framework unsurprisingly is tailored to how clinicians might think about cancer treatments. ASCO explains that the framework's first two net health benefit elements—clinical benefit (expressed in terms of overall survival, slowed disease progression, and proportion of patients responding to the medication) and toxicity are the type of standard outcomes oncologists are accustomed to from the clinical literature.[6p1] Still, ASCO notes that its framework is also

Box 7.1 How the ASCO Framework Computes Its Net Benefit Score

For cancer treatments, ASCO's framework compares a drug's monthly cost to its net health benefit score. The net health benefit score is the sum of three contributions: (1) clinical benefit, (2) toxicity, and (3) "bonus" points.

Clinical Benefit

Clinical benefit reflects a drug's mortality impact if available (100 times the percent reduction), its impact on disease progression as a second choice (80 times the percent reduction), or its response rate (70 times the response rate) as a last resort. For example, a drug that reduces mortality by 25% has a clinical benefit of $0.25 \times 100 = 25$ points. The multiplicative factors of 100, 80, and 70 have no firm basis, even if their relative sizes have face validity, as reduced mortality is judged to be inherently more important than slowed disease progression, which in turn, is more important than the response rate (the proportion of patients whose cancer declines after therapy).

Toxicity

ASCO quantifies toxicity in terms of an adverse effect index (higher values are less favorable), multiplied by -20. ASCO's adverse effect index reflects the number of effects, as well as their severity and frequency. Each more severe (non-fatal, Grade 3 or 4) effect—such as anemia—contributes 2 points if it affects at least 5% of patients, and 1.5 points otherwise. Each less severe (Grade 1 or 2) effect—such as nausea or diarrhea—contributes 1 point if it affects at least 10% of patients, and half a point otherwise. A drug with an adverse effect index 25% higher than the alternative's receives $-20 \times 25\% = -5$ points. A drug with an adverse effect index 50% *lower* than the alternative's receives $-20 \times -50\% = +10$ points.

Bonus

The ASCO framework awards up to three bonuses. First, a drug that extends the "tail of the curve" survival earns 20 bonus points. Extending the "tail of the curve" survival means the drug must at least double the probability of surviving for an "extended period of time," where "an extended period of time" means twice the median survival period. For example, if half the population receiving an "old" therapy lives at least 12 months, "extended survival" is twice as long, or 24 months. If, for example, a new treatment doubles the proportion of patients living for at least 24 months from 5% to 10%, it earns those 20 bonus points. Second, a drug that reduces patient cancer symptoms earns 10 bonus points. Finally, a drug earns another 10 bonus points if it reduces how frequently patients must receive treatment.

Source: Schnipper, L.E., Davidson, N.E., Wollins, D.S., Blayney, D.W., Dicker, A.P., Ganz, P.A., Hoverman, J.R., Langdon, R., Lyman, G.H., Meropol, N.J., Mulvey, T., Newcomer, L., Peppercorn, J., Polite, B., Raghavan, D., Rossi, G., Saltz, L., Schrag, D., Smith, T.J., Yu, P.P., . . . Schilsky, R.L. 2016. "Updating the American Society of Clinical Oncology value framework: Revisions and reflections in response to comments received." *Journal of Clinical Oncology* 34 (24): 2925–2934. https://doi.org/ 10.1200/JCO.2016.68.2518.

meant to aid patient decisions. Elements comprising the framework's "bonus score" reflect "convenience of receiving therapy, . . . [and] quality of life,"[5,6] elements that ASCO characterizes as "patient-reported outcomes." ASCO concludes that "the [net health benefit] represents the very elements that patients seek to understand as they consider treatment options and that most oncologists use to make treatment recommendations."[6p3]

In one sense, the extinction metaphor described in this chapter's introduction is somewhat exaggerated when it comes to the ASCO framework, which continues to appear in review articles: between 2016 and early 2020, the academic literature added approximately 30 articles mentioning "ASCO" and "value framework."[7] A closer look at those articles, however, reveals that while the ASCO framework has its enthusiasts, it seems to have little influence on the estimation of appropriate cancer drug prices. Some articles have explored how the ASCO framework's net health benefit score compares to scores produced by other value frameworks or whether different experts would independently award similar ASCO framework value scores for a particular drug (i.e., whether the ASCO framework is "reliable").[8,9] No US payer (e.g., an insurance company or government health plan) has publicly declared it will use the ASCO framework to help determine its selection of drug therapies or how much they are willing to pay.

Even articles with titles that suggest use of the ASCO framework disappoint. For example, one, entitled "Anticancer Drugs Approved by the Food and Drug Administration for Gastrointestinal Malignancies: Clinical Benefit and Price Considerations" reports prices and ASCO framework net health benefit scores for different classes of cancer drugs. It even points to the absence of a correlation between net health benefit scores and drug prices and notes that, relative to their price, some drug classes deliver more benefits (measured in terms of ASCO framework points) than others. But the article does not identify *appropriate* prices for the reviewed drugs.[10]

Why do the ASCO framework articles refrain from articulating value-based prices for cancer drugs? Perhaps because the framework's main purpose is to assist shared decision-making between patients and clinicians. To ASCO's credit, their framework has components for many salient characteristics that patients and their doctors must consider. But even audiences who might want to use the ASCO framework to quantify a drug's value find they cannot because of the framework's design.

There are multiple challenges with the framework's construction, including its presentation of a drug's total monthly cost. If the intent is to inform patient–clinician shared decisions, it would have been preferable to include a patient's out-of-pocket spending, which can depend on the type of insurance the patient has and whether the patient can take the drug orally or if it must be administered in a hospital or doctor's office. Beyond that, the root of the difficulty lies in the lack of clarity around how much an ASCO "net health benefit point" is worth. As challenging as it is to estimate what people would pay for a life-year or QALY, a "net health benefit point" is even more abstract. The ASCO scale is inexplicit because, as described earlier, it represents an amalgamation of judgments about treatment attributes—survival, toxicity, frequency of administration, palliation, and so on—that are themselves difficult to compare. Moreover, ASCO expresses a drug's performance on each of these attributes in terms of subscores and in a rather arbitrary manner (see Box 7.1). It then combines these subscores using arbitrary weights. For example, ASCO assumes that survival benefits can contribute up to 100 points to a drug's net health benefit score and that its comparative toxicity can increase or reduce the score by up to 20 points. That design implies that the best possible survival benefit is five times more valuable than avoiding the worst possible toxicity. Clinicians (and, more specifically, the experts ASCO assembled to create their framework) may judge these relative weights to have "face validity." But because that judgment is a hunch—as are other judgments underlying the ASCO framework, using the framework to estimate an appropriate price for a drug lacks rigor and credibility. While more "valuable" drugs tend to have more ASCO points, it remains unclear how much each point is worth—or even how each point's value could be estimated.

DrugAbacus

The Drug Pricing Lab at New York City's Memorial Sloan Kettering Cancer Center focuses on "the development of rational approaches to drug pricing and health insurance coverage that sustain innovation while ensuring patient access and affordability."[11] The lab describes DrugAbacus, which it maintains, as an "interactive tool [that] takes more than 50 cancer drugs and lets [the user] compare the company's price to one based on value."[11] This explicit comparison of price and value seems to address the ASCO framework's missing element.

And yet decision makers have not seemed to use DrugAbacus for coverage or pricing determinations. A Google search reveals no evidence that payers or other decision makers employ DrugAbacus to assess coverage or drug prices. Moreover, only seven academic articles (published through April 2020) mention DrugAbacus, and even then only in the context of comparing different frameworks, not for the assessment of value for specific drugs. Given that DrugAbacus reports a recommended price for each drug, why have decision makers apparently eschewed it? The fact that DrugAbacus uses cost-per-life-year ratios to quantify benefits –essentially mirroring ICER's methodology— makes its lack of popularity particularly curious given ICER's prominence.

Several aspects of DrugAbacus may explain its limited influence. First, the methodology is less transparent than ICER's. Whereas ICER describes its methods and even provides some access to its computer models, DrugAbacus provides relatively little information on its methods, such as what evidence it considers for each drug assessment or how it synthesizes information from different studies. As a result, the DrugAbacus assessments can seem to have a "black box" quality.

Second, as with the ASCO framework, the scope is limited to cancer treatments. The tool does not extend to therapies for other conditions of concern to payers, including drugs to treat widely prevalent infectious disease—like hepatitis C—and high-priced therapies for rare, chronic, life-threatening conditions, like cystic fibrosis, hemophilia, and Duchenne muscular dystrophy.

Third, although the "life years gained" benefit measure used by DrugAbacus resembles ICER's quality adjusted life year, DrugAbacus applies a series of "adjustment factors" that can introduce a double counting of benefits. For example, DrugAbacus scales up value for drugs that have a "novel mechanism of action"—meaning that they attack disease in new and innovative ways. But why should life years gained because of a drug's novel mechanism of action be worth more than life years gained because of some other attribute of the drug (e.g., fewer fatal adverse side effects)? Scaling up life years gained due to novelty amounts to awarding credit twice for the same benefit.

Finally, some of the adjustment factors are difficult to interpret. For example, DrugAbacus scales down a drug's benefit by as much as 30% to account for its toxicity. Hence, a highly toxic treatment that extends life for

10 years can have the same value as a non-toxic drug that extends life for seven years—that is, reflecting the full application of a 30% deduction to the original 10-year benefit). A drug that extends life for 10 years but is *half* as toxic has the same value as a non-toxic drug that extends life for 8.5 years—that is, reflecting *half* the application of the 30% deduction (or 15%) to the original 10-year benefit. The problem with this formulation is that DrugAbacus does not clearly explain the rationale for its "toxicity yardstick." For example, what does it mean for one drug to be "half as toxic" as another? Without defining this measure, DrugAbacus cannot meaningfully trade off toxicity and life years and hence cannot place a value on different levels of toxicity.

Other Frameworks

Other organizations have also promulgated drug value frameworks. The ACC/AHA framework classifies each therapy based on a comparison of its benefits and risks, the quality of the therapy's supporting evidence, and its cost-effectiveness, with ratios below (more favorable than) $50,000 per QALY indicating "high value," ratios from $50,000 to $150,000 per QALY indicating "intermediate value," and ratios exceeding $150,000 per QALY indicating "low value."[12] The ACC/AHA framework resembles ICER's in many respects (see Chapter 6 of this volume), although unlike ICER, the organizations behind the framework do not conduct their own independent assessments of new (and existing) therapies. Moreover, it is focused only on interventions for cardiovascular disease, reflecting the interests of its membership. Also, few ACC/AHA assessments have been conducted using this framework, whereas ICER regularly publishes assessments of high-profile drugs, including those for cardiovascular conditions.

The NCCN "Evidence Blocks" framework has five components: efficacy, safety, quality of evidence, consistency of evidence, and affordability. Assessments grade each component on a 1-to-5 scale. For example, the affordability component has five levels: (a) very expensive, (b) expensive, (c) moderately expensive, (d) inexpensive, and (e) very inexpensive. But NCCN provides no criteria to further describe these five categories, making it difficult to determine what price is appropriate for a therapy. Indeed, analyses have indicated a lack of correlation between NCCN's affordability levels and drug prices.[13]

ICER's Niche

Why have other frameworks failed to displace or even challenge ICER? ASCO's net health benefit point measure embeds obscure value judgments (e.g., the importance of survival gains compared to drug side effects). That makes it difficult to understand what the framework's net health benefit score should be worth. DrugAbacus estimates life years but scales them to account for other attributes—such as novelty—that do not clearly relate to therapeutic value or that seem to introduce double counting. The ACC/AHA framework relies on a cost-effectiveness platform but has not been used to analyze the drugs of greatest concern to payers. The NCCN framework reports a drug's "affordability" but does not explain how affordability should be assessed. Yet another entrant, the Patient-Perspective Value Framework, amounts to a checklist of attributes but does not provide an easy or intuitive way to translate those attributes into an acceptable price.[14-16]

By building the cost-per-QALY into the foundation of its framework, ICER estimates a drug's value based on widely accepted therapeutic attributes— namely, the contribution to length and quality of life. That conceptually straightforward approach to value assessment, together with its allowance for other considerations beyond cost-effectiveness and the resources it has injected into conducting assessments, has made ICER the dominant framework when it comes to evaluating drugs in the United States.

References

1. Blake, K. 2018. "On the origins of 'The March of Progress.'" *Washington University.* Accessed January 27, 2021. https://sites.wustl.edu/prosper/on-the-origins-of-the-march-of-progress/.
2. Neumann, P.J., and Weinstein, M.C. 2010. "Legislating against use of cost-effectiveness information." *New England Journal of Medicine* 363 (16): 1495–1497. https://doi.org/10.1056/NEJMp1007168.
3. Neumann, P.J., and Cohen, J.T. 2015. "Measuring the value of prescription drugs." *New England Journal of Medicine* 373 (27): 2595–2597. https://doi.org/10.1056/NEJMp1512009.
4. Goodman, C., Villarivera, C., Riposo, J., and Beam, E. 2016. "Comparison of value assessment frameworks using the National Pharmaceutical Council's guiding practice for patient-centered value assessment." *The Lewin Group.* http://www.lewin.com/content/dam/Lewin/Resources/Comparison-of-Value-Assessment-Frameworks.pdf.
5. Schnipper, L.E., Davidson, N.E., Wollins, D.S., Tyne, C., Blayney, D.W., Blum, D., Dicker, A.P., Ganz, P.A., Hoverman, J.R., Langdon, R., Lyman, G.H., Meropol, N.J., Mulvey, T., Newcomer, L., Peppercorn, J., Polite, B., Raghavan, D., Rossi, G., Saltz, L., Schrag, D., Smith, T.J., Yu, P.P., Hudis, C.A., and Schilsky, R.L. 2015. "American Society of Clinical

Oncology statement: A conceptual framework to assess the value of cancer treatment options." *Journal of Clinical Oncology* 33 (23): 2563–2577. https://doi.org/10.1200/JCO.2015.61.6706.

6. Schnipper, L.E., Davidson, N.E., Wollins, D.S., Blayney, D.W., Dicker, A.P., Ganz, P.A., Hoverman, J.R., Langdon, R., Lyman, G.H., Meropol, N.J., Mulvey, T., Newcomer, L., Peppercorn, J., Polite, B., Raghavan, D., Rossi, G., Saltz, L., Schrag, D., Smith, T.J., Yu, P.P., Hudis, C.A., Vose, J.M., and Schilsky, R.L. 2016. "Updating the American Society of Clinical Oncology value framework: Revisions and reflections in response to comments received." *Journal of Clinical Oncology* 34 (24): 2925–2934. https://doi.org/10.1200/JCO.2016.68.2518.

7. Brogan, A.P., Hogue, S.L., Vekaria, R.M., Reynolds, I., and Coukell, A. 2019. "Understanding payer perspectives on value in the use of pharmaceuticals in the United States." *Journal of Managed Care & Specialty Pharmacy* 25 (12): 1319–1327. https://doi.org/10.18553/jmcp.2019.25.12.1319.

8. Cheng, S., McDonald, E.J., Cheung, M.C., Arciero, V.S., Qureshi, M., Jiang, D., Ezeife, D., Sabharwal, M., Chambers, A., Han, D., Leighl, N., Sabarre, K.-A., and Chan, K.K.W. 2017. "Do the American Society of Clinical Oncology value framework and the European Society of Medical Oncology magnitude of clinical benefit scale measure the same construct of clinical benefit?" *Journal of Clinical Oncology* 35 (24): 2764–2771. https://doi.org/10.1200/JCO.2016.71.6894.

9. Del Paggio, J.C., Cheng, S., Booth, C.M., Cheung, M.C., and Chan, K.K.W. 2018. "Reliability of oncology value framework outputs: Concordance between independent research groups." *JNCI Cancer Spectrum* 2 (3): pky050–pky050. https://doi.org/10.1093/jncics/pky050.

10. Jiang, D.M., Chan, K.K.W., Jang, R.W., Booth, C., Liu, G., Amir, E., Mason, R., Everest, L., and Elimova, E. 2019. "Anticancer drugs approved by the Food and Drug Administration for gastrointestinal malignancies: Clinical benefit and price considerations." *Cancer Medicine* 8 (4): 1584–1593. https://doi.org/10.1002/cam4.2058.

11. "About the Drug Pricing Lab." n.d. *Drug Pricing Lab: Memorial Sloan Kettering.* Accessed January 27, 2021. https://drugpricinglab.org/about/.

12. Sorenson, C., Lavezzari, G., Daniel, G., Burkholder, R., Boutin, M., Pezalla, E., Sanders, G., and McClellan, M. 2017. "Advancing value assessment in the United States: A multistakeholder perspective." *Value in Health* 20 (2): 299–307. https://doi.org/10.1016/j.jval.2016.11.030.

13. Mitchell, A.P., Dey, P., Ohn, J.A., Tabatabai, S.M., Curry, M.A., and Bach, P.B. 2020. "The accuracy and usefulness of the National Comprehensive Cancer Network evidence blocks affordability rating." *PharmacoEconomics* 38 (7): 737–745. https://doi.org/10.1007/s40273-020-00901-x.

14. Seidman, J. 2017. "Avalere and FasterCures release Patient-Perspective Value Framework to incorporate patient preferences into healthcare treatment decisions." *Avalere.* Accessed January 27, 2021. https://avalere.com/press-releases/avalere-and-fastercures-release-patient-perspective-value-framework-to-incorporate-patient-preferences-into-healthcare-treatment-decisions.

15. Seidman, J., and Leinwand, B. 2018. "Avalere releases Patient-Perspective Value Framework scoring methodology report." *Avalere.* Accessed January 27, 2021. https://avalere.com/insights/avalere-releases-patient-perspective-value-framework-scoring-methodology-report.

16. Cohen, J.T., Ollendorf, D.A., and Neumann, P.J. 2018. "Will ICER's response to attacks on the QALY quiet the critics?." *Center for the Evaluation of Value and Risk in Health, Tufts Medical Center.* Accessed January 27, 2021. https://cevr.tuftsmedicalcenter.org/news/2018/will-icers-response-to-attacks-on-the-qaly-quiet-the-critics.

8

Do Drugs for Special Populations Warrant Higher Prices?

I think about the sheer number of people who pulled together just to save my sorry ass, and I can barely comprehend it. My crewmates sacrificed a year of their lives to come back for me. Countless people at NASA worked day and night . . . the cost for my survival must have been hundreds of millions of dollars. All to save one dorky botanist. Why bother?

—**Mark Watney,** *The Martian*

Rescue Me

In Andy Weir's novel, *The Martian*, NASA sacrifices time, equipment, and gobs of money to save a single crew member who is accidentally stranded on Mars.[1] Wouldn't it have been better for the agency, with countless other projects and people to serve, to refrain from the rescue, mourn this loss, direct its efforts toward preventing similar accidents in the future, and continue its planned agenda? That would have represented a better use of resources, and ultimately saved more lives.

For NASA, saving Mark Watney, *The Martian*'s titular character, involved an application of what bioethicist Albert R. Jonsen termed the "rule of rescue," the social imperative that prompts efforts to save individuals facing imminent but potentially avoidable death, with little regard for the associated expense or likelihood of success.[2] On the evening news and silver screen, we have become familiar with its usage, in Herculean efforts to save a toddler who tumbled down a well, miners stranded underground, or a youth soccer team trapped in a cave.[3-5] A critical feature is that subjects are *identifiable*, their individuality often amplified through media coverage. The moral instinct to act in such situations seems pure and unimpeachable. But devoting resources to aid identifiable individuals inescapably means fewer resources for unseen or underappreciated others at risk or in need of care.

The Right Price. Peter J. Neumann, Joshua T. Cohen, and Daniel A. Ollendorf, Oxford University Press (2021).
© Peter J. Neumann, Joshua T. Cohen, and Daniel A. Ollendorf. DOI: 10.1093/oso/9780197512883.003.0008

The rule of rescue also lurks behind many health policy decisions. The Orphan Drug Act of 1983, which promotes the development of drugs to treat diseases afflicting small numbers of patients, provides an example (see Box 2.3 in Chapter 2 of this volume). Manufacturers of orphan drugs receive financial incentives to develop products for rare conditions and face relaxed standards for the data they generate in support of their regulatory submissions.[6] The drug industry has benefited from the limited competition and higher drug prices that have resulted.

Whether such exceptions are justified—for drugs treating rare diseases or other conditions or for populations singled out for their distinctiveness—is an enduring and complex topic in value measurement. The issue has provoked debates among economists, ethicists, and policymakers. Some surveys suggest that people generally want to prioritize resources for treatments that address severe diseases (i.e., those with a high degree of morbidity or reduced life expectancy), even if doing so is not cost-effective.[7] On the other hand, such measures can detract from the goal of maximizing population health.[8]

It is perhaps unsurprising that historically, US payers have placed few restrictions on orphan drugs, even those with exorbitant prices. A 2013 survey found that while most US private payers had cost concerns and monitored the orphan drug pipeline to anticipate budgetary consequences, few actively managed these products.[9] A 2019 study of US commercial payer practices found that the rarer the disease, the less likely the restrictions on related drug therapies.[10] Despite their fiscal challenges and the costly outlays, state Medicaid attempts to restrict orphan drug use to patients with the most severe or advanced disease have often been reversed after legal challenges.[6]

HTA bodies that focus on efficiency have been challenged by orphan drugs (see Box 8.1). In applying its cost-effectiveness threshold, England and Wales' National Institute for Health and Care Excellence (NICE) has made exceptions for orphan drugs, using a benchmark of £100,000 (about $125,000) per QALY gained, roughly three to five times higher (less stringent) than its usual standard.[11] NICE further favors therapies that confer large QALY gains. For a new drug expected to provide 30 additional QALYs per person treated, for example, NICE has used a benchmark that corresponds to approximately £300,000 per QALY.[12] In a nod to budgetary considerations and system-wide fairness concerns, NICE has restricted drugs eligible for such adjustments to those treating "ultra-rare" diseases, defined to be conditions affecting fewer than 600 people in England and Wales).

Other HTA organizations have acknowledged the special nature of rare diseases (e.g., the small sample sizes in orphan drug trials that make detection of a clinical benefit more difficult and often great uncertainty about the drug's

Box 8.1 When a Very Expensive New Drug Can Save Money: ICER's Assessment of Hemophilia Treatment

In the early 1960s, the Warriner family was enjoying Thanksgiving dinner when their one-year-old son Mark fell off his grandfather's lap and sliced his gum against the table. The cut bled for a week.[1] Doctors diagnosed Mark with hemophilia, an X-chromosome linked mutation that causes a deficiency in a protein involved in blood clotting.

When Mark was born, children with hemophilia often did not survive into their 20s. Scientists struggled to understand the disease. Just a few decades earlier, snake venom and peanuts were used to aid in blood clotting. Growing up, Mark was forbidden from playing baseball or football, as even a bump or bruise could cause swelling that would cripple his joints. In the 1950s, doctors had discovered that they could temporarily restore the missing clotting factors in hemophilia patients by transfusing fresh, frozen plasma into them. But the transfusion process required days because clotting factors in the plasma were present at only low concentrations.[2] Mark spent a good part of his childhood in the hospital because he required multiday transfusions whenever he experienced a bleed.

The development of freeze-dried clotting factor concentrates easily stored as a powder transformed hemophilia care in the 1960s.[3] Instead of requiring hospitalization with every bleed, Mark could now remain at home where his mother could inject him with the new treatment. In the 1980s, hemophilia management suffered a setback because of HIV contamination of the blood supply. As many as half of all people with hemophilia and 90% of those with severe hemophilia contracted HIV from clotting factors produced from contaminated blood products.[4] By the 1990s, treatment had become safer because of more stringent blood screening protocols and because prophylaxis with synthetic clotting factors reduced the need for infusions from multiple times per week to once weekly or even less frequently. However, the new regimen brought an extraordinary cost: $613,000 annually on average, twice that of treatment that would only be required "on demand."[5]

Nonetheless, studies found that despite its high price, prophylaxis was cost-effective compared to on-demand treatment because it reduced clotting factor consumption, the number of bleeding episodes, and the risk of future disability from joint damage.[6,7] One study of infant boys with hemophilia showed that 93% of those who received prophylaxis had normal joints at age six, compared to 55% of boys in the on-demand therapy group.[8] Further complicating matters was the fact that roughly 25% to 30% of patients develop antibodies—called "inhibitors"—to clotting factor VIII or IX; this development requires treatment with bypassing agents (BPAs) that can themselves cost $300,000 to $2.5 million per year.[9-11] For all of these reasons, hemophilia became the costliest disease among 2010 Medicare beneficiaries, with up to 99% of direct costs attributable to factor replacement therapy.

With this clinical backdrop, ICER undertook an evaluation in 2018 of emicizumab-kxwh (Hemlibra®, Roche/Genentech), a new once-weekly prophylactic treatment for hemophilia A with a list price of $482,000 for the first year and $448,000 annually thereafter.[11,12] Emicizumab is a new kind of antibody that essentially mimics the missing clotting factor. In contrast to intravenous injections for clotting factor and BPA prophylaxis several times per week, emicizumab requires administration only once every 1 to 4 weeks (depending on the patient's body weight and the severity of their disease) and can be self-administered.[13] ICER concluded that even with life-time costs for emicizumab and associated care totaling $19 million, the treatment both improves health and saves money compared to either BPA prophylaxis or to no prophylaxis.[11] In particular, lifetime BPA prophylaxis treatment had a staggering projected cost of $99 million.

The ICER review raised questions about emicizumab, however. One was whether comparing it to BPA prophylaxis was appropriate. After all, because BPA prophylaxis was itself not cost-effective (at a lifetime cost of $99 million, even giving it credit for an entire lifetime in perfect health would still work out to $1 million or more per QALY), it made therapies compared to it look like they confer very good value. The more general point was that cost-effectiveness could be validly assessed only by comparing the therapy in question to other therapies that were themselves cost-effective. Using a cost-ineffective therapy as the comparator set an inappropriately "low bar."

A second question was whether it would be "fair" for the manufacturer to set a price that "captured" all of the downstream savings their product created for the healthcare system.[14] Why not split the savings in some way between the manufacturer and the rest of society?

A cure for hemophilia may now be on the horizon, promising patients a life free of painful bleeding episodes. Wall Street analysts have speculated that the gene therapy, valoctocogene roxaparvovec (BioMarin Pharmaceutical, Inc.), which continues development after the FDA rejected the company's initial application for approval in August 2020, could command record-high prices of $2 to $3 million.[15,16] Other pharmaceutical companies have their own gene therapies under development.

In a 2019 report on what it termed "single or short-term transformative therapies," ICER called for consideration of a hypothetical "shared savings" arrangement between drug companies and healthcare payers that would ensure adequate financial incentives for drug manufacturers to develop new products that reduced societal costs.[17] Evocative of Medicare's shared savings model for accountable care organizations, in which a network of providers who coordinate care for a group of beneficiaries share the savings with Medicare, drug companies would receive a portion of cost savings generated by their products.[18]

While a "shared savings" approach does not affect ICER's base-case cost-effectiveness analysis, which serves as the basis for its recommended value-based price, it does have implications for the amount a drug company might actually charge in the marketplace. It sends a signal that even if a drug does achieve substantial savings by obviating the need for an existing, expensive treatment, the manufacturer may not be rewarded for that benefit, particularly if the earlier products being replaced did not represent good value in the first place.[19]

[1] Banken, R., Rind, D., Cramer, G., Synnott, P.G., Chapman, R., Khan, S., Pearson, S.D., Carlson, J., Zimmerman, M., and Lubinga, S.J. 2018. "Voretigene Neparvovec for Biallelic RPE65—mediated retinal disease: Effectiveness and value." *Institute for Clinical and Economic Review*. https://icer.org/wp-content/uploads/2020/10/MWCEPAC_VORETIGENE_FINAL_EVIDENCE_REPORT_02142018.pdf.

[2] Lincoln, J.L. 2014, March. "Home treatment eases burden of hemophilia." *Philadelphia Bulletin*. Accessed July 15, 2020. https://www.hemophiliafed.org/news-stories/2014/03/mid-late-1960s-hemophilia-treatment/.

[3] "History of bleeding disorders." *National Hemophilia Foundation*. Accessed January 27, 2021. https://www.hemophilia.org/Bleeding-Disorders/History-of-Bleeding-Disorders.

[4] "The history of hemophilia." n.d. *The hemophilia, von Willebrand disease & platelet disorders handbook*. Accessed July 15, 2020. https://www.hog.org/handbook/article/1/3/the-history-of-hemophilia.

[5] "HIV/AIDS." 2020. *National Hemophilia Foundation*. https://www.hemophilia.org/Bleeding-Disorders/Blood-Safety/HIVAIDS.

[6] Earnshaw, S.R., Graham, C.N., McDade, C.L., Spears, J.B., and Kessler, C.M. 2015. "Factor VIII alloantibody inhibitors: Cost analysis of immune tolerance induction vs. prophylaxis and on-demand with bypass treatment." *Haemophilia* 21 (3): 310–319. https://doi.org/10.1111/hae.12621.

[7] Henry, N., Jovanovic, J., Schlueter, M., Kritikou, P., Wilson, K., and Myren, K.J. 2018. "Cost-utility analysis of life-long prophylaxis with recombinant factor VIIIFc vs recombinant factor VIII for the management of severe hemophilia A in Sweden." *Journal of Medical Economics* 21 (4): 318–325. https://doi.org/10.1080/13696998.2017.1405816.

[8] Thorat, T., Neumann, P.J., and Chambers, J.D. 2018. "Hemophilia burden of disease: A systematic review of the cost-utility literature for hemophilia." *Journal of Managed Care & Specialty Pharmacy* 24 (7): 632–642. https://doi.org/10.18553/jmcp.2018.24.7.632.

[9] Aledort, L.M., Haschmeyer, R.H., and Pettersson, H. 1994. "A longitudinal study of orthopaedic outcomes for severe factor-VIII-deficient haemophiliacs." *Journal of Internal Medicine* 236 (4): 391–399. https://doi.org/10.1111/j.1365-2796.1994.tb00815.x.

[10] Leissinger, C., Gringeri, A., Antmen, B., Berntorp, E., Biasoli, C., Carpenter, S., Cortesi, P., Jo, H., Kavakli, K., Lassila, R., Morfini, M., Negrier, C., Rocino, A., Schramm, W., Serban, M., Uscatescu, M.V., Windyga, J., Zulfikar, B., and Mantovani, L. 2011. "Anti-inhibitor coagulant complex prophylaxis in hemophilia with inhibitors." *New England Journal of Medicine* 365 (18): 1684–1692. https://doi.org/10.1056/NEJMoa1104435.

[11] Rota, M., Cortesi, P.A., Steinitz-Trost, K.N., Reininger, A.J., Gringeri, A., and Mantovani, L.G. 2017. "Meta-analysis on incidence of inhibitors in patients with haemophilia A treated with recombinant factor VIII products." *Blood Coagulation and Fibrinolysis* 28 (8): 627–637. https://doi.org/10.1097/MBC.0000000000000647.

[12] "Emicizumab for hemophilia A with inhibitors: Effectiveness and value final evidence report." 2018, April 16, *Institute for Clinical and Economic Review*. https://icer.org/wp-content/uploads/2020/10/ICER_Hemophilia_Final_Evidence_Report_041618.pdf.

[13] Rodriguez-Merchan, E.C., and Valentino, L.A. 2019. "Emicizumab: Review of the literature and critical appraisal." *Haemophilia* 25 (1): 11–20. https://doi.org/10.1111/hae.13641.

[14] "HEMLIBRA: Prescribing information." 2018. *Genentech*. https://www.gene.com/download/pdf/hemlibra_prescribing.pdf.

[15] "ICER finalizes method adaptations for assessing potential cures and other high-impact single or short-term therapies." 2019, November 12. *Institute for Clinical and Economic Review*. https://icer.org/news-insights/press-releases/final_potential_cures_methods/.

[16] Hopkins, J.S. "BioMarin explores pricing experimental gene therapy at $2 million to $3 million." *The Wall Street Journal*. Accessed July 15, 2020. https://www.wsj.com/articles/biomarin-explores-pricing-experimental-gene-therapy-at-2-million-to-3-million-11579190318#.

[17] Terry, M. 2020. "FDA turns down BioMarin's hemophilia A gene therapy." *Biospace*. https://www.biospace.com/article/fda-rejects-biomarin-s-hemophilia-a-gene-therapy.

[18] "Value assessment methods and pricing recommendations for potential cures: A technical brief." August 6, 2019. *Institute for Clinical and Economic Review*. https://icer.org/wp-content/uploads/2020/10/Valuing-a-Cure-Technical-Brief.pdf.

[19] "Shared savings program." *U.S. Centers for Medicare & Medicaid Services*. Last modified May 1, 2020. Accessed July 15, 2020. https://www.cms.gov/Medicare/Medicare-Fee-for-Service-Payment/sharedsavingsprogram/about.

long-term effects) but have avoided designation of separate cost-effectiveness benchmarks for drugs treating these conditions. ICER's 2017–2019 value framework for ultra-rare diseases is an exception. That framework, which addresses treatments for diseases affecting fewer than 10,000 Americans, called for sensitivity analyses that would judge a therapy's value by comparing its cost-effectiveness ratio to a series of benchmarks ranging as high as $500,000 per QALY (however, the value-based price range—$100,000 to $150,000 per QALY—remained the same as for common conditions).[13] Notably, ICER's 2020–2023 framework eliminated this practice and instead subjects its cost-effectiveness estimates for all conditions to benchmarks ranging from $50,000 to $200,000 per QALY.[14] Other authorities (e.g., those in France, Germany, and the Canadian province of Ontario) have ignored or downplayed cost-effectiveness criteria for orphan drugs and focused instead on clinical data and budgetary considerations.[6]

The Emperor of All Maladies: What Makes Cancer So Special?

Global cancer drug sales reached $100 billion in 2015[15] in large part because both new and established cancer drugs were routinely priced at several hundred thousand dollars per year. By 2018, 6 of the top 10 best-selling drugs worldwide were cancer therapies.[16] Their premium pricing has often pushed the cost-effectiveness ratios for these drugs well above conventional benchmarks.

Consider lenalidomide (Revlimid°; Celgene), indicated for multiple myeloma. The drug has its origins in the 1950s as the sedative thalidomide, which had been widely prescribed off-label to pregnant woman to combat morning sickness before data emerged linking the product to severe birth defects.[17] The accumulating evidence led the US Food and Drug Administration (FDA) to deny the drug approval to treat morning sickness in the early 1960s, despite pressure from the manufacturer. The incident, which stirred a re-examination of FDA's review processes and ultimately led to their overhaul in the Kefauver–Harris Drug Amendments Act of 1962,[18] seemed to spell the end for thalidomide. In the 1990s, however, researchers discovered that thalidomide's restriction of blood-vessel growth, the same activity that had caused the horrific birth defects, also seemed to stunt the growth of certain cancerous tumors. The drug was reborn as Thalomid° and approved to treat multiple myeloma in 1998. The FDA approved Revlimid in late 2005 as a somewhat more potent and less toxic form of thalidomide, and the drug is now a mainstay of multiple myeloma treatment. Its list price is $280,000 for a year's supply (or approximately $770 per pill).[19]

Why do cancer drugs command such high prices? For one, the disease remains a leading health concern, the second leading cause of death in the United States after heart disease.[20] That concern persists even though incidence rates for many cancers (and their associated deaths) have declined due to reductions in smoking, more widespread screening and early detection, and novel treatment approaches, including careful surveillance that have transformed some cancers into manageable, quasi-chronic conditions.[21,22] Drugs targeting other deadly diseases with the same degree of efficacy do not command the same high pricing that cancer drugs command.

In an effort to explain why cancer drugs have particularly high prices, researchers often point to the idea that cancer is a particularly dreaded disease.[23,24] Fear of cancer can motivate decisions, with what can seem like scant regard for the potential benefits, risks, and costs involved. Consider the man in his 50s, diagnosed with a low-risk, slow-growing prostate cancer that he is much more likely to die *with* rather than *from*, who nonetheless opts to have his prostate surgically removed despite the risk of sexual dysfunction and other long-term complications. Or the case of Sandra Lee, the celebrity TV chef, who chose bilateral radical mastectomy after a diagnosis of ductal carcinoma in situ, a noninvasive cluster of abnormal cells in a milk duct that has a low chance of spreading to the breast.[25] Such decisions are invariably complex and emotionally wrenching, but they illustrate how much value individuals sometimes place on addressing cancer.

The dread of cancer is a worldwide phenomenon. In many countries, efforts by national health systems to tamp down on rising cancer drug prices has met stiff resistance and complaints about impeded access to needed new medicines.[26] In England and Wales, patients and clinicians have sought immediate access to newly approved cancer drugs such as trastuzumab (Herceptin®; Roche/Genentech) to treat HER2-positive breast cancer.[27] NICE's lengthy review process, and its potential to say "no" to what it perceived to be marginally beneficial therapies, has angered citizens.[28p121] Media reports have described patients selling homes or emptying savings accounts to pay for new drugs that had received negative assessments or had yet to be reviewed.[29] By the end of the 2000s, NICE faced mounting criticisms over its denial of various high-priced cancer drugs that the agency deemed cost-*in*effective. Moreover, research indicated that the United Kingdom spent much less per year on cancer drugs than did peer group countries.[28p105]

The concern over access to cancer medications caused NICE to revise its procedures to recognize the elevated value people may place on fighting diseases posing an imminent threat to life. While not reserved for cancer, NICE has applied the "end-of-life" criteria almost exclusively to oncology drugs. The criteria allowed for exceptions to its usual cost-effectiveness benchmark range of £20,000 to £30,000 (about $35,000 to $50,000) per QALY for patients expected to live fewer than two years without a new treatment, although NICE restricted these exceptions to cases satisfying two criteria. First, NICE required evidence that the new treatment would extend life by at least three months. Second, the disease could affect only small numbers of patients. NICE provided "extra credit" for drugs that produced added health gains at the end of a patient's life, benefiting many cancer therapies, which tend to confer such gains.[30]

NICE took additional steps to increase access to cancer drugs that did not satisfy conventional cost-effectiveness criteria. In the run-up to the 2010 national elections, the government announced a new Cancer Drugs Fund with an annual budget of roughly £200 million. The fund's intent was to pay for drugs with evidence of positive clinical benefit but unfavorable cost-effectiveness. The initiative provided a temporary political salve but how much it helped population health was unclear. Because it prevented the National Health Service (NHS) from wielding cost-effectiveness criteria to pressure drug companies to reduce their prices, cancer drug costs soon depleted the fund's resources, and authorities were forced to reduce the number of products covered.[31] Moreover, absent a cost-effectiveness benchmark, drugs with limited clinical evidence received coverage. An analysis of the fund's drugs listed from 2010 to 2015 found that only one third provided meaningful clinical benefit.

During this period, the NHS spent in excess of £1 billion on these mostly marginal drugs, equal to one year's worth of system-wide *total* cancer drug spending.[31]

In the ensuing years, the NHS worked to find an intermediate approach for cancer drugs by limiting wasteful spending without re-imposing its original cost-effectiveness criteria. In 2016, it overhauled the Cancer Drugs Fund to address the evidence limitations and budget shortfalls. Under the new arrangement, treatments with evidence that NICE deemed promising but insufficient could receive fund resources for up to two years while additional information, including data on the real-world experience of patients, was collected.[32] After the two-year period, NICE would then consider whether to revise its guidance, conduct another review, or reject a drug's coverage.

Canada also created a special health technology assessment (HTA) process for cancer drugs designed to expand the criteria considered beyond cost-effectiveness to also include input from patient groups. To help speed the review process, Canada permits cancer drugs to undergo an HTA *before* receiving regulatory approval.[33] Some research has demonstrated that the separate process has reduced review time.[34] Decisions to approve or reject a new therapy tend to be made on clinical rather than economic grounds,[35] although in some cases cost-effectiveness does play a role. In those cases, the government generally funds cancer drugs with cost-effectiveness ratios up to about CAN$140,000 per QALY ($110,000 per QALY in US dollars) unconditionally. At cost-effectiveness ratios above that level, however, the government's approval becomes conditional on efforts to "improve cost-effectiveness"— efforts that likely include behind the scenes discounts or additional consideration of data on long-term safety and/or efficacy.[36]

Children Are Our Future

"There can be no keener revelation of a society's soul than the way in which it treats its children," said Nelson Mandela. That sentiment is particularly salient in the face of the many grave and life-threatening conditions that affect children, including serious genetic disorders detected at birth or shortly thereafter. While research may reveal mixed opinions on whether resources should be prioritized for rare diseases, people overwhelmingly favor singling out children for special consideration.[37s–39]

The special status children hold might itself put pressure on regulatory authorities to approve treatments for this population. The lack of supporting data compounds the challenge for regulators, payers, and prescribers. Clinical trials of drugs tend to recruit adults only, and once approved, many drugs do not carry separate approvals for pediatric conditions, even when they are used in children. Limited evidence on drug performance in children persists, despite rules granting pharmaceutical companies added market exclusivity when they conduct studies demonstrating their drugs work in children.[40] In many cases, physicians are left to prescribe drugs "off label" to children, without a good understanding of how the benefits and risks of these drugs may vary by a patient's age and stage of development.[40]

Data quality also complicates health technology assessment for interventions to treat children. Nonetheless, there seems to have been little "need" to establish special criteria for conducting cost-effectiveness analyses of treatments targeting children. First, expensive interventions can often satisfy conventional cost-effectiveness criteria because younger individuals have more potential to gain QALYs. For example, a life-saving drug for a 10-year-old might save 70 life years, whereas treating a 60-year-old gains only 20 life years.[41] Indeed, many interventions producing the greatest QALY gains are for children. Some CAR-T treatments, as well as gene therapy for spinal muscular atrophy, for example, have relatively favorable cost-effectiveness ratios despite high prices (see Chapter 1 of this volume and Box 8.2).[42,43]

Cost-effectiveness analyses of treatments for children can produce favorable ratios even when they "discount" (i.e., down-weight) the value of health benefits accrued in the distant future (see Box 4.3 in Chapter 4 of this volume). For example, using a 3% annual rate makes 70 life years saved for a 10-year-old equal in value to 30 discounted years—a 58% reduction. Discounting has a smaller impact on the value of health gains in adults. For example, discounting at a 3% annual rate makes 20 life years saved for a treated 60-year-old equal in value to 15 discounted years, a 25% reduction.

The second factor mitigating the need for child-specific cost-effectiveness criteria is the fact that children generally do not suffer from the chronic and expensive-to-treat conditions (e.g., cancer, Alzheimer's disease, cardiovascular disease) that afflict older adults. As a result, healthcare spending on children represents a limited portion of total healthcare spending. In 2013, healthcare spending on children up to age 19 amounted to $233.5 billion, or about 8% of the national total of $2.875 trillion that year.[44] Hence, in the aggregate, shifting resources to children for certain childhood afflictions has a relatively small effect on overall spending.

Finally, severe pediatric conditions tend to overlap with rare disease and cancer indications, for which exceptions to the standard cost-effectiveness criteria already exist, as previously described in this chapter. It is perhaps for these reasons that despite the emotionally charged nature of evaluations

Box 8.2 Valuing a $2.1 Million Gene Therapy

Shortly after returning home from the hospital with their newborn, Levi, Nathan Hoot, a physician, and his wife, Leah, could not shake the sense that something was not quite right about their son's fussiness and low muscle mass. When he was three and a half months old, Levi was diagnosed with type 1 spinal muscular atrophy (SMA).[1]

SMA is a rare degenerative disease caused by a mutation in the survival motor neuron gene 1 that affects the nervous system and leads to loss of movement. The disease has four main subtypes that differ by severity and age of onset. Type 1 SMA, also called infantile onset SMA, is the most common and severe. Children with type 1 SMA are often unable to lift their heads or achieve other physical milestones. Most ultimately require ventilation and do not live past age two.[42]

The FDA approved the first drug for SMA, nusinersen, (Spinraza®; Biogen Idec), in 2016. Spinraza's price ($750,000 the first year of treatment and $375,000 for each year thereafter) and limited clinical evidence supporting its effectiveness raised eyebrows. But the Hoots figured they had no alternatives, and Levi did not have much time; by four months old, he had already lost the ability to swallow. Doctors initiated treatment in the hope of forestalling further decline. Fast forward to 24 months, an age at which 90% of infants with type 1 SMA would have progressed to ventilation or death. Levi is able to sit upright next to his brother while watching cartoons. He is learning to recite the alphabet and to count.[2] Without Spinraza, it is likely he would have suffered respiratory failure and never spoken his first words.

Nonetheless, health economists raised questions. ICER would eventually conclude that Spinraza was not cost-effective at its listed price.[42] Many health insurers restricted coverage of the therapy to the most severe SMA cases.[a] In its most favorable scenario, ICER estimated Spinraza's cost-effectiveness to be $709,000 per QALY for patients diagnosed before they exhibited symptoms and recommended a 83% to 90% discount on Spinraza's price.[42]

In 2019, the second therapy approved by FDA to treat SMA generated more headlines. With its $2.1 million price tag, onasemnogene abeparvovec (Zolgensma®; Novartis AG/AveXis) was labeled the world's most expensive drug. A 60-minute Zolgensma infusion costs more than ten 2018 Lamborghini Huracans,[3] a 78-foot Abacus yacht,[4] or a 24-acre private island in the Bahamas.[5] But ICER's evaluation of Zolgensma was more favorable than its review of Spinraza. ICER estimated in its primary analysis that Zolgensma, when used in patients with type 1 SMA, would provide nearly 9 more QALYs than Spinraza (12.23 vs. 3.24). When each treatment was compared to the previous standard of care, Zolgensma's cost-effectiveness ratio of

$243,000 per QALY was much more favorable than Spinraza's ratio of $1.1 million per QALY.[42]

Prior to its approval in 2019, Zolgensma's manufacturer, Novartis AG/AveXis, had floated a potential price range of $1.5 million to $5 million for the product.[6] The final $2.1 million price was justified as being 50% less than the 10-year cost of disease management with Spinraza. It was also not far from ICER's value-based price range of $1.1 to $1.9 million.[7]

The available evidence for Spinraza and Zolgensma highlighted evidence limitations common in assessments of drugs for rare diseases, including small patient populations and the lack of clinical studies with a control group. In its evaluation, ICER acknowledged these challenges and encouraged payers to address the uncertainty by negotiating agreements that tie payment to ongoing data collection that would confirm enduring clinical benefits (see Chapter 9 of this volume). Nevertheless, ICER gave Zolgensma the benefit of the doubt by assuming that there would be no regression in motor function improvements over time. ICER also suggested that, in addition to considering the drug's effect on mortality and permanent ventilation, evaluations consider outcomes, such as rolling over, head control, or the six-minute walk test, which might better capture short-term benefits and better characterize improvements in children with later-onset disease who rarely require ventilation.

ICER's evaluation demonstrated that even the highest priced therapy in the world can be cost-effective (or reasonably close) if it provides substantial benefit. But the assessment also underscored the considerable uncertainty surrounding its use. Zolgensma's pivotal clinical trial was a study with no control group and with an enrollment of only 12 infants who had type 1 SMA and received a high dose of the therapy. While all of the patients were alive without requiring permanent ventilation after 24 months—a remarkable result—the therapy's long-term safety and whether its clinical benefits will endure remain unknown.[42]

The uncertainty of the long-term benefits for these high-cost therapies make them good candidates for contracting arrangements that tie payment to performance (see Section 9.4 in Chapter 9 of this volume). Several countries including Brazil, the United Kingdom, and the United States have reported the use of outcomes-based payment models for Spinraza and Zolgensma, although limited information is available about the precise nature of many of these agreements.[8] In the United States, for example, Massachusetts, one of the few states with federal approval from the Centers for Medicare and Medicaid to negotiate value-based contracts, reached an agreement to pay slightly less than $2 million for Zolgensma. Installments will be extended over five years and refunds issued if patients do not achieve certain clinical milestones.[9,10]

[1] Cohen, J.T., Neumann, P.J., and Ollendorf, D.A. 2020, May 20. "Valuing And pricing remdesivir: Should drug makers get paid for helping us get back to work?" *Health Affairs*. https://www. healthaffairs.org/do/10.1377/hblog20200518.966027/full/

[2] Hoot, N.R. 2019. "Nusinersen for type 1 spinal muscular atrophy: A father's perspective." *Pediatrics*: e20190226. https://doi.org/10.1542/peds.2019-0226.

[3] "Understanding spinal muscular atrophy (SMA)." n.d. *Novartis*. https://www. novartis.com/our-company/novartis-pharmaceuticals/novartis-gene-therapies/ understanding-spinal-muscular-atrophy-sma.

[4] "Lamborghini models." n.d. *TrueCar*. Accessed January 27, 2021. https://www.truecar.com/prices-new/lamborghini/.

[5] "2018 Abacus 78." n.d. *YachtWorld*. Accessed January 27, 2021. https://www.yachtworld.com/ boats/2018/abacus-78-3234538/.

[6] "A natural paradise in the beautiful Bahamas." n.d. *VLADI Private Islands*. Accessed January 27, 2021. https://www.vladi-private-islands.de/en/islands-for-sale/caribbean/bahamas/low-cay/.

[7] Lovelace, B.J., and LaVito, A. 2019. "FDA approves Novartis' $2.1 million gene therapy—making it the world's most expensive drug." *CNBC*. Accessed January 27, 2021. https://www.cnbc.com/2019/05/ 24/fda-approves-novartis-2-million-spinal-muscular-atrophy-gene-therapy.html.

[8] "ICER comments on the FDA approval of Zolgensma for the treatment of spinal muscular atrophy." 2019. *Institute for Clinical and Economic Review*. Accessed July 24, 2020. https://icer.org/news-insights/ press-releases/icer_comment_on_zolgensma_approval/.

[9] Performance Based Risk Sharing (PBRS) Database. 2020. *University of Washington School of Pharmacy*. https://sop.washington.edu/

[10] Bebinger, M. 2020. "Mass. outlines deal for a $2 million drug: Only if it works." *WBUR, CommonHealth*. Accessed January 27, 2021. https://www.wbur.org/commonhealth/2020/02/07/ massachusetts-masshealth-zolgensma-cost-control.

[a] Authors analysis of the Tufts Medical Center Specialty Drug and Evidence Coverage database, June 2020.

involving drugs for children, HTA organizations have not explicitly carved out special cases or priority status for pediatric populations. In short, there seems to be a sense that traditional cost-effectiveness approaches can accommodate treatments for pediatric conditions in most cases.

Cell and Gene Therapies

Although they tend to target rare diseases, cancers, and pediatric illness, for which many HTA bodies have already adopted accommodations, cell and gene therapies introduce additional distinct challenges for economic evaluation.[45] First, their high development and manufacturing costs—augmented by the challenge of scaling up specialized processes—make these therapies expensive. Extremely high costs suggest high prices that might rule out the prospect that cost-effectiveness analysis will find these therapies to reflect good value. Second, the quality of the information characterizing risks and benefits is limited. Clinical trials frequently involve a small number of subjects and lack randomized control groups. That complicates estimation of value. Finally, a "fair" evaluation is critical, as these therapies often offer the prospect of a "cure," transforming potential death sentences into manageable conditions. As one 2019 commentary noted, "taken individually, none of these characteristics is exclusive to gene therapy. . . . Rather, it is the *confluence* of these various characteristics in the case of gene therapy that leads to specific methodological challenges."[45]

Still, it is unclear why conventional cost-effectiveness analysis cannot accommodate such treatments. Even therapies with premium prices may be judged to have good value if they produce sufficient health gains (see Box 8.2). Assessments of other treatments for once-fatal conditions, such as HIV, have not received exceptions, nor have many other "curative" interventions, such as certain surgical procedures. Still, the idea that "curative" therapies require special status has taken hold.

In 2019 ICER, in collaboration with NICE and the Canadian Agency for Drugs and Technologies in Health, developed principles for "single- or short-term transformative therapies," noting that these treatments may warrant special consideration because of added uncertainty, particularly with regard to long-term effects.[46] ICER's report also discussed scenario analyses that would involve "sharing savings" with the health system. The adjustments aimed to address the following concerns. First, unlike traditional drugs for which society reaps savings after a drug's market exclusivity expires and inexpensive generic copies drive prices down, cell and gene therapies are unlikely to face substantial generic competition. Second, the government tends to contribute substantially to research and development costs for these treatments, raising questions about how much of the therapy's value (in the form of revenue) should ultimately flow to the manufacturer. Allocating a share of the savings to the health system reduces costs to taxpayers, companies, and payers, but such allocations also reduce incentives for drug manufacturers to develop drugs that decrease healthcare system costs.

ICER has developed an approach for these therapies. To address the limited quality of the clinical data, it will include optimistic and conservative scenarios about long-term consequences and an assessment of how long the therapy's clinical benefits must persist to keep the cost-effectiveness ratio below $150,000 per QALY.[47] ICER will also allow its expert panels that vote on therapy value to go beyond conventional value attributes—like length and quality of life. One attribute, termed the "value of hope" considers the prospect, even if limited, that treatment will lead to a complete and durable cure (see Chapter 9 of this volume).[48] Another attribute, termed "real option value," involves the possibility that access to advanced therapies extend life enough for an individual to benefit from a future innovation (see Chapter 9 of this volume).

How Much Does a Drug's Value Depend on the Disease or Population Treated?

As part of its assessment process, ICER convenes expert panels who vote on whether each drug under review represents low, intermediate, or high value. Cost-effectiveness evidence feeds into their deliberations, but they also consider the drug's clinical evidence, and two qualitative sets of considerations that ICER has referred to as "other benefits and disadvantages," and "contextual considerations" (see Box 8.3).

If cost-effectiveness were the only factor that matters to ICER committee members, then their votes would align perfectly with that measure: committee members would vote uniformly for a "high value" designation for drugs with favorable cost-effectiveness and give a "low value" designation for drugs with an unfavorable designation. Committee members would vote to designate as "intermediate value" drugs with cost-effectiveness ratios in the middle. Any deviations from this alignment would point to the influence of considerations other than cost-effectiveness when it comes to how people—in this case, the members of the ICER committees—think about drug value.[8,49]

We previously tabulated 721 committee member votes cast in reviews of 60 treatments assessed by ICER from December 2014 through February 2020.[8,49] Of these 60 treatments, 13 targeted cancer and 5 treated ultra-rare conditions. Figure 8.1 summarizes these votes across five cost-effectiveness categories, ranging from most favorable at the far left (drugs that save money and improve health) to least favorable at the far right (drugs that improve health at a cost of $500,000 or more per QALY saved). In each category, the portion of the bar that is green corresponds to the proportion of votes cast for a designation of "high value" for drugs in that category; the portion of the bar that is yellow corresponds to the proportion of votes cast for a designation of "intermediate value" for drugs in that category; and, finally, the portion of the bar that is red corresponds to the proportion of votes cast for a designation of "low value" for drugs in that category.

As expected, green, high-value designation votes are most prevalent for drugs with the most favorable cost-effectiveness (i.e., the bar to the far left). Green, high-value designation votes are most prevalent in the "favorable cost-effectiveness" categories toward the left, whereas red, low-value designation votes are most prevalent in the "unfavorable cost-effectiveness" categories toward the right. But cost-effectiveness alone did not determine how committee members voted. For example, for drugs that saved money (first bar at the far left) while improving health, around 10% of the votes were for a low-value designation (red). Only a little more than half of the votes were

Box 8.3 Qualitative Factors Considered by ICER's Expert Panels

Other benefits and disadvantages

This intervention provides significant direct patient health benefits that are not adequately captured by the QALY.

This intervention offers reduced complexity that will significantly improve patient outcomes.

This intervention will reduce important health disparities across racial, ethnic, gender, socio-economic, or regional categories.

This intervention will significantly reduce caregiver or broader family burden

This intervention offers a novel mechanism of action or approach that will allow successful treatment of many patients for whom other available treatments have failed.

This intervention will have a significant impact on improving return to work and/or overall productivity.

There are other important benefits or disadvantages that should have an important role in judgments of the value of this intervention.

Contextual considerations

This intervention is intended for the care of individuals with a condition of particularly high severity in terms of impact on length of life and/or quality of care.

This intervention is intended for the care of individuals with a condition that represents a particularly high lifetime burden of illness.

This intervention is the first to offer any improvement for patients with this condition.

Compared to "the comparator," there is significant uncertainty about the long-term risk of serious side effects of this intervention.

Compared to "the comparator," there is significant uncertainty about the magnitude or durability of the long-term benefits of this intervention.

There are additional contextual considerations that should have an important role in judgments of the value of this intervention.

Note: Categories as stipulated in ICER's 2017–2019 value assessment framework.

Source: Overview of the ICER value assessment framework and update for 2017–2019. 2018. Institute for Clinical and Economic Review. https://icer.org/wp-content/uploads/2020/10/ICER-value-assessment-framework-Updated-050818.pdf.

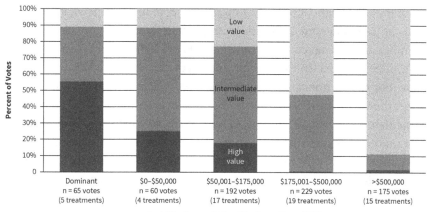

Figure 8.1: Distribution of ICER Committee Votes by Treatment Cost-Effectiveness Ratios, December 2014 through February 2020

Abbreviations: ICER=Institute for Clinical and Economic Review. Dominant means an intervention saves money and gains QALYs (improves health).

Notes: From December 2014 to February 2020, ICER convened 45 committees to review 152 treatments. Among the 152 treatments, ICER reported a cost-per-QALY estimate and held a committee vote on value in 60 cases. We analyzed the 721 individual committee member votes (for "high", "intermediate" or "low" value) on these 60 therapies. For cases in which ICER reported cost-effectiveness as a range, we used the midpoint. For conditions such as obesity, for which ICER separately analyzed four types of bariatric surgery but held one collective vote for the four interventions, we averaged the individual cost-effectiveness estimates. An online supplemental table provides a breakdown of committee votes by treatment disease-target type (cancer vs. non-cancer).

Source: Authors' analysis of publicly available ICER committee votes (https://icer.org/). Earlier versions of this figure appeared in Neumann PJ, Silver MC, Cohen JT, "Should a drug's value depend on the disease or population it treats? Insights from ICER's value assessments," *Health Affairs* blog, November 6, 2018 and Cohen JT, Silver MC, Ollendorf DA, Neumann PJ, "Does the Institute for Clinical and Economic Review Revise Its Findings in Response to Industry Comments?," *Value in Health*, December, 2019.

for a high-value designation (green). At the far right of the figure, close examination reveals that some committee members cast a vote for a high-value designation even though drugs in this category have cost-effectiveness ratios exceeding $500,000 per QALY, a level that widely exceeds widely recognized benchmarks indicative of what a QALY is worth.[50]

Despite these deviations, and despite the evidence described earlier in this chapter, there is limited evidence to support the idea that committee members place an especially high value on drugs that treat rare diseases. Of five therapies for ultra-rare conditions represented in Figure 8.1—all of which had unfavorable cost-effectiveness ratios exceeding $500,000 per QALY (far right category in the figure), committee members designated four as low value.

On the other hand, committee members seem to be somewhat more generous in their assessment of cancer drugs than they are of noncancer drugs. For nine cancer drugs costing from $175,000 to $500,000 per QALY, 63% of the committee member votes were for intermediate value and 37% were for low value. For the 10 noncancer drugs with cost-effectiveness ratios in the same range, the voting proportions were roughly reversed: 37% of the votes for intermediate value and 62% for low value. Committee member comments shed light on other factors that swayed their votes. For the one ultra-rare therapy that garnered any high-value votes (voretigene neparvovec [Luxturna˚; Spark Therapeutics, Inc.] to treat a genetic disorder that causes blindness starting in childhood—see Box 6.4 in Chapter 6 of this volume), favorably inclined committee members mentioned the treatment's novel "mechanism of action."[51p69] In other cases where committee members voted for high value despite unfavorable cost-effectiveness, the factors they mentioned as influential included reduced caregiver burden, improved productivity, and substantial disease severity. In cases where committee members voted for low value despite favorable cost-effectiveness, factors they mentioned as influential included a lack of evidence, uncertain benefits compared to alternative therapies, and safety concerns. These results reveal the struggles that ICER's committees—and society at large—face when judging whether a drug's price reflects reasonable value. The votes suggest that cost-effectiveness represents a reasonably good proxy for value, at least as judged by ICER's committees: they tend to designate as high or at least intermediate value drugs priced so that they have favorable cost effectiveness ratios; they tend to designate as low value drugs priced so that they have unfavorable cost-effectiveness ratios. Even in the case of treatments for ultra-rare conditions and cancer, the committee members tended to stick with low-value designations for drugs priced so that their cost-effectiveness ratios are unfavorable. Still, the ICER committee votes suggest that while cost-effectiveness is a useful starting point for assessing value, other factors may play a role, and sometimes carry important weight in votes and recommendations.

References

1. Weir, A. 2014. *The Martian*. Crown.
2. Jonsen, A.R. 1986. "Bentham in a box: Technology assessment and health care allocation." *The Journal of Law, Medicine & Ethics* 14 (3-4): 172–174. https://doi.org/doi:10.1111/j.1748-720X.1986.tb00974.x.
3. "'Baby Jessica' McClure rescued from Midland, Texas well on October 16, 1987." 2019. *6ABC*. https://6abc.com/baby-jessica-rescuing-saving-from-well-mcclure/5622578/.

4. "Chile's mine rescue: Plucked from the bowels of the earth." 2010, October 14. *The Economist.* https://www.economist.com/the-americas/2010/10/14/plucked-from-the-bowels-of-the-earth.

5. Beech, H., Paddock, R.C., and Suhartono, M. 2018, July 12. "'Still can't believe it worked': The story of the Thailand cave rescue." *The New York Times.* https://www.nytimes.com/2018/07/12/world/asia/thailand-cave-rescue-seals.html.

6. Ollendorf, D.A., Chapman, R.H., and Pearson, S.D. 2018. "Evaluating and valuing drugs for rare conditions: No easy answers." *Value in Health* 21 (5): 547–552. https://doi.org/10.1016/j.jval.2018.01.008.

7. Taylor, M., Chilton, S., Ronaldson, S., Metcalf, H., and Nielsen, J.S. 2017. "Comparing increments in utility of health: An individual-based approach." *Value in Health* 20 (2): 224–229. https://doi.org/10.1016/j.jval.2016.12.009.

8. Neumann, P.J., Silver, M.C., and Cohen, J.T. 2018, November 6. "Should a drug's value depend on the disease or population it treats? Insights from ICER's value assessments." *Health Affairs.* https://doi.org/10.1377/hblog20181105.38350.

9. Handfield, R., and Feldstein, J. 2013. "Insurance companies' perspectives on the orphan drug pipeline." *American Health & Drug Benefits* 6 (9). http://www.ahdbonline.com/issues/2013/november-december-2013-vol-6-no-9/1623-insurance-companies-perspectives-on-the-orphan-drug-pipeline.

10. Chambers, J.D., Panzer, A.D., Kim, D.D., Margaretos, N.M., and Neumann, P.J. 2019. "Variation in US private health plans' coverage of orphan drugs." *The American Journal of Managed Care* 25 (10): 508–512.

11. National Institute for Health and Care Excellence, National Health Service England. 2016. "Proposals for changes to the arrangements for evaluating and funding drugs and other health technologies appraised through NICE's technology appraisal and highly specialized technologies programmes." https://www.nice.org.uk/Media/Default/About/what-we-do/our-programmes/technology-appraisals/NICE_NHSE_TA_and_HST_consultation_document.pdf.

12. National Health Service England, National Institute for Health and Care Excellence. 2017, March 15. "NICE and NHS England consultation on changes to the arrangements for evaluating and funding drugs and other health technologies assessed through NICE's technology appraisal and highly specialized technologies programmes." https://www.nice.org.uk/Media/Default/About/what-we-do/NICE-guidance/NICE-technology-appraisals/board-paper-TA-HST-consultation-mar-17-HST-only.pdf.

13. "Modifications to the ICER value assessment framework for treatments for ultra-rare diseases." 2017. Institute for Clinical and Economic Review. https://icer.org/wp-content/uploads/2020/10/ICER_URD_Framework_Adapt_013120.pdf.

14. "2020-2023 Value Assessment Framework." 2020. Institute for Clinical and Economic Review. https://icer.org/wp-content/uploads/2020/10/ICER_2020_2023_VAF_102220.pdf.

15. Herper, M. 2015, May 5. "The cancer drug market just hit $100 billion and could jump 50% in four years." *Forbes.* https://www.forbes.com/sites/matthewherper/2015/05/05/cancer-drug-sales-approach-100-billion-and-could-increase-50-by-2018/?sh=557c94032dc6

16. Brooks, M. 2019. "Cancer drugs dominate top 10 best-selling drugs in 2018." *Medscape.* Accessed January 27, 2021. https://www.medscape.com/viewarticle/910600.

17. Sunday Times (London). 1979. *Suffer the children: The story of thalidomide.* New York: Viking Press.

18. Fintel, B., Samaras, A.T., and Carias, E. 2009. "The thalidomide tragedy: Lessons for drug safety and regulation." *Helix.* Accessed January 27, 2021. https://helix.northwestern.edu/article/thalidomide-tragedy-lessons-drug-safety-and-regulation.

19. IBM Micromedex® REDBOOK®. 2020. Greenwood Village, Colorado, CO: IBM Watson Health.

20. National Center for Health Statistics. "Leading causes of death." *Centers for Disease Control and Prevention.* Last modified January 12, 2021. Accessed January 27, 2021. https://www.cdc.gov/nchs/fastats/leading-causes-of-death.htm.

21. Chopra, D. 2018. "Optimistic thoughts about cancer—for real." *SF Gate.* Accessed January 27, 2021. https://www.sfgate.com/opinion/chopra/article/Optimistic-Thoughts-About-Cancer-For-Real-11719628.php.

22. Chopra, D. 2018. "Ending the dread of cancer." *SF Gate.* Accessed January 27, 2021. https://www.sfgate.com/opinion/chopra/article/Ending-the-Dread-of-Cancer-11738735.php.

23. Ozga, M., Aghajanian, C., Virtue, S., McDonnell, G., Jhanwar, S., Hichenberg, S., and Sulimanoff, I. 2015. "A systematic review of ovarian cancer and fear of recurrence." *Palliative & Supportive Care* 13: 1–10. https://doi.org/10.1017/S1478951515000127.

24. Heyhoe, J., Reynolds, C., and Lawton, R. 2020. "The early diagnosis of cancer in primary care: A qualitative exploration of the patient's role and acceptable safety-netting strategies." *European Journal of Cancer Care* 29 (1): e13195. https://doi.org/10.1111/ecc.13195.

25. Baxter, N.N., Virnig, B.A., Durham, S.B., and Tuttle, T.M. 2004. "Trends in the treatment of ductal carcinoma in situ of the breast." *Journal of National Cancer Institute* 96 (6): 443–448. https://doi.org/10.1093/jnci/djh069.

26. Martinalbo, J., Bowen, D., Camarero, J., Chapelin, M., Démolis, P., Foggi, P., Jonsson, B., Llinares, J., Moreau, A., O'Connor, D., Oliveira, J., Vamvakas, S., and Pignatti, F. 2016. "Early market access of cancer drugs in the EU." *Annals of Oncology* 27 (1): 96–105. https://doi.org/10.1093/annonc/mdv506.

27. "NICE and Herceptin." 2005. *King's Fund.* https://www.kingsfund.org.uk/sites/default/files/Herceptin%20policy%20position.pdf.

28. Timmins, N., Rawlins, M., and Appleby, J. 2016. *A terrible beauty: A short history of NICE.* London: Health Intervention and Technology Assessment Program.

29. Faden, R.R., Chalkidou, K., Appleby, J., Waters, H.R., and Leider, J.P. 2009. "Expensive cancer drugs: A comparison between the United States and the United Kingdom." *The Milbank Quarterly* 87 (4): 789–819. https://doi.org/10.1111/j.1468-0009.2009.00579.x.

30. "Appraising life-extending, end of life treatments." 2009. *National Institute for Health and Care Excellence.* https://www.nice.org.uk/guidance/gid-tag387/documents/appraising-life-extending-end-of-life-treatments-paper2.

31. Aggarwal, A., Fojo, T., Chamberlain, C., Davis, C., and Sullivan, R. 2017. "Do patient access schemes for high-cost cancer drugs deliver value to society? Lessons from the NHS Cancer Drugs Fund." *Annals of Oncology* 28 (8): 1738–1750. https://doi.org/10.1093/annonc/mdx110.

32. "Appraisal and funding of cancer drugs from July 2016 (including the new Cancer Drugs Fund)." 2016. *NHS England.* https://www.england.nhs.uk/wp-content/uploads/2013/04/cdf-sop.pdf.

33. "Process in brief." n.d. *Canadian Agency for Drugs and Technologies in Health.* https://cadth.ca/pcodr/process-in-brief.

34. Srikanthan, A., Mai, H., Penner, N., Amir, E., Laupacis, A., Sabharwal, M., and Chan, K.K.W. 2016. "Impact of pCODR on cancer drug funding decisions. CADTH Symposium 2016." *Canadian Agency for Drugs and Technologies in Health. Pan-Candian Oncology Drug Review.* https://www.cadth.ca/sites/default/files/symp-2016/presentations/april11-2016/Concurrent-Session-B7-Amirrtha-Srikanthan.pdf.

35. Skedgel, C., Wranik, D., and Hu, M. 2018. "The relative importance of clinical, economic, patient values and feasibility criteria in cancer drug reimbursement in Canada: A

revealed preferences analysis of recommendations of the Pan-Canadian Oncology Drug Review 2011–2017." *PharmacoEconomics* 36 (4): 467–475. https://doi.org/10.1007/s40273-018-0610-0.

36. Andersen, S.K., Penner, N., Chambers, A., Trudeau, M.E., Chan, K.K.W., and Cheung, M.C. 2019. "Conditional approval of cancer drugs in Canada: Accountability and impact on public funding." *Current Oncology* 26 (1): e100–e105. https://doi.org/10.3747/co.26.4397.

37. Bowling, A. 1996. "Health care rationing: The public's debate." *BMJ* 312 (7032): 670. https://doi.org/10.1136/bmj.312.7032.670.

38. Nicod, E., and Kanavos, P. 2016. "Scientific and social value judgments for orphan drugs in health technology assessment." *International Journal of Technology Assessment in Health Care* 32 (4): 218–232. https://doi.org/10.1017/S0266462316000416.

39. Reckers-Droog, V., van Exel, J., and Brouwer, W. 2018. "Who should receive treatment? An empirical enquiry into the relationship between societal views and preferences concerning healthcare priority setting." *PloS One* 13 (6): e0198761–e0198761. https://doi.org/10.1371/journal.pone.0198761.

40. Sutcliffe, A.G. 2003. "Testing new pharmaceutical products in children." *BMJ (Clinical Research Ed.)* 326 (7380): 64–65. https://doi.org/10.1136/bmj.326.7380.64.

41. Schwappach, D.L.B. 2002. "Resource allocation, social values and the QALY: A review of the debate and empirical evidence." *Health Expectations* 5 (3): 210–222. https://doi.org/10.1046/j.1369-6513.2002.00182.x.

42. Tice, J.A., Walsh, J.M.E., Otuonye, I., Chapman, R., Kumar, V., Seidner, M., Ollendorf, D.A., and Pearson, S.D. 2018. *Chimeric antigen receptor T-cell therapy for B-cell cancers: Effectiveness and value. Institute for Clinical and Economic Review.* https://icer.org/wp-content/uploads/2020/10/ICER_CAR_T_Final_Evidence_Report_032318.pdf.

43. Ellis, A.G., Mickle, K., Herron-Smith, S., Kumar, V.M., Ciancolo, L., Seidner, M., Rind, D., and Pearson, S.D. 2019. "Spinraza® and Zolgensma® for spinal muscular atrophy: Effectiveness and value." *Institute for Clinical and Economic Review.* https://icer.org/wp-content/uploads/2020/10/ICER_SMA_Final_Evidence_Report_110220.pdf.

44. Bui, A.L., Dieleman, J.L., Hamavid, H., Birger, M., Chapin, A., Duber, H.C., Horst, C., Reynolds, A., Squires, E., Chung, P.J., and Murray, C.J.L. 2017. "Spending on children's personal health care in the United States, 1996–2013." *JAMA Pediatrics* 171 (2): 181–189. https://doi.org/10.1001/jamapediatrics.2016.4086.

45. Drummond, M.F., Neumann, P.J., Sullivan, S.D., Fricke, F.-U., Tunis, S., Dabbous, O., and Toumi, M. 2019. "Analytic considerations in applying a general economic evaluation reference case to gene therapy." *Value in Health* 22 (6): 661–668. https://doi.org/10.1016/j.jval.2019.03.012.

46. "Value assessment methods for 'single or short-term transformative therapies' (SSTs)." 2019. *Institute for Clinical and Economic Review.* https://icer.org/wp-content/uploads/2020/10/ICER_SST_ProposedAdaptations_080619-2.pdf.

47. Cohen, J.T., Chambers, J.D., Silver, M.C., Lin, P.-J., and Neumann, P.J. 2019, September 4. "Putting the costs and benefits of new gene therapies into perspective." *Health Affairs.* https://doi.org/10.1377/hblog20190827.553404. https://www.healthaffairs.org/do/10.1377/hblog20190827.553404/full/.

48. Lakdawalla, D.N., Doshi, J.A., Garrison, L.P., Jr., Phelps, C.E., Basu, A., and Danzon, P.M. 2018. "Defining elements of value in health care—a health economics approach: An ISPOR Special Task Force report." *Value in Health* 21 (2): 131–139. https://doi.org/10.1016/j.jval.2017.12.007.

49. Cohen, J.T., Silver, M.C., Ollendorf, D.A., and Neumann, P.J. 2019. "Does the Institute for Clinical and Economic Review revise its findings in response to industry comments?" *Value in Health* 22 (12): 1396–1401. https://doi.org/10.1016/j.jval.2019.08.003.
50. Neumann, P.J., Cohen, J.T., and Weinstein, M.C. 2014. "Updating cost-effectiveness—the curious resilience of the $50,000-per-QALY threshold." *New England Journal of Medicine* 371 (9): 796–797. https://doi.org/10.1056/NEJMp1405158.

PART III
GETTING TO VALUE-BASED PRICING
FOR DRUGS

9

Improving Value Measurement

Assessing the value of drugs (and other health technologies) attracts a lot of interest. The International Society for Pharmacoeconomics and Outcomes Research (ISPOR) holds meetings on multiple continents every year and claims some 20,000 members in 110 countries.[1] Another professional society, Health Technology Assessment International, boasts 37 nonprofit organizational members, many of which are government agencies charged with assessing the value of drugs and other healthcare technologies.[2] The field supports numerous academic journals. The original Panel on Cost-Effectiveness in Health and Medicine in 1996 produced a book-long volume on the state of the field and recommendations for standard practices.[3] The updated and expanded revision authored by the Second Panel ran to over 500 pages.[4]

Why all the attention? One factor is the desire among health economists to achieve consistency in methods because incongruous measurement muddles comparisons. One drug may have a more favorable cost-effectiveness ratio than another, but the difference may simply reflect methodological inconsistencies across studies rather than genuinely better value for the drug.

More crucially, as Chapter 3 of this volume argued, a drug's price should correspond to its value to ensure the most advantageous allocation of resources. It follows that value measurement itself should be accurate. Errors that creep into drug value calculations can result in overpayment for drugs that deliver too little or errant market signals to drug companies discouraging them from investing in the most beneficial innovation. This chapter addresses what needs to be done to make value assessment as accurate as possible.

Ensuring That Value Reflects All That Matters: Elevating the Societal Perspective

As Chapter 4 of this volume described, a value assessment's "perspective" dictates which elements it includes. The "healthcare sector" perspective limits consideration to the patient's health and to costs incurred by the healthcare

The Right Price. Peter J. Neumann, Joshua T. Cohen, and Daniel A. Ollendorf, Oxford University Press (2021).
© Peter J. Neumann, Joshua T. Cohen, and Daniel A. Ollendorf. DOI: 10.1093/oso/9780197512883.003.0009

system—meaning, for example, that for an elderly patient, the cost of a home health aide (an expense to the healthcare payer) is *in*, but caregiving time spent by a family caregiver (*not* an expense to the healthcare payer) is *out*. The broader societal perspective accounts for everything that matters to somebody, so the value of the family caregiver's time is included, as are many other potential impacts, including effects of an intervention on worker productivity, a student's school performance, or even the justice system (e.g., due to the consequences of illicit drug use).

The healthcare sector perspective has several advantages. First, because many existing cost-effectiveness analyses employ this perspective, using it in new assessments facilitates comparisons.[5] Second, it focuses on factors of concern to payers—key decision makers in the United States—who underwrite risks and set their premiums based on healthcare expenditures. Third, as the Institute for Clinical and Economic Review (ICER) has argued (see Chapter 6 of this volume), including all the societal perspective components makes assessments far more extensive and can introduce numerous uncertain assumptions. ICER has also argued that the societal perspective is ethically questionable because it places less value on restoring the health of people without paid employment. Advocates for the societal perspective caution, however, that the healthcare sector perspective omits important outcomes and that, despite its convenience and alignment with the agenda of one constituency (payers), it provides the "wrong" answer from the perspective of most everyone else.

In recent years, the field has worked to find a compromise. Whereas the original 1996 Panel on Cost Effectiveness in Health and Medicine recommended use of the societal perspective for all assessments, the Second Panel in 2016 recommended that the healthcare sector and societal perspectives share top billing. A review of 45 sets of national guidelines found that 30 prioritized the healthcare sector (or payer) perspective, 12 prioritized a societal perspective, and the remaining 3 gave equal billing to both perspectives.[5] Meanwhile, ICER has moved toward greater recognition of the societal perspective. While its 2017–2019 framework included the societal perspective as a "co-base case" only for drugs targeting ultra-rare diseases, its 2020–2023 framework includes the societal perspective as a co-base case for *all* assessments for which societal impacts might be substantial.

This evolution raises two questions. First, how often do analyses use a societal perspective? A survey of the academic literature found that historically only 18% of cost-effectiveness analyses have employed a societal perspective, and use has declined somewhat over time.[5] Importantly, the survey classified studies generously, crediting a study for taking the societal perspective if it included a single element beyond those classified as part of the healthcare sector. Only 11% of published cost-effectiveness analyses have tracked productivity impacts, and 6%, caregiver time.

Second, how much does use of the societal perspective matter? Because it involves more effort and introduces uncertainty, perhaps analysts tend to avoid the societal perspective because it usually does not have a sizeable impact on a drug's estimated cost-effectiveness ratio. For 68 studies that reported cost-effectiveness ratios computed from both the healthcare sector and societal perspective, the previously mentioned review found that ratios computed using the societal perspective (median of about $23,000 per QALY) were modestly more favorable (lower) than corresponding ratios computed using the healthcare sector perspective (about $30,000 per QALY). In short, published cost-effectiveness analyses typically afford the societal perspective limited attention, but where analysts report results using both perspectives, the societal perspective seems to have a modestly beneficial impact. In general, comparisons suggest that using the societal perspective often makes little material difference.

Ostensibly, ICER walks a fine line, using a societal perspective only when its impact would make a difference. One indication of how this strategy would develop in practice came in early May 2020, two months into the COVID-19 pandemic, when the US Food and Drug Administration (FDA) granted emergency use authorization for remdesivir, the antiviral treatment developed by Gilead Sciences.[6] The FDA's actions followed release of preliminary results of a National Institutes of Health (NIH) study showing that in a placebo-controlled study of 1,063 hospitalized subjects with advanced COVID-19 disease, remdesivir reduced recovery time from a median of 15 days to 11 days.[7] Moreover, the drug decreased mortality from 11.9% to 7.1%, although this result fell just shy of statistical significance.

ICER soon weighed in, recommending that, based on its mortality reduction, remdesivir should be priced at about $4,500 for a 10-day course.[8] Importantly, ICER rejected consideration of societal benefits, stating, "Policymakers would view it inappropriate to set a price for a treatment for COVID-19 to capture the potential broader economic benefits associated with future economic recovery."[8] As the authors of this book wrote at the time, this decision seemed "a glaring omission."[9] Even ignoring any mortality benefit, the NIH study indicated that remdesivir would reduce the time COVID-19 patients would require care in hospital intensive care units. That clinical benefit could alleviate pressure on a key resource choke point, reducing the chance that the health system would become overwhelmed by severely ill patients. As that was one of the main reasons for implementing costly social distancing measures in the first place, remdesivir offered the prospect of more quickly relaxing those actions.

How much is it worth to return workers to their jobs and children to schools? Even recognizing the preliminary nature of the results and the modest magnitude of the clinical improvements, the societal benefits were potentially immense. While incorporating the entirety of this value into a drug's price would be impractical, failing to recognize any of this value missed an opportunity to encourage drug companies to develop therapies that confer not only clinical benefits, but also broader, nonhealth gains. We suggested that ICER report remdesivir's value with and without recognition of those societal benefits so that deliberations over an appropriate price could consider the resulting estimates along with other factors.

Having caused the most serious pandemic in a century, the novel coronavirus causing COVID-19 represents an unusual case. But it is certainly not the only condition for which therapies might have an outsized societal impact. In 2019, for example, the United Nations warned of the threat posed by drug-resistant bacterial infections. In calling for a series of steps, including incentives "to spur innovation in antimicrobial medicines," the UN described the threat as "catastrophic," noting,

> World Bank estimates that by 2030 up to 24 million people could be forced into extreme poverty, mainly in low-income countries, and annual economic damage as a result of antimicrobial resistance could be comparable to the shocks experienced during the 2008–2009 global financial crisis—but with no end in sight.[10]

Not recognizing these impacts when considering benefits conferred by interventions to mitigate antimicrobial resistance understates the value of these innovations. It is thus crucial to include these factors in our assessments and in turn incentivize more appropriately the development and implementation of antimicrobial medicines. Otherwise, we risk having them languish on the back burner until a crisis is upon us.

Critically, including societal benefits when estimating the value of a diagnostic, vaccine, or therapy does not mean that the manufacturer should capture the entire societal benefit. In all likelihood, paying a price reflecting the entire societal value for many innovations would not be feasible; nor would it be necessary to ensure an adequate signal for future innovations. But a societal perspective analysis can serve as useful information for pricing discussions, helping policymakers consider the full costs and benefits of products and the wide-ranging ramifications of their actions.[9]

Although infectious diseases offer a stark example of how health conditions can have broad nonhealth impacts, they are not unique. For example, conditions affecting people of working age influence productivity. One European study showed that over a six-month period, low back pain reduces worker productivity by €4,000 (approximately $4,600)[11] due to both absenteeism and "presenteeism" (reduced efficiency while at work).[12] In the United States, lost productivity due to major depressive disorder costs $100 billion per year, a sum similar to depression's healthcare sector costs (see Box 9.1).[13] Health conditions impose substantial costs on other sectors of the economy as well. The informal care delivered to patients with dementia who live at home would cost nearly $28,000 per year if it had to be performed by professional caregivers. Valued in terms of the foregone earnings of the informal caregivers, it is on average worth less, but is still substantial at approximately $13,000 per year.[14] As a final example, the cost of opioid use disorder to the criminal justice system in 2016 was estimated to total $7.8 billion, reflecting added expenses for police protection ($2.9 billion), judicial and legal expenditures ($1.3 billion), corrections and incarceration ($3.3 billion), and property loss ($0.3 billion).[15]

While using the societal perspective often has a modest impact on a medical therapy's estimated cost-effectiveness, in some cases (e.g., drugs for infectious diseases) societal considerations dominate. The health technology assessment community should commit to including societal considerations when they can matter. The Second Panel also recommended use of an "Impact Inventory" as a checklist and reporting template.[4] The inventory includes health outcomes and health sector costs, productivity, social services, education, housing, and the environment. Because inclusion of nonhealth elements adds complexity and uncertain assumptions, guidelines for conducting assessments should be flexible, directing analysts to focus on elements that can substantially influence the results.

QALYs: The Worst Way to Measure Health, Except for All the Others

The Metric Some People Love to Hate

If QALYs were a person, they might receive a lot of hate mail. People complain that QALYs are not patient-focused, that they are used as rationing tools by health insurers, and that putting numbers on people's health is dehumanizing.[16–18] "The entire superstructure of the QALY methodology is built

Box 9.1 Assessing Drugs for Mental Health: ICER's Assessment of Esketamine for Depression

Evaluating drugs for psychiatric conditions presents distinct challenges: the uncertain etiology and course of mental health disorders; the varied and unpredictable effects of interventions; the influence of cultural and social factors; and the stigma that can prevent timely diagnosis and treatment. Major depressive disorder, an emotionally crippling and physically disabling condition, presents a prime example.

Some 17 million Americans have experienced at least one major depressive episode, with often profound effects on their personal and professional lives.[1] Half of suicides in the United States are among individuals who suffer from major depression.[2] Management of major depressive disorder often involves psychotherapy and medications, but while antidepressants are effective in some people, they require considerable time to show benefit and often that benefit wanes, forcing patients to seek alternatives. For sufferers of the condition it is easy to lose hope.

Ashley Clayton, who was diagnosed with depression in middle school, knew this feeling well.[3] A 2019 profile in *Brain & Behavior* recounted her story.[3] Despite a history of trauma, self-harm, and suicide attempts, she became the first member of her family to attend college and then landed a research position in Yale's Department of Psychiatry. Although she had managed her symptoms with medication and psychotherapy, her condition worsened and she made the difficult decision take a partial medical leave from the work she found so rewarding. Ashley tried at least a dozen medications, several types of psychotherapy, and ultimately electroconvulsive therapy (ECT) or "shock" therapy, which can be highly effective but is reserved for the most severe cases because of its intensity and the potential for adverse effects on memory and cognition.[4] Her ECT sessions left her confused, and the mere act of preparing a peanut butter and jelly sandwich became daunting. Having exhausted conventional options, Ashley reached out to a colleague conducting research on a promising alternative.[3]

Ketamine is a recent entrant to the drug armamentarium for depression, after traveling a circuitous journey. First approved by the FDA in 1970 for use in general anesthesia,[5] ketamine found widespread application as a painkiller in combat situations and emergency rooms. It also gained notoriety as a party drug ("Special K") because it offered a "high" that seemed to have few long-term consequences and delivered what users described as a pleasant "out of body" experience.[6,7] After years of misuse and abuse, in the late 1990s the Drug Enforcement Agency labeled ketamine a controlled substance.[8]

However, clinical experimentation with ketamine continued, including research suggesting its promise in patients with major depression, even in those who had exhausted alternatives and contemplated suicide. Eager to try this new alternative, Ashley entered a clinical trial and received an intravenous infusion of ketamine just a week later. Afterward, she went home to sleep off the nausea and headache she experienced. When she awoke, she felt like a new person. She was able to sense pleasure and positive emotions that she had not experienced in years.

Other clinical studies, including randomized trials sponsored by the National Institute of Mental Health, reported similar results indicating that ketamine temporarily relieved depressive symptoms in 60% or more of patients who tried it.[9] Moreover, people typically experienced these improvements within hours of infusion (in contrast, most antidepressants take four to six weeks to show any effects). In addition, the treatment seemed safe, other than some patient reports of those temporary "out of body" effects and mild elevations in blood pressure.

While the studies generated hope for a field in need of better therapies, key obstacles stood in ketamine's path. For one, the compound must be administered via infusion by trained clinicians, thus limiting its use. For another, the drug was already generic, presenting a major challenge for any drug company seeking to profit from its development and approval for a new indication.

Enter Janssen, a pharmaceutical company owned by Johnson & Johnson, which sought to advance esketamine (Spravato®), a close molecular cousin of ketamine that could be delivered by nasal spray (although still by a trained clinician). After conducting its own clinical studies, Janssen submitted esketamine for review to the FDA in September 2018 as a therapy for treatment-resistant depression. Approval followed in March 2019. The prospect of the first breakthrough product for the disorder in a generation created considerable excitement. However, the supporting clinical evidence also generated concern.[10] The magnitude of esketamine's effect on depressive symptoms relative to placebo seemed modest—just a few points on a key depression scale. Furthermore, long-term safety data were lacking. Complicating matters was the fact that many patients in the clinical trial seemed able to discern whether they were taking esketamine or placebo due to those "out of body effects," thus raising questions about the integrity of the protocol, which called for subjects to be blinded to whether they received esketamine or placebo." And three patients committed suicide in the esketamine group, compared to none in the placebo group. Finally, there was the drug's list price of $35,000 to $50,000 per year, depending on the dosing schedule and number of sessions.

These costs and clinical uncertainties loomed large in ICER's assessment of esketamine in 2019. After considering the evidence, ICER estimated the cost-effectiveness of the product at around $200,000 per QALY. ICER concluded that esketamine's price would have to drop by 25% to 50% to satisfy conventional value benchmark criteria.[11] In addition, ICER determined that fewer than 20% of eligible patients could take esketamine before the drug's cumulative costs would exceed the organization's budget benchmark. (After undertaking its own assessment, the National Institute for Health and Care Excellence rejected the drug for England and Wales on grounds that the product's benefit in comparison to other antidepressants was unclear. The National Institute for Health and Care Excellence also highlighted the fact that the clinical trials supporting esketamine did not enroll patients whose depression was truly resistant to other therapies and that long-term outcomes were uncertain.)[12,13]

Janssen cried foul, criticizing several ICER assumptions, including the manner in which ICER characterized eligible patients (e.g., overestimating how long patients would remain on therapy thus incorrectly inflating cost estimates) and disregarding flexible dosing recommendations.[14] The company also noted that ICER failed to consider esketamine's broader benefits, including those highlighted by ICER's own advisory committee, such as its reduction of caregiver and family burden and its ability to help patients to return to work.

It is possible that ICER's QALY estimate did not effectively account for all of the treatment benefits that patients and their families care about (see the previous discussion). Patient advocates recommended the development of new outcome measures that incorporate all aspects of well-being, including productivity and caregiver "spillover" effects.[15]

ICER's esketamine evaluation also revealed the challenges drug companies face in supporting premium prices for therapies that affect quality of life rather than quality *and* length of life. In ICER's evaluation, use of esketamine resulted in 250 more depression-free days than conventional treatment, and the magnitude of its quality-of-life benefit, measured in QALYs, was 19 times larger than the QALY gain attributable to its improved survival benefit.

The addition of 250 depression-free days seems impressive, but it does not amount to a large gain when expressed in QALYs. For one, the ICER analysis spread this gain over a lifetime horizon, which it assumed would stretch 21 years into the future. Applying discounting to benefits accrued that far in the future noticeably diminishes its present value (see Chapter 4 of this volume). Second, the difference between a day with depression and a day without depression, while substantial, typically amounts to less of a QALY gain than an extension of survival (indeed, research suggests that in evaluating QALY gains, some people value length of life more highly than quality of life, although such preferences are complex and heterogeneous).[16,17] Taking into account both of these factors, ICER estimated that esketamine confers 0.19 additional QALYs over a lifetime, (i.e., about 70 quality-adjusted *days*).

ICER's evaluation also highlighted the need for drug companies to support claims that their products confer nonhealth benefits, such as a greater propensity to return to work or reduced caregiver burden.[18] Moreover, it underscores the need for drug developers to better anticipate and document the potential quality-of-life benefits that their drugs may confer. Their preparation must, for example, include more careful consideration of how sensitive their symptom scale or quality-of-life instrument is to the treatment benefit they hope to quantify. For example, to quantify esketamine's impact on quality of life, ICER used the primary outcome measures from the Phase III trial of esketamine (the Montgomery–Åsberg depression rating scale and the Patient Health Questionnaire-9), but those measures may not be sufficiently sensitive to the clinical benefits conferred by this drug.

[1] "Depression." National Alliance on Mental Illness. Accessed July 30. https://www.nami.org/About-Mental-Illness/Mental-Health-Conditions/Depression.

[2] "Suicide claims more lives than war, murder, and natural disasters combined." 2020. *The American Foundation for Suicide Prevention.* https://www.theovernight.org/index.cfm?fuseaction=cms.page&id=1034.

[3] Bhojani, F. 2019. "A recovery story: After every available option was exhausted, ketamine has enabled her life to resume." *Brain & Behavior Research Foundation.* Accessed July 23, 2020. https://www.bbrfoundation.org/blog/recovery-story-after-every-available-option-was-exhausted-ketamine-has-enabled-her-life-to-resume.

[4] "Electroconvulsive therapy (ECT)." n.d. *Mayo Clinic.* Accessed July 30, 2020. https://www.mayoclinic.org/tests-procedures/electroconvulsive-therapy/about/pac-20393894.

[5] "Drugs@FDA: FDA-approved drugs: New drug application (NDA): 016812." *US Food & Drug Administration.* https://www.accessdata.fda.gov/scripts/cder/daf/index.cfm?event=overview.process&ApplNo=016812.

[6] Velasquez-Manoff, M. 2018, May 8. "Ketamine stirs up hope—and controversy—as a depression drug." *Wired.* https://www.wired.com/story/ketamine-stirs-up-hope-controversy-as-a-depression-drug/

[7] Thielking, M. 2019, March 6. "FDA approves esketamine, the first major depression treatment to reach U.S. market in decades." *Scientific American.* https://www.scientificamerican.com/article/fda-approves-esketamine-the-first-major-depression-treatment-to-reach-u-s-market-in-decades/.

[8] Schedules of controlled substances: Placement of ketamine into schedule III. 64 Fed. Reg. 37673 (1999).

[9] "From street drug to depression therapy." 2018. *Harvard Health.* https://www.health.harvard.edu/mind-and-mood/from-street-drug-to-depression-therapy

[10] Huetteman, E. 2019, June 12. "FDA overlooked red flags in drugmaker's testing of new depression medicine." *Medscape.* https://www.medscape.com/viewarticle/914296.

[11] Atlas, S.J., Agboola, F., Fazioli, K., Kumar, V.M., Adair, E., Rind, D., and Pearson, S. 2019. "Esketamine for the treatment of treatment-resistant depression: Effectiveness and value." *Institute for Clinical and Economic Review.* https://icer.org/wp-content/uploads/2020/10/ICER_TRD_Final_Evidence_Report_062019.pdf.

[12] Smith, A. 2020, January 28. "Spravato rejected by NICE." *PharmaTimes.* Accessed July 30, 2020. http://www.pharmatimes.com/news/spravato_rejected_by_nice_1323580.

[13] McKee, S. 2020, September 3. "Janssen disappointed with second NICE no for Spravato." *PharmaTimes.* http://www.pharmatimes.com/news/janssen_disappointed_with_second_nice_no_for_spravato_1347797.

[14] Karkare, S., Le, H.H., Sheehan, J.J., Sliwa, J.K., Zhang, Q., and Barber, B. 2020. "Pitfalls of cost-effectiveness analysis in practice: A TRD case example in the United States with esketamine versus oral antidepressants." *Journal of Managed Care & Specialty Pharmacy* 26 (4): 568–569. https://doi.org/10.18553/jmcp.2020.26.4.568.

[15] "TRD: Public comment on draft report." 2019. *Institute for Clinical and Economic Review.* Accessed January 25, 2021. https://icer.org/wp-content/uploads/2020/10/ICER_TRD_Public_Comments_050919.pdf.

[16] Kozminski, M.A., Neumann, P.J., Nadler, E.S., Jankovic, A., and Ubel, P.A. 2010. "How long and how well: Oncologists' attitudes toward the relative value of life-prolonging v. quality of life-enhancing treatments." *Medical Decision Making* 31 (3): 380–385. https://doi.org/10.1177/0272989X10385847.

[17] Greenberg, D., Hammerman, A., Vinker, S., Shani, A., Yermiahu, Y., and Neumann, P.J. 2013. "Which is more valuable, longer survival or better quality of life? Israeli oncologists' and family physicians' attitudes toward the relative value of new cancer and congestive heart failure interventions." *Value in Health* 16 (5): 842–847. https://doi.org/10.1016/j.jval.2013.04.010.

[18] Cohen, J.T., Silver, M.C., Ollendorf, D.A., and Neumann, P.J. 2019. "Does the Institute for Clinical and Economic Review revise its findings in response to industry comments?" *Value in Health* 22 (12): 1396–1401. https://doi.org/10.1016/j.jval.2019.08.003.

upon philosophical sand," wrote one critic in 2019.[19] As we have seen, the use of cost-per-QALY ratios by payers to inform drug coverage and pricing decisions attracts intense opposition in some quarters. One patient advocacy organization in 2019 urged patients to sign a petition "to stop health insurers and policymakers from using ICER's methodology and the use of Quality Adjusted Life Years as a measure for the value of medicines."[20]

Still, QALYs endure because they perform a useful function, namely capturing in a single number a treatment's impact on life expectancy and quality of life and providing a standard for comparing the value of diverse interventions. A question going forward is whether we can preserve the QALY while improving upon its limitations.

Do QALYs Adequately Capture People's Health Preferences?

When people criticize QALYs for not being patient-centric, they are saying that decisions based on cost-per-QALY analyses do not reflect how people prefer to spend money to improve health. At first blush, the criticism may seem surprising. Surely, people care about life expectancy and quality of life, the two elements captured in QALYs. On the other hand, QALYs may not capture certain aspects of people's preferences. For example, QALYs may not reflect particular goals and priorities individuals have in treatment decisions, such as desiring a life-extending cancer therapy because it may increase their chance of attending an upcoming family wedding.[21] People may want to pay more for treatments for severe diseases, whether or not that is consistent with

QALY maximization.[22,23] QALYs do not inherently distinguish between a long period spent in a moderately diminished health state and a shorter period spent in a more severe health state.

Researchers have explored how QALYs may not capture people's attitudes toward risk and uncertainty when it comes to health and treatment decisions. Most treatment effects are uncertain; outcomes vary across individuals, and usually it is not possible to determine in advance whether a drug will work.[24] How individuals feel about treatments that affect their life expectancy and quality of life depends on their risk preferences, as well as their baseline health and their prospects. For example, people in poor health may place greater value on health gains.[25] Treatment at end of life may be valued more highly than conventional QALYs would suggest.[26] Health technology assessment bodies try to incorporate these sorts of preferences by using higher (more generous) cost-effectiveness benchmarks for treatments for life-threatening illnesses.[27]

Even if it does not improve outcomes on average, a new drug that that has more predictable benefits can add value in ways not captured by QALYs.[26] In similar fashion, a diagnostic test that reduces uncertainty may have value even if it does not change average outcomes by providing a "value of knowing" for patients, independent of the QALY gain from changes in care itself.[28]

Many individuals will place a premium on therapies that offer a small chance of substantial health gains, a phenomenon sometimes called "the value of hope."[29-31] For example, many patients would be willing to take a gamble on a risky but promising cancer drug, although a QALY-maximizing strategy would not recognize such preferences. Knowing that there is a possibility that one's life might be extended can enhance how a patient experiences the present by allowing them to anticipate future life events.

QALYs may also fail to capture the indirect value people derive from treatments that extend life expectancy and allow people to gain access to a new drug that becomes available after they would have otherwise died. In economist terms, they gain an "option" to use the new technology. This potential "option value" is unaccounted for in traditional cost-effectiveness analyses, but in theory could be estimated.[32] Some research has calculated that option value could add as much as 25% to conventional value estimates for breast cancer treatments.[26]

Finally, because health insurance typically pays for much of the cost of high-priced drugs, and people purchase insurance before they become ill, the ex ante (or "insurance") perspective is relevant. A new drug to treat COVID-19 not only improves the health of people with the condition, but also benefits everyone in the insurance pool by making them less fearful of becoming severely ill if they do contract the virus. The drug might also protect against substantial financial risk because it averts the expenses and lost income that could accompany a severe and prolonged illness.

In theory, QALY calculations could be expanded beyond length and quality of life to also reflect the sorts of elements as previously described and to "build a better QALY." Research on the matter is ongoing but might help in future drug valuation exercises. A task force convened by ISPOR not only argued that conventional cost-per-QALY analyses are a useful starting point but also called for broadening or augmenting the QALY.[26,33] Accounting for nontraditional elements means "a QALY is not a QALY"—in other words, not all QALYs are created equal, but will depend on the context and what preferences they incorporate.

In turn, different cost-per-QALY benchmarks may be applicable for different situations. One study suggested, for example, that cost-effectiveness benchmarks should be five times higher (more generous) for Alzheimer's disease than for peptic ulcer disease, whereas we currently treat them uniformly.[24] Importantly, though, if by building other elements into the QALY we increase the apparent number of QALYs that health technologies deliver, then our unchanged healthcare budget has fewer dollars to spend on gaining each of these QALYs. To live within our budget, the original cost-per-QALY value benchmark must become more stringent (i.e., it must decrease). In other words, we need to reconsider what resources society is willing to forego to obtain the "new" QALY.[34]

Are Decisions Based on QALYs Fair?

As Chapter 6 of this volume explained, a key objection to QALYs is that decisions based on them are "unfair." Rather than wishing to optimize the population's health (i.e., total QALYs), people also seek other goals, such as prioritizing the most severely ill, reducing health disparities, and avoiding discrimination on grounds of age, race, or disability (Chapter 12 in the Second Panel report).[35,36] When it comes to allocating healthcare spending, we all care about who gains and loses, not merely whether we maximize the total number of QALYs gained.[35] In the crowded intensive care unit, doctors prioritize ventilators for COVID-19 patients to those most in need and most likely to survive.[37] In allocating scarce livers for transplantation, policymakers balance the aggregate medical good with considerations of justice, such as equalizing the distribution of organs across geographic areas.[38,39] In many ways, decision makers puzzle over potential trade-offs between efficiency (e.g., maximizing the total number of QALYs gained) and equity (e.g., maximizing the chance that people have access to an intervention). This trade-off is perhaps nowhere as stark as in discussions of treatments for very rare and severe diseases (see Chapter 8 of this volume).[40]

Researchers have offered various strategies to address these concerns. Some have proposed modifying traditional cost-effectiveness analyses to account for ethical considerations—such as favoring the severely ill over the less severely ill (Chapter 12 in the Second Panel report).[36,41] In theory, one could elicit preferences for such priorities and then use different cost-per-QALY benchmarks for drugs treating different population subgroups.[41] For example, analyses might use a higher (more generous) benchmark of, say, $200,000 per QALY for a drug that extends life for patients with late-stage cancer. A question, though, is how to determine what value benchmarks should be used for different treatments and populations given the complex and diverse views people have about such matters and the lack of consensus in the field about appropriate methods (Chapter 12 in the Second Panel report).[36]

As we also saw in Chapter 6, ICER has begun supplementing its use of QALYs with the "equal value life year gained" (evLYG), a metric similar to QALYs, but in which any extensions to life as a result of treatment are valued at full health.[42] As a consequence, the evLYG does not discriminate against patients with disabilities or poor baseline health by designating years lived with their condition as "worth less" than years lived in typical health. But the evLYG can undervalue drugs that improve the quality of life of patients in addition to extending life. Another proposed QALY-modification is the "health years in total" (HYT), which attempts to overcome the discriminatory aspects of the QALY and the evLYG's failure to recognize quality-of-life gains from treatment.[43] The intuition is to both (a) recognize a fully valued year of life for every year a treatment extends survival, regardless of an individual's health state and (b) augment the valuation of added survival years with credit for any symptom improvements.

While the technical adjustments are complex, the separate counting of survival and symptom improvement value for the HYT approach can also be viewed as a double counting of benefits. Indeed, a treatment that extends life for one year and improves symptoms during that year will be credited with a gain of *more* than one HYT. This result makes sense in the context of the HYT methodology, but it complicates its interpretation. Moreover, it also means that a HYT gain usually exceeds the corresponding gain expressed in QALYs. As a result, a HYT is worth *less* than a QALY. The developers of this measure estimate that if a QALY is worth between $50,000 to $150,000, an HYT is worth $34,000 to $89,000.[43]

A different approach for addressing equity concerns presents information on the distributional consequences *alongside* traditional cost-per-QALY results. For example, an analysis might report on both the most efficient intervention (most favorable cost-effectiveness ratio) and on an alternative, less efficient but more equitable intervention. For both strategies, the analysis might report distributional information, and for the less efficient strategy, it might also report the number of QALYs sacrificed, relative to the most efficient strategy.[35]

"Distributional" and "extended cost-effectiveness analysis" techniques present information on how an intervention affects different socioeconomic groups.[44] These approaches broaden the scope of traditional evaluations to incorporate fairness concerns.[45,46] For example, two drugs with similar cost-effectiveness ratios may have very different consequences across income groups. An effective new drug—say, for HIV—may provide a disproportionate benefit to low-income and uninsured individuals by reducing their risk of financial distress due to health costs and by preventing illness-related impoverishment.[34,47] Such information might help policymakers identify appropriate drug prices (perhaps giving greater priority to drugs that help lower-income groups). One challenge with distributional or extended cost-effectiveness analysis is that they require individual financial burden data linked to specific illnesses and conditions, and that information may be difficult to obtain.

Numerous researchers have also proposed "multicriteria decision analysis," which involves identifying different attributes for drugs, assigning weights corresponding to their importance, and calculating aggregate scores.[48–50] This approach can account for multiple characteristics beyond those typically reflected in QALYs.

Multicriteria decision analysis remains an active area of inquiry and may help aid drug evaluations.[51] One review identified 58 attributes considered in resource allocation decisions, including factors pertaining to ethics (e.g., meeting needs of vulnerable populations), organizations (e.g., system capacity), and system-wide goals (e.g., supporting innovation and economic growth).[52] The method has been used to guide decisions in certain areas, such as vaccine policy (online appendix).[53]

Still, many conceptual and feasibility questions remain about who should assign the weights and how to combine them to calculate a value score.[34] Nor does multicriteria decision analysis provide a clear decision rule for allocating resources (e.g., to rank drugs when some perform better on certain dimensions and worse on others). Unlike cost-effectiveness analysis, multicriteria decision analysis explicitly accounts for attributes that matter to people, but it does not explicitly address budget constraints or opportunity costs.

Retaining and Improving the QALY

QALYs are simply a metric to quantify health. They can help address a difficult and unavoidable question: how to estimate and compare the benefits of what are often heterogeneous health interventions? By accounting for both longevity and quality of life, QALYs provide a useful, although imperfect, measurement standard. QALYs can help to guide health decisions, foster consistency and transparency, and provide a way to represent the output of the healthcare and public health systems.[16] Although no single number can ever fully capture the complexity of preferences for health, QALYs provide a useful point of departure for thinking about how to allocate scarce resources— whether the price for a new drug is reasonable or whether a health program is worth the investment. Without cost-per-QALY analyses, ICER's reports would lack a potent tool for benchmarking value and for calculating and defending a value-based price.

A philosopher and ethicist, Peter Singer, has observed (with apologies to Winston Churchill), QALYs may be the worst way to measure health, except for all of the others.[54] Many critics protest the use of QALYs but tend not to offer solutions beyond nebulous comments about the need to place patients at the forefront of decisions.[17,18] Moreover, alternatives to QALYs have their own ethical challenges because any decision rule for allocating resources is fraught with discriminatory implications.

QALYs will likely remain important because the need to understand comparative value will persist, a reality reflected in the ever-increasing number of published cost-per-QALY studies.[5] Conceptual issues will always remain.[16] An example is the question of whose preferences should form the basis of the quality-of-life weights used to construct QALYs: those of patients or members of the general population? Arguments for using patient preferences emphasize that individuals directly affected by and most experienced with a health state or disease can best provide responses. Arguments in favor of community-based preferences highlight the idea that health plan enrollees and taxpayers, as the ultimate payers of private and public healthcare, are best positioned to inform ex ante decisions about covered benefits as potential patients. Moreover, the preferences of society should matter in health resource allocation decisions, as health systems benefit all citizens. Complicating matters is that because some people (e.g., young children or older adults with Alzheimer's disease) cannot respond to preference elicitation questions, proxy respondents must be used. But which proxies? In what circumstances? These and other questions will continue to be debated and will likely never be fully resolved.

Research on approaches for enhancing and improving the QALY should be applauded and supported. In the meantime, policymakers can use conventional cost-per-QALY calculations as an input into deliberations while considering other factors, such as equity, that might not be well captured and by allowing input from patients in the review process. Without QALYs, health systems would still face difficult trade-offs. Decision makers would still confront and make difficult choices about paying for the healthcare that people need and desire. But they would lack a practical instrument to aid in the process.

Reality Check—Anticipating What Happens to Drug Costs When Drugs Go Generic

Cystic fibrosis is a genetic disease affecting a range of organs, including the liver, lungs, and pancreas, although most of its impacts stem from its pulmonary effects. The disease is caused by a defective gene for a protein called cystic fibrosis transmembrane conductance regulator (CFTR), which is crucial for maintaining salt and water balance in body tissues. Over time, cystic fibrosis produces an accumulation of thick mucus in the lungs that makes breathing more difficult and pulmonary infections more likely.

Historically, children born with cystic fibrosis could expect to live only around 20 years.[55] Over the years, screening and symptomatic treatment improved life expectancy somewhat. More recently, a series of drugs that increase the quantity or rectify the function of the CFTR protein have offered more dramatic improvements. Life expectancy has reached the high 30s for individuals with cystic fibrosis born and diagnosed in 2010, and projections suggest that it could reach the mid-50s if mortality continues to decline at the rate at which it fell from 2000 to 2010.[56]

ICER estimated that health benefits conferred by CFTR modulators amounted to a gain of from 5.0 to 6.1 QALYs per treated patient (even after "discounting" health benefits accruing decades in the future; see Box 4.2 in Chapter 4 of this volume).[57] Nonetheless, ICER concluded that because lifetime treatment costs could run into the millions of dollars, CFTR modulators were not cost-effective.

In response, Vertex Pharmaceuticals, the drugs' developer, argued that although treatment could last 40 years, ICER had made no allowance for the prospect of a drop in drug prices after their patents expired and generic competitors entered the marketplace.[58] Vertex also contended that for "small molecule" drugs like CFTR modulators—namely, drugs that would be relatively easy for other companies to manufacture—prices typically fall by 80% in the five years following their loss of market exclusivity.

ICER declined to alter their approach, contending that as a practical matter, it is difficult to predict the timing of generic drug entry because drug companies often engage in tactics to delay patent expirations (see Chapter 2), and that even after market exclusivity ends, the timing of generic introductions is uncertain.[59] ICER added that although loss of market exclusivity can substantially reduce prices, it might not do so for drugs treating diseases with relatively small populations, like cystic fibrosis, because the smaller market size attracts less generic competition.

ICER noted in response to Vertex, it "does not as a rule consider such 'dynamic pricing' approaches in its modeling unless there is known timing for patent expiry and certainty around expected changes in price."[59] Because future patent expiration dates and subsequent generic pricing are almost always uncertain, ICER's criteria seem to prohibit assumptions about price declines accompanying a drug's loss of patent protection. ICER's position creates a conflict between the imperative to measure drug value—and resulting net costs—as realistically as possible by accounting for future generic drug pricing, and the desire to avoid the highly uncertain and perhaps unrealistic assumptions that accompany efforts to anticipate long-term market dynamics.

How important are price changes driven by the introduction of generics? Some observers have emphasized that the genericization of drugs is the ultimate purpose of the pharmaceutical industry. Peter Kolchinsky, a virologist, biotechnology investor, and author of the 2019 book, *The Great American Drug Deal*, has explained, for example, "It is the destiny of nearly all new drugs to become as affordable and accessible as Zestril," a blood pressure medication originally introduced in 1987 and now prescribed as a generic drug 100 million times a year to Americans, for several dollars per patient each month.[60p23] Notably, generics now account for almost 90% of all prescriptions in the US.[61] Kolchinsky points to the "mountain of generic drugs"—from angiotensin-converting enzyme inhibitors (for high blood pressure) to statins (hyperlipidemia) to antiretrovirals (HIV) and others—that innovative brand-name pharmaceutical companies have created.[60pp17-28] New drugs start out as high-priced, brand-name products but, over the long term, they continue to provide the same benefits in perpetuity as substantially lower cost generics. Unlike, say, a coronary bypass surgery, which never "goes generic" and whose price remains high forever, drugs are a special commodity with transitorily high prices. And unlike a medical procedure, a drug is a "global public good" in that the product—and the knowledge it represents—can be used around the world.[62]

Viewed this way, drugs should be regarded more as an investment than an expense.[63] An assessment that assumes drug prices remain unchanged after patent expiration misses the key attribute that distinguishes drugs from other healthcare interventions, like surgeries or physical therapy. For drugs, the benefits continue long after the initial development is paid for; for other types of interventions, continued benefits depend on continued payments. To observers like Kolchinsky, ICER's omission of generic pricing is not a secondary issue, but a fundamental one that denies the central reality making drugs different from other medical treatments.

As we saw in Chapter 2 of this volume, the real world does not always conform to this ideal. Pharmaceutical companies have strong incentives to delay patent expiration, and they often act on them. As the National Academy of Sciences pointed out, the biopharmaceutical market is complex and confusing—characterized by limited competition, opacity about pricing methods, obscure financial arrangements, and perverse incentives.[64p170] As noted in Chapter 3 of this volume, generic-like "biosimilar" competition for biologics—complex molecular entities that are grown rather than synthesized artificially—has been slow to gain traction in the United States. Nor is Kolchinsky naïve to these realities. Indeed, he calls for a "Biotechnology Social Contract" to help ensure, among other things, that drugs lose their patent protection in a predictable way. He even favors strong government action—essentially a form of price controls—for drugs that "can't or won't go generic."[60pp93-109]

ICER officials might respond to Kolchinsky's position by pointing out that, as yet, the real world possesses no Biotechnology Social Contract. They might reasonably add that if one attempts to anticipate the impact of generic entry, there are also other aspects of drug pricing to recognize. For one, between a drug's launch and its eventual genericization, product prices typically increase. As just one example, the monthly cost of the erectile dysfunction drugs sildenafil (Viagra°) and tadalafil (Cialis°) nearly tripled during the six-year period between 2012 and 2017.[65] At the same time, the drugs' manufacturers successfully delayed the products' genericization (Viagra was approved by the FDA in 1998; Cialis, in 2004). Should these general tendencies also be factored into the drug's cost? Second, if assessments account for price reductions following a drug's patent expiration, they should also account for the possibility that any brand-name comparator drug (i.e., the therapy to which the new drug is compared) will go generic and experience a price reduction.

Finally, even if a drug does go generic and its price falls, follow-on innovation may lead to the creation of a new drug that displaces the original medication. Just as it would be unrealistic to assume a $500 investment in the next generation iPhone can be amortized over decades (because the purchaser will surely replace it with an improved device sooner), we cannot assume that a drug will continue to be used forever after it goes generic.

On the other hand, some drugs are used for decades despite the advent of follow-ons. Lipitor—in brand-name form and as the generic, "atorvastatin"—remains extremely popular a quarter century after its introduction.[66] Follow-on innovations have been developed for certain subgroups or to be used alongside statins.[67] Moreover, even if innovation displaces a drug, the original drug may have spurred that innovation and hence analysts might credit that product in part for the new innovation's value—rather than simply assuming that its benefit stream fades as its use phases out.

Setting aside the computational challenges, there is another argument against building anticipated price reductions into value assessments. The opposing position agrees that lower prices following the introduction of generics do indeed reduce a drug's cost over its entire life cycle. But it argues against giving the drug companies "credit" in their pricing policies for that eventual cost reduction.* From that view, the period following a drug's patent expiration is a period when "society," not the drug company, is entitled to capture the drug's surplus value. In other words, we should pretend that the drug's price never decreases because doing so prevents justification of a high price during its early years that would funnel generic price savings back to the drug company.

The problem with this position is that making drugs appear to be more costly than they actually are in the long run can cause a misallocation of healthcare resources. If drugs seem so expensive, we might divert resources to perform more hip replacement surgeries, rather than pay for a drug that could substitute for those replacements. Had we accounted for its true long-term average costs, we might have seen that the drug delivered better value than the surgery. That would not have been apparent had we pretended that the drug's price would not decrease following its genericization.

For these reasons, value assessments should reflect the anticipated impact of future price reductions following the introduction of a drug's generic competition. But for estimates to be realistic, the field needs reasonable assumptions for how drug prices react to the loss of exclusivity. Existing evidence reveals some patterns. For example, as ICER noted in the case of new cystic fibrosis

---

* Mark Sculpher, personal communication. March 18, 2020.

treatments, drugs for diseases with smaller populations tend to have fewer generic entrants, and when the number of generic competitors is small, the influence on prices can be limited. Furthermore, prices of biosimilars may not be substantially lower than the originator biologic, because manufacturing is complex and costly. More evidence would provide the information analysts need to build assumptions about generic pricing into their models, so that assessments can better reflect a drug's life cycle costs. That would be more realistic—and provide a better understanding of a drug's value—than simply ignoring this critical feature that sets drugs apart from other health interventions.

Accounting for Uncertainty: Dealing With Unknowable Unknowns

As challenging as it is to determine what elements analysts should consider in drug value assessment—the focus of this chapter thus far—actually measuring value presents its own difficulties because the information needed is incomplete. The clinical trials that support a drug's FDA approval help quantify its health benefits: the symptom relief, moderated disease progression, or mortality reduction. But characterizing value in terms of net costs incurred and QALYs gained also depends on knowing, among other things, the frequency and severity of adverse events, the preference weights to attach to treatment benefits and side effects (see Chapter 4 of this volume), and how therapy might offset downstream care costs.

Some of this information may be available at a drug's launch, because the clinical trials reviewed by FDA reported it. Other information—on care costs and preference weights for different health conditions—may be available because researchers collected it in earlier studies. But often, needed information is absent or is imprecise because, for example, the population included in clinical studies may differ from the individuals who actually take the drug (e.g., the study population may be younger and healthier), or the duration of follow-up in the trial may be much shorter than the lifetime time horizon that most economic models employ.

So much uncertainty can make value assessments seem pointless. But while uncertainty can impede exact estimates of a drug's costs and QALY gains, it need not present an insurmountable obstacle. For example, even if we can only narrow our estimate of a drug's cost-effectiveness to between $10,000 and $25,000 per QALY, we can still be reasonably confident the drug reflects good value by conventional standards because, as described in Chapter 4 of this volume, a QALY is worth at least $50,000 (in the United States). Similarly, if a drug improves health at a cost of $500,000 to $1 million a QALY, we can be reasonably confident it represents poor value. In short, we can sometimes determine whether a drug is a good or bad buy even if we do not know exactly how good or bad a deal it is.

Because it may be sufficient to know whether a drug's cost-effectiveness ratio exceeds or falls below a value benchmark, researchers routinely employ sensitivity analysis to determine whether alternative, plausible assumptions can shift the ratio so that it crosses the value benchmark. To illustrate, suppose a new drug costs $30,000 more than the drug it purports to replace. The new drug's benefits are uncertain, with a gain between 0.05 and 0.10 QALYs. If we assume pessimistically that the new drug gains only 0.05 QALYs, its cost-effectiveness ratio is $30,000 per 0.05 QALYs gained—that is, $\frac{\$30,000}{0.05\ QALYs}$, or $600,000 per QALY. On the other hand, if we assume optimistically that the drug gains 0.10 QALYs, its cost-effectiveness ratio is $30,000 per 0.10 QALYs gained—that is, $\frac{\$30,000}{0.10\ QALYs}$, or $300,000 per QALY. No matter what plausible assumption we adopt for the magnitude of the drug's QALY gain, the drug "buys" QALYs at a price of at least $300,000. Even assuming a QALY is worth $150,000, QALYs gained by this drug are expensive. While the drug's exact value remains unknown, its price should raise red flags with decision makers.

We can extend this example to more realistic situations with multiple uncertain quantities (see Box 9.2). More sophisticated methods can identify not only the range of plausible cost-effectiveness ratios, but which ratio values are most likely. Moreover, these methods can help identify which of the knowledge gaps contribute most to the cost-effectiveness ratio's uncertainty and hence what kind of research would most efficiently narrow that uncertainty (see Box 9.3).

Ideally, these methods help signal to decision makers whether the drug price is a good or bad deal or, short of that, identify key data gaps that, if addressed, could help resolve ambiguous cases. Even if the key information gaps can be identified, however, it may require considerable time to gather the needed information. For example, for drugs that treat chronic conditions— like Alzheimer's disease or heart disease—a key question is how long a drug will continue to work, often referred to as the "durability" of the drug's effect. While we would like to know the drug's long-term effects, pivotal clinical trials typically follow patients for a relatively short period of time, say six months or one year. For that reason, value assessments of gene therapies (treatments

Box 9.2 One-Way Sensitivity Analysis

A "one-way" sensitivity analysis investigates the influence of each uncertain quantity in a value assessment, one variable at a time. Initially, the analysis sets all of these quantities to the analyst's "best guess" or "base case" values. Then it might assign the most optimistic, plausible value to the first quantity and, leaving other quantities at their base case values, recalculate the drug's cost-effectiveness ratio. Next, the analysis assigns the most pessimistic, plausible value to the first quantity and again recalculates the drug's cost-effectiveness ratio. The difference between these two cost-effectiveness ratios represents the influence of the first uncertain quantity.

The analysis then returns the first quantity to its base case value and conducts the optimistic–pessimistic computations for the second uncertain quantity, recording its influence on the cost-effectiveness ratio. The analysis conducts this pair of computations for all uncertain quantities. After computing the low-end (optimistic) and high-end (pessimistic) cost-effectiveness ratios for each uncertain quantity, the results can be arranged by degree of influence.

Consider ICER's 2017 analysis that compared poly ADP ribose polymerase inhibitors to standard of care for ovarian cancer.[1] In their cost-effectiveness analysis of rucaparib (Rubraca®) to provide maintenance therapy for patients with platinum-sensitive disease, ICER examined the influence of 11 uncertain quantities. The assumed utility preference weight for the "progressed cancer" health state for patients on standard of care treatment contributed more uncertainty than any other parameters. Assigning this quantity its most "optimistic" plausible value (0.55) while holding other quantities equal to their base case values produces a cost-effectiveness ratio of about $217,000 per QALY gained. Substituting the most pessimistic plausible value (0.80) increases the ratio to more than $1 million per QALY gained.

The second most influential quantity is the utility weight for the "progressed cancer" health state for patients taking the active therapy, rucaparib. Assigning the most optimistic value (0.55) produces an estimated cost-effectiveness ratio of $254,000, while replacing that quantity with the most pessimistic plausible value (0.80) inflates the cost-effectiveness ratio to $745,000.

Figure 9.1, which displays the influence of 5 of the 11 uncertain assumptions analyzed by ICER, is instructive. First, none of the alternative assumption values reduces the cost-effectiveness ratio for rucaparib below $217,000 per QALY gained. At the time ICER wrote this report, it generally regarded drugs to be of low value if they improved health at a cost exceeding $175,000 per QALY gained. Hence, despite the uncertainty, ICER could be relatively confident that for this patient population, this therapy was not favorably cost-effective by conventional standards. Second, the sensitivity analysis indicates that the utility weights for patients with "progressed cancer"—receiving

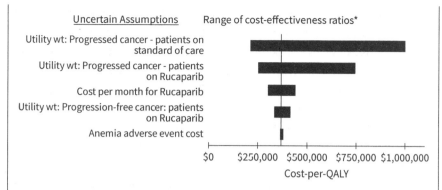

Figure 9.1: One-way sensitivity analysis illustrating the influence of assumptions on the cost-effectiveness of poly ADP ribose polymerase (PARP) inhibitors to standard of care (SOC) for maintenance therapy of platinum-sensitive ovarian cancer

* Based on ICER's analysis of Poly ADP-Ribose Polymerase (PARP) Inhibitors for Ovarian Cancer (Figure E3 on p. 142).[1] Each horizontal bar represents the range cost-effectiveness estimates produced by varying the corresponding assumption, one at a time, between its minimum and maximum plausible value. The vertical line represents to the cost-effectiveness estimate corresponding to use of ICER's base case assumptions.

Source: Samal, L., Ollendorf, D.A., Synnott, P.G., Cramer, G., Chapman, R., Kumar, V., Khan, S., and Pearson, S.D. 2017. Poly ADP-ribose polymerase (PARP) inhibitors for ovarian cancer: effectiveness and value. Institute for Clinical and Economic Review. http://icerorg.wpengine.com/wp-content/uploads/2020/10/MWCEPAC_OVARIAN_FINAL_EVIDENCE_REPORT_10112017-1.pdf.

either standard of care or rucaparib (active therapy) treatment—were the most important sources of uncertainty. That makes better information for these quantities potentially helpful.

Although one-way sensitivity analysis provides useful insights, it has limitations. First, while it indicates the range of cost-effectiveness ratios corresponding to optimistic and pessimistic estimates for each uncertain quantity, it reveals nothing about the relative *plausibility* of alternative cost-effectiveness ratio estimates. Typically, the ratio incorporating "base case" estimates for uncertain quantities is more plausible than ratios calculated using pessimistic or optimistic values. But by how much?

Second, one-way sensitivity analysis examines how each uncertain assumption *individually* influences cost-effectiveness ratios. It says nothing about how, for example, using pessimistic values for two assumptions simultaneously would influence ratios—or how a ratio's value would be influenced by using optimistic values for two assumptions at the same time. The problem with investigating these sorts of combinations is that there are loads of possibilities. The example at hand involves 11 assumptions (the figure here displays the influence of only five assumptions). If each has an optimistic, base case, and a pessimistic value, there are more than 177,000 combinations, making it infeasible to examine all of the possibilities. Moreover, inspecting the resulting range of cost-effectiveness estimates is unlikely to be useful because the calculated cost-effectiveness ratio corresponding to use of all of the pessimistic assumptions will likely be highly unfavorable while the calculated cost-effectiveness ratio corresponding to use of all of the optimistic assumptions will be highly favorable. Neither of these extremes is likely, but the analysis does not provide information about the plausibility of the ratios between these extremes. Knowing that a drug's cost-effectiveness ratio may be very unfavorable, very favorable, or somewhere in between does not by itself provide decision makers with much actionable information.

[1] Samal, L., Ollendorf, D.A., Synnott, P.G., Cramer, G., Chapman, R., Kumar, V., Khan, S., and Pearson, S.D. 2017. "Poly ADP-ribose polymerase (PARP) inhibitors for ovarian cancer: Effectiveness and value." *Institute for Clinical and Economic Review.* Accessed January 25, 2021. http://icerorg. wpengine.com/wp-content/uploads/2020/10/MWCEPAC_OVARIAN_FINAL_EVIDENCE_ REPORT_10112017-1.pdf.

that manipulate how genes function in a patient—such as Luxturna, which treats a congenital vision disease, as described in Box 6.4 in Chapter 6 of this volume) make assumptions about the therapy's projected benefits over the patient's lifetime.[68] Uncertainty analyses might conclude that, given optimistic assumptions, the drug confers high value, while under pessimistic assumptions, it confers low value. That much ambiguity makes the assessment unhelpful because it is impossible to rule out the chance that the drug reflects either a good or a bad deal.

What to do? Decision makers might prefer to wait for results from long-term clinical studies, but for pricing and coverage purposes, they need to know a drug's value when it is approved. Adopting optimistic assumptions in the absence of data can result in overpayment for drugs that ultimately fail to deliver. But using pessimistic assumptions sends a signal to future drug developers that they will receive limited payment for therapies addressing chronic, long-term conditions and thus provide less of an incentive to invest in treatments for these conditions.

Rather than insisting on establishing a drug's value at its launch, payers and drug developers can instead agree to update value estimates (and price) as new information becomes available. Because these arrangements may reduce payment to the drug company if its therapy falls short of expectations, they are sometimes referred to as "performance-based, risk-sharing agreements."[69] Examples include

- A discount to the payer if a drug fails to reduce cholesterol levels at least as much as observed in clinical trials;

Box 9.3 Probabilistic Sensitivity Analysis

To address the challenge posed by multiple uncertain assumptions, researchers have developed "probabilistic sensitivity analysis" (PSA). This approach involves choosing at random a value for each uncertain quantity, with the most plausible values for each uncertain quantity having the highest probability of being selected. For each set of uncertain quantities chosen, PSA calculates the corresponding cost-effectiveness ratio. Repeating these steps many times creates a large set of ratio estimates. Ratios corresponding to plausible input combinations will appear most often. Thus, the analysis characterizes not only the range of possible cost-effectiveness ratios but also their plausibility. PSAs also shed light on which assumptions contribute the most uncertainty to the estimated cost-effectiveness ratio, and how much improved knowledge of those assumptions will reduce the ratio's uncertainty.

Being able to describe the plausibility of alternative cost-effectiveness ratios can help decision makers. For example, even if extreme values for the ratios cannot be completely ruled out, PSA results often show that the ratio is very likely to be on one side of the QALY value benchmark (e.g., $100,000 per QALY) or the other. In addition, identifying the most important sources of uncertainty can help decision makers prioritize research to reduce uncertainty as efficiently as possible. Because of its usefulness, many consensus groups—including the Second Panel on Cost-Effectiveness in Health and Medicine—recommend PSA.[1]

Still, PSA has its limitations. Importantly, it requires quantification of the plausibility of alternative values for each uncertain assumption. Even identifying the bounds on plausible ranges can be difficult, let alone determining how plausible alternative values are within those ranges (i.e., describing a quantity's probability distribution).

As a thought experiment, if one were interested in estimating the number of people who annually climb Mt. Marcy, New York State's highest peak (a favorite hike of one of this book's authors), how might one develop a probability distribution for that value? We could consider plausible ranges for the number of available hiking days during the summer season, what fraction of those days has "good" weather, how many people hike on good versus bad weather days, and so forth. But how does one meaningfully assign probabilities to alternative estimates for the proportion of, say, good weather days during the summer? Or for the number of hikers on good versus bad weather days? If the distributions we assign to each quantity do not represent our knowledge, they do not describe our views regarding the plausibility of the alternatives.

Estimating quantities more removed from our experience is even more difficult. For example, the sun creates energy by fusing hydrogen atoms to create helium; the resulting helium atom has a mass that is slightly less than the mass of the component inputs to this reaction, with the "missing" mass transformed into energy via Albert Einstein's famous equation, $E = mc^2$. How many tons of hydrogen does the sun transform into helium each second (a process that has been ongoing for about 5 billion years)? For most people, the only possible answer to this question (absent Googling the topic) is a very wide distribution over which all values may seem as plausible as any of the others (i.e., the value distribution may be close to "uniform").

If a cost-effectiveness ratio is similarly uncertain, then characterizing its distribution amounts to conceding that it spans a wide range of possible values and that we have no insight as to which values within that range are most plausible. In short, while uncertainty analysis provides a means of characterizing what we know about a drug's cost-effectiveness, it does not replace missing knowledge. If information is limited, we are left concluding that a drug may or may not have good value, without even knowing which of those possibilities is most likely.

[1] Sculpher, M.J., Basu, A., Kuntz, K.M., and Meltzer, D.O. 2017. "Reflecting uncertainty in cost-effectiveness analysis." In *Cost-effectiveness in health and medicine*, edited by P.J. Neumann, G.D. Sanders, L.B. Russell, J.E. Siegel and T.G. Ganiats, 289–318. New York: Oxford University Press.

- A price reduction for a drug if it does not reduce a key diabetes biomarker (hemoglobin A1c levels) as much as a competing drug; and
- Rebates if patients with diabetes who receive a drug fail to meet treatment goals and require additional therapy.

Use of these and similar arrangements is on the rise in the United States and abroad.[70,71] One report found 62 publicly announced such agreements in the United States during the 2010s (through mid-2019).[72] Still, one might have expected more such agreements given the number of opportunities for them (the modest number may also reflect underreporting, as many agreements are proprietary). In part, limited use of these agreements may reflect regulatory challenges. For example, use of risk-sharing agreements could trigger other Medicare and Medicaid pricing requirements that could further lower prices for those payers (which drug companies would oppose). They might also conflict with laws that prohibit payments that could be regarded as "kickbacks" to insurance companies.[70] Agreements might also depend on impermissible discussions by drug companies about off-label drug uses.

Data collection challenges can also be substantial, including identification of relevant outcomes that can be readily tracked; establishment of protocols to measure these outcomes; development of infrastructure to facilitate timely data collection; and for some diseases, follow-up time that extends beyond the duration of pricing agreements between manufacturers and payers.[73]

While it is impossible to produce all of the data optimally available to reduce uncertainty, certain steps can make it more common. First, the federal government should revise regulations without unduly damaging the safeguards they embody (the Trump administration released one such proposal in mid-2020).[74] Second, payers and drug developers should make collection of data to assess a drug's value a standard part of the drug development process. That means identifying relevant outcomes and determining how to use those outcomes to estimate value, building the collection of needed information into trials conducted to support a drug's approval, and developing infrastructure to facilitate data collection after a drug receives approval.

Who Should Measure Drug Value?

As discussed in Chapter 5 of this volume, the history of government-led health technology assessment in the United States is one of advances, disappointments, and sidesteps. Unlike many countries, the United States lacks a single, centralized body to evaluate drug value. Still, the fragmented American healthcare system continues to maintain an ecosystem of assessment activities in various public and private bodies. For example, the Veterans Administration evaluates drugs for patients it serves. The Advisory Committee on Immunization Practices evaluates vaccines. The US Preventive Services Task Force issues advice on the evidence supporting preventive services. The Centers for Medicare and Medicaid Services evaluates "big-ticket" items affecting Medicare beneficiaries. Other agencies, such as the Centers for Disease Control and Prevention and the Agency for Healthcare Research and Quality (AHRQ), have their own congressionally mandated responsibilities. Private health plans conduct evaluations to serve their own populations.

A natural question is whether a new federal health technology assessment body is needed. A new agency could bring the legitimacy, funding, and broad perspective that other bodies may lack. To be sure, there are many issues to consider regarding the appropriate scope, placement, structure, governance, and resource demands of any new agency, as well as how such an entity would interact with stakeholders, how transparent and participatory it would be, and whether its recommendations would be advisory or mandatory.

Federal efforts in this area have always faced stiff headwinds, and these seem likely to persist. One possibility is to augment the health technology assessment activities of government agencies such as the AHRQ (or quasi-government ones, such as the Patient-Centered Outcomes Research Institute [PCORI]), giving them authority to consider the cost-effectiveness and budget impact of drugs. However, given the political climate, it is difficult to imagine political support to extend the authority of these bodies to making judgments regarding "fair" prices (see Box 9.4).

Prospects for a private-sector health technology assessment organization seem more promising. One possibility is for the government to rely on ICER for reviews of drugs and other technologies. ICER could remain in the private sector, supported by foundation and other private (and/or public) funding sources, and its assessments used as inputs into public payer coverage decisions. There is precedent for such arrangements, as ICER has occasionally tailored its evaluations to public payer needs. In 2012, for example, ICER assessed the evidence on treatments for diabetic macular edema to inform the Medicare Evidence Development and Coverage Advisory Committee (MedCAC) decision on the topic and provided testimony at the public MedCAC meeting.[75] In 2020, the Department of Veterans Affairs commissioned ICER to assess the use of trained service dogs to treat veterans with posttraumatic stress disorder.[76]

The idea would also face challenges. Having the Center for Medicare and Medicaid Services formally use ICER assessments would create political opposition. The approach may also force changes to ICER's governance or voting panels to include broader representation (e.g., the pharmaceutical industry currently has no representation on ICER's governance board or voting committees).

Some observers have championed a government "certifying agency" for health technology assessment organizations that have satisfied criteria for the quality of their methods, reporting, and processes.[77] One can imagine a "dashboard" of standardized metrics that assessment groups would display for each review. The dashboard could include information on a drug's clinical benefits and risks, cost-effectiveness, budget impact, and contextual elements (e.g., the impact of treatments on improving worker productivity), which would facilitate side-by-side comparisons. Certifying entities could include AHRQ, PCORI, or the MedCAC. An analog of this approach is the Federal Aviation Administration's certification of private consultants who determine the airworthiness of aircraft based on stringent criteria issued by the Federal Aviation Administration.

Government certification of health technology assessment organizations would help build legitimacy but is by itself insufficient. Instead, all stakeholders must believe that the reported findings reflect a credible, objective, transparent, participatory, and fair process. In many scientific endeavors, a careful

Box 9.4 Should the Federal Government Evaluate a Drug's cost-Effectiveness? PCORI as a Cautionary Tale

The Affordable Care Act (ACA) of 2010 created the Patient-Centered Outcomes Research Institute (PCORI), an independent, nonprofit, nongovernmental organization, to conduct comparative-effectiveness research but prohibited this institute from developing or using cost-per-QALY benchmarks.[1] The ACA specifically forbade the use of cost-per-QALY "as a threshold" (the term health economists use to refer to value benchmarks). The precise intent of this language was never entirely clear. One could interpret it to mean that the PCORI, or its contractors or grantees, could still calculate cost-per-QALY ratios as long as they did not then compare those ratios to a benchmark (e.g., $100,000 per QALY). Comparing cost-per-QALY ratios across interventions could still be useful to decision makers even without invocation of an explicit benchmark. However, the ACA's language on cost-per-QALY analyses, as well as its mandate for the Institute to focus on clinical comparative effectiveness research, meant that the PCORI would not conduct or fund cost-effectiveness analyses at all.

In some ways, the ACA's language, a bow to critics of "big government" healthcare and the soon-to-be clichéd "death panels," was not entirely surprising. Prior attempts to increase government funding for comparative and cost-effectiveness research had failed or been curtailed. For example, legislation proposed in 2003 would have authorized $75 million in annual appropriations—$50 million for NIH and $25 million for AHRQ—to conduct and publish studies of the comparative effectiveness and cost-effectiveness of drugs accounting for a high level of expenditures or used by individuals in federally funded health programs.[2] Further, the bill would have required the AHRQ to develop standards for the design and conduct of cost-effectiveness analyses, and it stipulated that only methodologically sound studies would be considered. The bill was never advanced due to pressure from the drug industry, however.[3] The 2003 Medicare drug legislation granted AHRQ authority to conduct comparative effectiveness and cost-effectiveness research but explicitly forbade the Centers for Medicare & Medicaid Services from using this information to withhold coverage of new drugs.

The prohibition on cost-per-QALY analyses also reflected long-standing concerns that such studies discriminate based on age and disability, favoring younger and healthier populations who have more potential QALYs to gain (see previous discussion). Enacting the ACA was already a monumental political lift, and it seemed politically expedient to rid the controversial new institute of any mission resembling that of Britain's National Institute for Health and Care Excellence. To further mollify critics, the new institute was labeled "patient-centered" and the law stipulated that the findings of PCORI-sponsored research could not be construed as mandates for practice guidelines, coverage recommendations, payment, or policy recommendations.

Over the past decade, the PCORI has funded a wide variety of research projects.[4] Still, the prohibition on cost-effectiveness information has been unfortunate. A ban on valuing life extension presents its own ethical dilemmas. Taken literally, it means that spending resources to extend by a month the life of a 100-year-old person who is in a vegetative state cannot be valued differently from spending resources to extend the life of a child by many healthy years. Although the ACA may have sought to avert discrimination, it instead helped to perpetuate the current system of implicit rationing and hidden biases.

Ideally, the prohibition against cost-effectiveness analysis would be lifted, allowing the PCORI, with its stable funding stream (from federal appropriations and a fee assessed on private insurance and self-insured health plans) to conduct and fund cost-effectiveness analyses of new drugs and other services.[1] Without such a policy, there is no clearly articulated policy for coordinating cost-effectiveness research across government agencies. While the federal government conducts or sponsors some research in sundry places, it is not directed toward specific decision makers. There is little effort toward prioritization to understand whether we are asking the right questions and focusing on the right problems. In theory, the PCORI could fulfill those roles.

The PCORI's experience is another cautionary tale. In late 2019, the organization was reauthorized for 10 years.[5] When it comes to supporting economic analyses, the reauthorization suggests some additional flexibility for the PCORI in evaluating economic outcomes in that PCORI-funded research can examine issues pertaining to patient costs. But the prohibition on cost-effectiveness analysis remains.

[1] Neumann, P.J., and Weinstein, M.C. 2010. "Legislating against use of cost-effectiveness information." *New England Journal of Medicine* 363 (16): 1495–1497. https://doi.org/10.1056/NEJMp1007168.

[2] H.R. 2356—Prescription Drug Comparative Effectiveness Act of 2003. 108th Congr. (2003).

[3] Pear, R. 2003, June 1. "Drug companies increase spending on efforts to lobby congress and governments." *The New York Times.* Accessed August 19, 2020. https://www.nytimes.com/2003/06/01/us/drug-companies-increase-spending-on-efforts-to-lobby-congress-and-governments.html.

[4] "PCORI at age eight: Progress, impact, and more to do." 2018. *Patient-Centered Outcomes Research Institute.* Accessed July 24, 2020. https://www.pcori.org/blog/pcori-age-eight-progress-impact-and-more-do.

[5]S.2891—Patient Centered Outcomes Research Institute Reauthorization Act. 116th Congr. (2019).

description of one's methods provides enough information to convince others that the reported work is free of errors or bias. The sin qua non of science is provision of sufficient detail to allow others to reproduce the original work and confirm that they produce the same results as the initial investigators. We

Box 9.5 The Value of Open-Source Models

Although it is unusual for authors publishing cost-effectiveness analyses to also publish the "source code" (a model's human-readable computer instructions) for their simulations,[1] some commentators—including some of the authors of this book—have advocated for more openness. This box describes their position, as articulated in a commentary in the *Annals of Internal Medicine*.[78]

The argument in favor of openness drew inspiration from an article published in 2005 by John Ioannidis, a professor of medicine and epidemiology at Stanford University. In that article Ioannidis famously argued that in biomedical research, because of conflicts of interest, underpowered study designs, and journal editor biases that favor publication of positive results, "most published research findings are false."[2]

The *Annals* commentary[78] noted that questions of credibility likewise pertain to cost-effectiveness analysis in healthcare. Indeed, such analyses face additional challenges because they involve projections beyond randomized controlled trials to longer-term outcomes not captured during trials. These projections typically rely on computer models to simulate "hypothetical trials" that have not or cannot be conducted.

Providing enough methodological detail to allow other scientists to reproduce an experiment is the hallmark of empirical science. It serves as a check on the "ubiquity of error"—the possibility "that mistakes and self-delusion can creep in absolutely anywhere."[3p9] The conventional notion is that a scientific finding is accepted only if other scientists can independently reproduce the results. The same basic principle applies to computational science (e.g., simulation modeling used in cost-effectiveness analyses). In this case, the *Annals* commentary argued that the best way to ensure reproducibility is to release the computer program source code.

The *Annals* commentary advanced additional reasons why the medical community should embrace open publication of the simulation source code used in cost-effectiveness analyses. First, such openness facilitates updates to reflect changing conditions. An assessment of a diabetes prevention drug, for example, will require incorporating new information that emerges about a drug's safety and efficacy, and any changes to its price or information about the therapy to which it is being compared. Realistically, the original model developers will not have the funding or interest to continually update their models.

Second, open publication of models can reduce duplication of effort, particularly in developing countries. Analysts and decision makers in those countries typically lack resources to create their own simulation models.[4] Making source code available can facilitate the customization of cost-effectiveness analyses to their local conditions. Third, open model publication would also accelerate new uses of simulation models. For example, it would expedite model use for individualized treatment decisions based on a person's risk factors.

The commentary acknowledged that open publication faces challenges. Third parties might revise models in ways that are scientifically invalid to promote their interests. If the revised versions are held to the "open publication" standard, however, such manipulation would likely be detected, and the attendant claims would fail to gain credibility. This sort of unsolicited, crowd-sourced review has worked well, albeit with some challenges, to mitigate publication abuses in Wikipedia, for example.

There is also the question of intellectual property rights. Free distribution of model source code could reduce incentives to further work. On the other hand, open publication of source code could increase its value by raising visibility. The *Annals* commentary argued that, perhaps more important, routine open publication of simulation models could finally elevate this type of work to the status of "science," ultimately boosting its credibility. That, combined with the potential for extending the utility of the underlying simulation models, could enhance the value of the services offered by the original model authors while informing health policy and individual care decisions for the greater good.

---

[1] Emerson, J., Bacon, R., Kent, A., Neumann, P.J., and Cohen, J.T. 2019. "Publication of decision model source code: Attitudes of health economics authors." *Pharmacoeconomics* 37 (11): 1409–1410. https://doi.org/10.1007/s40273-019-00796-3.

[2] Ioannidis, J.P.A. 2005. "Why most published research findings are false." *PLOS Medicine* 2 (8): e124. https://doi.org/10.1371/journal.pmed.0020124.

[3] Donoho, D.L., Maleki, A., Rahman, I.U., Shahram, M., and Stodden, V. 2009. "Reproducible research in computational harmonic analysis." *Computing in Science & Engineering* 11 (1): 8–18. https://doi.org/10.1109/MCSE.2009.15.

[4] Teerawattananon, Y., Tantivess, S., Yamabhai, I., Tritasavit, N., Walker, D.G., Cohen, J.T., and Neumann, P.J. 2016. "The influence of cost-per-DALY information in health prioritisation and desirable features for a registry: A survey of health policy experts in Vietnam, India and Bangladesh." *Health Research Policy and Systems* 14 (1): 86. https://doi.org/10.1186/s12961-016-0156-6.

---

have argued that for value assessment, simply describing the computer simulation models used to project costs and health outcomes is insufficient because doing so does not provide enough detail to eliminate ambiguity and facilitate reproduction of the original work (see Box 9.5). Health technology assessment organizations should also publish the computer "source code" (i.e., the computer model's human-readable instructions).[78] That information would make it possible for others to reproduce the original work and then investigate the impact of alternative assumptions on the model's projections. Because others could conduct their own sensitivity analyses, they would not be dependent on the original authors' judgments about which plausible alternative assumptions are worthy of testing. If a model's predictions prove robust following a good "kicking of the tires" by outsiders, the model would gain credibility.

Stakeholders must also believe that the assessment organization's *process* is legitimate. A private organization—such as ICER—enhances its legitimacy in assessing benefits and costs that are matters of scientific judgment when external parties have an opportunity to present counter arguments to ICER's analysis. On the other hand, ICER, like other private assessment organizations, lacks standing for the purpose of deciding how much people are willing to pay for health (QALYs). This kind of value judgment is properly left to the public and private health plans that are accountable to the populations for which they are making these judgments. The implication is that private health technology assessment organizations can legitimately *report* cost-effectiveness estimates but should refrain from drawing conclusions about whether that ratio represents "good" or "bad" value and what price should be charged to align a drug's cost with value.

References

1. "Our members." *International Society for Pharmacoeconomics and Outcomes Research.* Accessed June 28, 2020. https://www.ispor.org/about/our-members.
2. "Organizational members." *Health Technology Assessment international.* Accessed June 5, 2020. https://htai.org/membership/organizational-members/.
3. Gold, M.E., Siegel, J.E., Russell, L.B., and Weinstein, M.C. 1996. *Cost-effectiveness in health and medicine* (1st ed.). New York: Oxford University Press.
4. Neumann, P.J., Sanders, G.D., Russell, L.B., Siegel, J.E., and Ganiats, T.G. 2017. *Cost-effectiveness in health and medicine* (2nd ed.). New York: Oxford University Press.
5. Kim, D.D., Silver, M.C., Kunst, N., Cohen, J.T., Ollendorf, D.A., and Neumann, P.J. 2020. "Perspective and costing in cost-effectiveness analysis, 1974–2018." *PharmacoEconomics* 38, 1135–1145. https://doi.org/10.1007/s40273-020-00942-2.
6. Hilton, D.M. 2020. "Letter to Ashley Rhoades, Senior Associate, Regulatory Affairs, Gilead Sciences, Inc." *U.S. Food & Drug Administration.*
7. Beigel, J.H., Tomashek, K.M., Dodd, L.E., Mehta, A.K., Zingman, B.S., Kalil, A.C., Hohmann, E., Chu, H.Y., Luetkemeyer, A., Kline, S., Lopez de Castilla, D., Finberg, R.W., Dierberg, K., Tapson, V., Hsieh, L., Patterson, T.F., Paredes, R., Sweeney, D.A., Short, W.R., Touloumi, G., . . . Lane, H.C. 2020. "Remdesivir for the treatment of covid-19—preliminary report." *New England Journal of Medicine* 383: 1813–1826. https://doi.org/10.1056/NEJMoa2007764.
8. Whittington, M.D., and Campbell, J.D. 2020. "Alternative pricing models for remdesivir and other potential treatments for COVID-19." *Institute for Clinical and Economic Review.* Accessed January 25, 2021. https://icer.org/wp-content/uploads/2020/10/ICER-COVID_Initial_Abstract_05012020.pdf

9. Cohen, J.T., Neumann, P.J., and Ollendorf, D.A. 2020, May 20. "Valuing and pricing remdesivir: Should drug makers get paid for helping us get back to work?" *Health Affairs*. https://www.healthaffairs.org/do/10.1377/hblog20200518.966027/full/.

10. "No time to wait: Securing the future from drug-resistant infections: Report to the secretary-general of the United Nations." 2019. *Interagency Coordination Group on Antimicrobial Resistance*. https://www.who.int/antimicrobial-resistance/interagency-coordination-group/IACG_final_report_EN.pdf?ua=1.

11. "Euro to US dollar spot exchange rates for 2019." *ExchangeRates*. Last modified July 27, 2020. Accessed July 5, 2020. https://www.exchangerates.org.uk/EUR-USD-spot-exchange-rates-history-2019.html.

12. Dutmer, A.L., Schiphorst Preuper, H.R., Soer, R., Brouwer, S., Bültmann, U., Dijkstra, P.U., Coppes, M.H., Stegeman, P., Buskens, E., van Asselt, A.D.I., Wolff, A.P., and Reneman, M.F. 2019. "Personal and societal impact of low back pain: The Groningen spine cohort." *Spine* 44 (24): E1443–E1451. https://doi.org/10.1097/brs.0000000000003174.

13. Greenberg, P.E., Fournier, A.-A., Sisitsky, T., Pike, C.T., and Kessler, R.C. 2015. "The economic burden of adults with major depressive disorder in the United States (2005 and 2010)." *Journal of Clinical Psychiatry* 76 (2): 155–162.

14. Hurd, M.D., Martorell, P., Delavande, A., Mullen, K.J., and Langa, K.M. 2013. "Monetary costs of dementia in the United States." *New England Journal of Medicine* 368 (14): 1326–1334. https://doi.org/10.1056/NEJMsa1204629.

15. Rhyan, C.N. 2017. "The potential societal benefit of eliminating opioid overdoses, deaths, and substance use disorders exceeds $95 billion per year." *Center for Value in Health Care*. https://altarum.org/sites/default/files/uploaded-publication-files/Research-Brief_Opioid-Epidemic-Economic-Burden.pdf.

16. Neumann, P.J., and Cohen, J.T. 2018. "QALYs in 2018—advantages and concerns." *JAMA* 319 (24): 2473–2474. https://doi.org/10.1001/jama.2018.6072.

17. Perfetto, E.M. 2018. "ISPOR's initiative on US value assessment frameworks: A missed opportunity for ISPOR and patients." *Value in Health* 21 (2): 169–170. https://doi.org/10.1016/j.jval.2017.12.002.

18. Coelho, T. 2018. "Congress must protect health care access from being denied based on flawed analysis." *The Hill*. Accessed May 15, 2020. https://thehill.com/opinion/healthcare/379351-congress-must-protect-patients-from-being-denied-access-to-care-based-on.

19. Smith, W.S. 2019. "The U.S. shouldn't use the 'QALY' in drug cost-effectiveness reviews." *STAT*. Accessed July 19, 2020. https://www.statnews.com/2019/02/22/qaly-drug-effectiveness-reviews/.

20. "ICER uses QALYs to evaluate health care. Here's why that's bad for patients." 2019. *ICERWatch*. Accessed July 19, 2020. https://icerwatch.org/icer-qaly-bad-for-patients/.

21. Doshi, J.A., Sonet, E.M., Puckett, J.T., and Glick, H. 2018, March 19. "The need for a new patient-centered decision tool for value-based treatment choices in oncology." *Health Affairs*. http://healthaffairs.org/do/10.1377/hblog20180309.241877/full/.

22. Nord, E., Richardson, J., Street, A., Kuhse, H., and Singer, P. 1995. "Maximizing health benefits vs egalitarianism: An Australian survey of health issues." *Social Science & Medicine* 41 (10): 1429–1437. https://doi.org/10.1016/0277-9536(95)00121-M.

23. Linley, W.G., and Hughes, D.A. 2013. "Societal views on NICE, cancer drugs fund and value-based pricing criteria for prioritising medicines: A cross-sectional survey of 4118 adults in Great Britain." *Health Economics* 22 (8): 948–964. https://doi.org/10.1002/hec.2872.

24. Lakdawalla, D.N., and Phelps, C.E. 2020. "Health technology assessment with risk aversion in health." *Journal of Health Economics* 72: 102346. https://doi.org/10.1016/j.jhealeco.2020.102346.

25. Taylor, M., Chilton, S., Ronaldson, S., Metcalf, H., and Nielsen, J.S. 2017. "Comparing increments in utility of health: An individual-based approach." *Value in Health* 20 (2): 224–229. https://doi.org/10.1016/j.jval.2016.12.009.

26. Lakdawalla, D.N., Doshi, J.A., Garrison, L.P., Jr., Phelps, C.E., Basu, A., and Danzon, P.M. 2018. "Defining elements of value in health care—a health economics approach: An ISPOR Special Task Force report." *Value in Health* 21 (2): 131–139. https://doi.org/10.1016/j.jval.2017.12.007.

27. "End of life care for adults." 2011. *National Institute for Health and Care Excellence*. Last modified March 7, 2017. Accessed July 24, 2020. https://www.nice.org.uk/guidance/qs13.

28. Neumann, P.J., Cohen, J.T., Hammitt, J.K., Concannon, T.W., Auerbach, H.R., Fang, C., and Kent, D.M. 2012. "Willingness-to-pay for predictive tests with no immediate treatment implications: A survey of US residents." *Health Economics* 21 (3): 238–251. https://doi.org/10.1002/hec.1704.

29. Lakdawalla, D.N., Romley, J.A., Sanchez, Y., Maclean, J.R., Penrod, J.R., and Philipson, T. 2012. "How cancer patients value hope and the implications for cost-effectiveness assessments of high-cost cancer therapies." *Health Affairs* 31 (4). https://doi.org/10.1377/hlthaff.2011.1300.

30. Lin, P.-J., Concannon, T.W., Greenberg, D., Cohen, J.T., Rossi, G., Hille, J., Auerbach, H.R., Fang, C.-H., Nadler, E.S., and Neumann, P.J. 2013. "Does framing of cancer survival affect perceived value of care? A willingness-to-pay survey of US residents." *Expert Review of Pharmacoeconomics & Outcomes Research* 13 (4): 513–522. https://doi.org/10.1586/14737167.2013.814948.

31. Shafrin, J., Schwartz, T.T., Okoro, T., and Romley, J.A. 2017. "Patient versus physician valuation of durable survival gains: Implications for value framework assessments." *Value in Health* 20 (2): 217–223. https://doi.org/10.1016/j.jval.2016.11.028.

32. Snider, J.T., Romley, J.A., Vogt, W.B., and Philipson, T.J. 2012. "The option value of innovation." *Forum for Health Economics & Policy* 15 (2). https://doi.org/10.1515/1558-9544.1306.

33. Garrison, L.P., Pauly, M.V., Willke, R.J., and Neumann, P.J. 2018. "An overview of value, perspective, and decision context—a health economics approach: An ISPOR special task force report." *Value in Health* 21 (2): 124–130. https://doi.org/10.1016/j.jval.2017.12.006.

34. Phelps, C.E., Lakdawalla, D.N., Basu, A., Drummond, M.F., Towse, A., and Danzon, P.M. 2018. "Approaches to aggregation and decision making—a health economics approach: An ISPOR special task force report." *Value in Health* 21 (2): 146–154. https://doi.org/10.1016/j.jval.2017.12.010.

35. Cookson, R., Mirelman, A.J., Griffin, S., Asaria, M., Dawkins, B., Norheim, O.F., Verguet, S., and J. Culyer, A. 2017. "Using cost-effectiveness analysis to address health equity concerns." *Value in Health* 20 (2): 206–212. https://doi.org/10.1016/j.jval.2016.11.027.

36. Brock, D.W., Daniels, N., Neumann, P.J., and Siegel, J.E. 2017. "Ethical and distributive considerations." In *Cost-effectiveness in health and medicine*, edited by P.J. Neumann, G.D. Sanders, L.B. Russell, J.E. Siegel and T.G. Ganiats, 319–342. New York: Oxford University Press.

37. Truog, R.D., Mitchell, C., and Daley, G.Q. 2020. "The toughest triage: Allocating Ventilators in a pandemic." *New England Journal of Medicine* 382 (21): 1973–1975. https://doi.org/10.1056/NEJMp2005689.

38. "Ethical principles in the allocation of human organs." 2015. *U.S. Department of Health & Human Services*. https://optn.transplant.hrsa.gov/resources/ethics/ethical-principles-in-the-allocation-of-human-organs/.

39. Ladin, K., and Hanto, D.W. 2017. "Are geographic differences in transplantation inherently wrong?" *Current Opinion in Organ Transplantation* 22 (2): 174–178 https://journals.lww.com/co-transplantation/Fulltext/2017/04000/Are_geographic_differences_in_transplantation.15.aspx.

40. Verguet, S. 2013. "Efficient and equitable HIV prevention: A case study of male circumcision in South Africa." *Cost Effectiveness and Resource Allocation* 11 (1): 1. https://doi.org/10.1186/1478-7547-11-1.

41. Nord, E. 2015. "Cost-value analysis of health interventions: Introduction and update on methods and preference data." *PharmacoEconomics* 33 (2): 89–95. https://doi.org/10.1007/s40273-014-0212-4.

42. "Cost-effectiveness, the QALY, and the evLYG." n.d. *Institute for Clinical and Economic Review*. Accessed January 25, 2021. https://icer.org/our-approach/methods-process/cost-effectiveness-the-qaly-and-the-evlyg/.

43. Basu, A., Carlson, J., and Veenstra, D. 2020. "Health years in total: A new health objective function for cost-effectiveness analysis." *Value in Health* 23 (1): 96–103. https://doi.org/10.1016/j.jval.2019.10.014.

44. Shafrin, J., and Venkatachalam, M. 2020, July 15. "Creating incentives to narrow the gap in health outcomes: Expanding value assessment to incorporate health inequality." *Health Affairs*. https://www.healthaffairs.org/do/10.1377/hblog20200708.876257/full/.

45. Verguet, S., Laxminarayan, R., and Jamison, D.T. 2015. "Universal public finance of tuberculosis treatment in India: An extended cost-effectiveness analysis." *Health Economics* 24 (3): 318–332. https://doi.org/10.1002/hec.3019.

46. Asaria, M., Griffin, S., and Cookson, R. 2016. "Distributional cost-effectiveness analysis: A tutorial." *Medical Decision Making* 36 (1): 8–19.

47. Verguet, S., Kim, J.J., and Jamison, D.T. 2016. "Extended cost-effectiveness analysis for health policy assessment: A tutorial." *PharmacoEconomics* 34 (9): 913–923. https://link.springer.com/article/10.1007/s40273-016-0414-z.

48. Devlin, N.J., and Sussex, J. 2011. "Incorporating multiple criteria in HTA: Methods and processes." *Office of Health Economics*. https://www.ohe.org/publications/incorporating-multiple-criteria-hta-methods-and-processes#.

49. Marsh, K., Lanitis, T., Neasham, D., Orfanos, P., and Caro, J. 2014. "Assessing the value of healthcare interventions using multi-criteria decision analysis: A review of the literature." *PharmacoEconomics* 32 (4): 345–365. https://doi.org/10.1007/s40273-014-0135-0.

50. Nord, E. 2018. "Beyond QALYs: Multi-criteria based estimation of maximum willingness to pay for health technologies." *The European Journal of Health Economics* 19 (2): 267–275. https://doi.org/10.1007/s10198-017-0882-x.

51. Angelis, A., Linch, M., Montibeller, G., Molina-Lopez, T., Zawada, A., Orzel, K., Arickx, F., Espin, J., and Kanavos, P. 2020. "Multiple criteria decision analysis for HTA across four EU member states: Piloting the advance value framework." *Social Science & Medicine* 246: 112595. https://doi.org/10.1016/j.socscimed.2019.112595.

52. Guindo, L.A., Wagner, M., Baltussen, R., Rindress, D., van Til, J., Kind, P., and Goetghebeur, M.M. 2012. "From efficacy to equity: Literature review of decision criteria for resource allocation and healthcare decisionmaking." *Cost Effectiveness and Resource Allocation* 10 (1): 9. https://doi.org/10.1186/1478-7547-10-9.

53. Neumann, P.J., Kim, D.D., Trikalinos, T.A., Sculpher, M.J., Salomon, J.A., Prosser, L.A., Owens, D.K., Meltzer, D.O., Kuntz, K.M., Krahn, M., Feeny, D., Basu, A., Russell, L.B., Siegel, J.E., Ganiats, T.G., and Sanders, G.D. 2018. "Future directions for cost-effectiveness analyses in health and medicine." *Medical Decision Making* 38 (7): 767–777. https://doi.org/10.1177/0272989X18798833.

54. Singer, P. 2009. Why we must ration health care. *The New York Times Magazine.* https://www.nytimes.com/2009/07/19/magazine/19healthcare-t.html.
55. Brayshaw, S. 2019. "Cystic fibrosis: Life expectancy." *National Jewish Health.* Accessed August 18, 2020. https://www.nationaljewish.org/conditions/cystic-fibrosis-cf/life-expectancy.
56. MacKenzie, T., Gifford, A.H., Sabadosa, K.A., Quinton, H.B., Knapp, E.A., Goss, C.H., and Marshall, B.C. 2014. "Longevity of patients with cystic fibrosis in 2000 to 2010 and beyond: Survival analysis of the cystic fibrosis foundation patient registry." *Annals of Internal Medicine* 161 (4): 233–241. https://doi.org/10.7326/M13-0636.
57. Balk, E.M., Trikalinos, T.A., Mickle, K., Cramer, G., Chapman, R., Khan, S., Ollendorf, D.A., and Pearson, S.D. 2018. "Modulator treatments for cystic fibrosis: Effectiveness and value." *Institute for Clinical and Economic Review.* Accessed January 25, 2021. https://icer.org/wp-content/uploads/2020/09/CF_Final_Evidence_Report_06082018.pdf.
58. Cahill, J.R. 2018. "Re: Response to ICER draft evidence report by Vertex Pharmaceuticals concerning ivacaftor (KALYDECO®), lumacaftor/ivacaftor (ORKAMBI®), and tezacaftor/ivacaftor (SYMDEKO™)." *Institute for Clinical and Economic Review.* Accessed January 25, 2021. https://icer.org/wp-content/uploads/2020/09/CF_Draft_Report_Public_Comments_04242018.pdf.
59. "Cystic fibrosis: Response to public comments on draft evidence report." 2018. *Institute for Clinical and Economic Review.* Accessed January 25, 2021. https://icer.org/wp-content/uploads/2020/09/Cystic_Fibrosis_Response_to_Comments_05032018.pdf.
60. Kolchinsky, P. 2019. *The great American drug deal.* Boston: Evelexa Press.
61. "The case for competition." 2019. *Association of Accessible Medicines.* https://accessiblemeds.org/sites/default/files/2019-09/AAM-2019-Generic-Biosimilars-Access-and-Savings-US-Report-WEB.pdf.
62. Garrison, L.P., and Towse, A. 2017. "Value-based pricing and reimbursement in personalised healthcare: Introduction to the basic health economics." *Journal of Personalized Medicine* 7 (3): 10. https://doi.org/10.3390/jpm7030010.
63. Goldman, D., and Jena, A.B. 2017. "Value-based drug pricing makes sense, but is difficult to pull off." *USC Schaeffer: Leonard D. Schaeffer Center for Health Policy & Economics.* https://healthpolicy.usc.edu/article/value-based-drug-pricing-makes-sense-but-is-difficult-to-pull-off/.
64. National Academies of Sciences, E., and Medicine. 2018. *Making medicines affordable: A national imperative,* edited by N.R. Augustine, G. Madhavan, and S.J. Nass. Washington, DC: The National Academies Press.
65. Wineinger, N.E., Zhang, Y., and Topol, E.J. 2019. "Trends in prices of popular brand-name prescription drugs in the United States." *JAMA Network Open* 2 (5): e194791. https://doi.org/10.1001/jamanetworkopen.2019.4791.
66. Liu, A. 2018. "From old behemoth Lipitor to new king Humira: Best-selling U.S. drugs over 25 years." *Fierce Pharma.* https://www.fiercepharma.com/pharma/from-old-behemoth-lipitor-to-new-king-humira-u-s-best-selling-drugs-over-25-years#:~:text=Though.
67. Crismaru, I., Pantea Stoian, A., and Bratu, O.G., et al. 2020. "Low-density lipoprotein cholesterol lowering treatment: The current approach." *Lipids in Health and Disease* 19. https://lipidworld.biomedcentral.com/articles/10.1186/s12944-020-01275-x.
68. Cohen, J.T., Chambers, J.D., Silver, M.C., Lin, P.-J., and Neumann, P.J. 2019, September 4. "Putting the costs and benefits of new gene therapies into perspective." *Health Affairs Blog: Considering Health Spending.* https://www.healthaffairs.org/do/10.1377/hblog20190827.553404/full/.
69. Yu, J.S., Chin, L., Oh, J., and Farias, J. 2017. "Performance-based risk-sharing arrangements for pharmaceutical products in the United States: A systematic review." *Journal of*

Managed Care & Specialty Pharmacy 23 (10): 1028–1040. https://doi.org/10.18553/jmcp.2017.23.10.1028.

70. Goodman, C., Villarivera, C., Gregor, K., and van Bavel, J. 2019. "Regulatory, policy, and operational considerations for outcomes-based risk-sharing agreements in the U.S. market: Opportunities for reform." *Journal of Managed Care & Specialty Pharmacy* 25 (11): 1174–1181. https://doi.org/10.18553/jmcp.2019.19167.

71. Carlson, J.J., Gries, K.S., Yeung, K., Sullivan, S.D., and Garrison, L.P., Jr. 2014. "Current status and trends in performance-based risk-sharing arrangements between healthcare payers and medical product manufacturers." *Applied Health Economics and Health Policy* 12 (3): 231–238. https://doi.org/10.1007/s40258-014-0093-x.

72. PhRMA. 2019, June 7. "Value-based contracts: 2009–Q2 2019." http://phrma-docs.phrma.org/files/dmfile/PhRMA_ValueBasedContracts_Q2_2019.pdf.

73. Neumann, P.J., Chambers, J.D., Simon, F., and Meckley, L.M. 2011. "Risk-sharing arrangements that link payment for drugs to health outcomes are proving hard to implement." *Health Affairs* 30 (12): 2329–2337. https://doi.org/10.1377/hlthaff.2010.1147.

74. Centers for Medicare & Medicaid Services. 2020. "Medicaid program; establishing minimum standards in Medicaid state drug utilization review (DUR) and supporting value-based purchasing (VBP) for drugs covered in Medicaid, revising Medicaid drug rebate and third party liability (TPL) requirements." *Department of Health and Human Services.* https://s3.amazonaws.com/public-inspection.federalregister.gov/2020-12970.pdf.

75. Ollendorf, D.A., Migliaccio-Walle, K., Colby, J.A., and Pearson, S.D. 2012. "Anti-vascular endothelial growth factor treatment for diabetic macular edema." *Institute for Clinical and Economic Review.* Accessed January 25, 2021. https://www.cms.gov/Medicare/Coverage/DeterminationProcess/downloads/id85TA.pdf.

76. "ICER to assess cost-effectiveness of trained service dogs for Americans with PTSD." 2020. *Institute for Clinical and Economic Review.* https://icer.org/announcements/ptsd_service_dogs_announcement/.

77. Phelps, C.E. 2020. "A new centralized HTA assessment organization: Need, purposes, governance, and funding." University of Rochester working paper.

78. Cohen, J.T., Neumann, P.J., and Wong, J.B. 2017. "A call for open-source cost-effectiveness analysis." *Annals of Internal Medicine* 167 (6): 432–433. https://doi.org/10.7326/M17-1153. https://www.acpjournals.org/doi/abs/10.7326/M17-1153.

10
Aligning Prices With Value

Two Views on Prices

"Obscure Model Puts a Price on Good Health and Drives Down Drug Costs,"
proclaimed a 2019 *Wall Street Journal* headline.[1] The "obscure model" referred to cost effectiveness analyses conducted by the Institute for Clinical
and Economic Review (ICER). The headline seemed to confirm the faith of
ICER's supporters that value measurement could slow the onslaught of drug
price increases.

ICER's findings, some of which appear in Table 6.1 in Chapter 6 of this
book, seem to support the cause. To be sure, the organization has occasionally
concluded that even some pricey treatments (e.g., emicizumab to treat hemophilia A) can save money because they replace even costlier therapies. But
many of the drugs listed in Table 6.1 have cost-effectiveness ratios above conventional value benchmarks ($100,000 or $150,000 per quality-adjusted life-
year gained [QALY]). Reducing prices to meet those standards could make
drugs more affordable, while simultaneously preserving sufficient pricing signals to future innovators. As the Laura and John Arnold Foundation declared
when announcing its second round of support for ICER in 2017, "ICER
can help stakeholders build a system in which payers, policymakers, drug
manufacturers, and others collaborate to bring new drugs to market in a way
that allows for optimal patient access, without creating unsustainable strains
on health care budgets."[2]

As we have seen, ICER's assessments can be controversial. Most receive substantial criticism, usually from drug companies. But even if we parked those
objections and imagined that everyone agreed that ICER correctly measured
drug value and that pharmaceutical companies set prices accordingly, key
challenges posed by drug costs would remain.

As Chapter 3 of this volume explained, few of the popular proposals to address drug costs mention specific valuation approaches like cost-effectiveness
analysis, and those that do tend to list it as a secondary component. Many

The Right Price. Peter J. Neumann, Joshua T. Cohen, and Daniel A. Ollendorf, Oxford University Press (2021).
© Peter J. Neumann, Joshua T. Cohen, and Daniel A. Ollendorf. DOI: 10.1093/oso/9780197512883.003.0010

stakeholders seem to reject value assessment as a key remedy or argue that it represents an incomplete solution because it does not address fundamental issues of access and affordability. Revisiting Table 6.1 in Chapter 6 of this volume, it is clear that even the value-based prices remain out of reach for the vast majority of Americans.

If there existed a Rorschach test for drug prices, it might conjure one of two images. Some people might perceive prices as a compass directing companies to invest in products that people value most. Aligning prices with value is akin to a "true north" orientation of the compass's arrow. Failure to link prices with value sends misleading signals to drug producers.

Others might regard drug prices as a wall preventing patients from accessing the drugs they need. For them, the barrier should be as low as possible. But aligning prices with value might have little effect in lowering the wall. How then to accomplish that goal?

Cost-Plus Pricing to Maximize Access

Focusing on access rather than value does not, of course, mean lowering drug prices to zero. One option for improving affordability is "cost-plus" or "cost recovery" pricing in which product manufacturers are reimbursed to cover their production and distribution costs, and, possibly, their added research and development (R&D) costs.[3,4] Reimbursement may also include a mutually agreed upon "fair profit" mark-up. The idea has obvious appeal: in times of crisis, governments might take exceptional actions such as paying essential producers with cost-plus pricing to ensure access to treatments, tests, or vaccines at low cost for millions of Americans who need them.[5] Even in normal times, such pricing is appealing, as it assures that manufacturers can cover their costs, while prohibiting exploitative "excess" profits.

The concept is not new. Federal contracts from the Department of Defense, Centers for Disease Control and Prevention, and other agencies often follow a "cost-reimbursable" arrangement.[6] The War Powers Act and its successor, the Defense Production Act, allow the president broad authority to redirect domestic production during times of crisis.[7] Governments have deployed cost-recovery models in low- and middle-income settings for decades,[8] enabling cash-strapped health systems to provide access to treatments and manufacturers to receive predictable revenues without risking operating losses.[8] But cost recovery models have seldom been used for drugs in the United States. One exception is a rarely used US Food and Drug Administration (FDA) provision to cover the cost of investigational drugs to allow clinical trial continuation.[9] Another is FDA's authority to grant orphan drug designation to therapies for common conditions if it determines sales will not cover costs.[10]

Some have argued for a cost-recovery pricing system as a way to limit drug costs. But the model has limitations. For one, the approach requires an estimation of costs, which can be difficult to calculate (e.g., a company's research investment on an early compound may generate knowledge that leads to a follow-on compound, but how to apportion the costs?). More important, this approach might not succeed in reducing cost growth. The Centers for Medicare and Medicaid Services (CMS) abandoned its cost-plus reimbursement of hospitals in the early 1980s because hospital spending grew rapidly after the creation of the Medicare program in 1965.[11] That outcome should not surprise. If hospitals, drug companies, or other parties know that their costs will be reimbursed, they have little incentive to restrain expenses. Critically, because cost-plus pricing guarantees payment regardless of a therapy's effects on health outcomes, it provides drug firms less incentive to produce game-changing products. For drug companies, a less risky and still lucrative strategy is to invest in "safer" products that can easily win FDA approval even if they do little to improve health.

Payments Without a Per-Person Price

If tempering drug price increases by reimbursing costs can backfire, perhaps the access problem can be addressed by altering the system that pays drug companies for each patient treated.

Prizes

One alternative to per-patient pricing is a "prize model," whereby companies that invent drugs meeting prespecified criteria receive a large, upfront payment from the government. Because drug developers have no marketing exclusivity under a prize system, other suppliers can quickly enter the marketplace, with ensuing competition driving a drug's price to affordable levels.[12p171] That competition and the resulting low prices obviate the need to assess value for the purpose of setting a price. A variant on this approach, called the Health Impact Fund, rewards innovators based on how much health their drug confers, while holding prices to the cost of manufacturing over the long term.[13] The priority review voucher program, created by Congress in

2007, is yet another kind of award-based approach; under the program, companies that develop drugs for neglected or rare pediatric diseases receive a bonus priority review voucher to be used for another drug.[14]

The prize approach offers two potential advantages. First, it may improve patient access to drugs by reducing prices.[15] Second, whereas traditional approaches reward drug firms via total sales and thus tend to provide incentives for companies to focus on diseases affecting large populations, prizes facilitate more fine-tuned government control over incentives. For example, the government can grant rewards in areas with weak incentives for companies to invest (e.g., new antibiotics, treatments for diseases affecting small populations, or critical therapies, vaccines, and diagnostics for a possible future pandemic).[4,15]

But implementation of a monetary prize involves a number of logistical complications, such as ensuring that the government sufficiently finances a prize fund, and coordinating prizes and intellectual prize rights in different countries. For instance, if the United States awards a prize for a new drug, can generic manufacturers sell copies of the drug in other countries that do not participate in the prize system?[16pp153–173] Prize models also reduce incentives for companies to invest in ongoing, incremental product improvements or in product marketing and educational campaigns.[17]

Even if these issues could be addressed, a prize-granting scheme must still determine how big a reward should be granted for each new drug. To encourage companies to' work on the most beneficial drugs, bigger prizes should be awarded for drugs that confer greater benefits. Indeed, to properly incentivize drug discovery and development, the size of the prize should correspond to the value of the drug's benefit. Measuring that value depends on accounting for the drug's impact on quality and length of life, as well as other effects, such as offsets to future care costs. In short, prize models do not sidestep the need to measure value; they simply shift the terms.

The "Netflix" Model

Five years after the introduction of highly effective treatments for hepatitis C in 2013, only 15% of the infected population had access.[18] The therapies' limited use stemmed in part from the dependence of many eligible patients on budget-constrained state Medicaid programs or prison healthcare systems. Despite the large number of potential customers, drug companies did not reduce prices to expand access, apparently because they could maximize profits by treating a small number of people at high per-person prices. As a remedy, some policymakers proposed a "subscription model" as an alternative.

A subscription approach addresses access problems by replacing per-person payments with a single fee to cover the entire population, regardless of how many people ultimately receive treatment.[19] The arrangement is often termed the "Netflix model" after the video streaming service, which charges a fixed monthly fee no matter how many movies or television shows a subscriber views.[19] And as Netflix makes "binge viewing" more prevalent than if viewers paid an incremental fee for each film or TV series episode viewed, a subscription drug plan can make drugs more widely accessible. Because the subscriber pays no additional fee for each movie or episode, they keep viewing. Similarly, under a subscription drug plan, even people who place limited value on a drug—or have limited capacity to pay for it—will use it because they incur no (or very little) incremental cost. Crucially, as Box 10.1 illustrates, compared to per-person pricing, a subscription approach can increase access without diminishing the drug company's financial return and hence without weakening incentives for companies to invest in the development of similar drugs in the future.

As described in Box 10.1, the subscription drug model improves access only under certain conditions. First, the amount people can afford to pay for the drug must vary so much that over a range of prices, some people would acquire the drug while others cannot. If everyone could afford the same amount, the drug company would set that amount as the drug's price, everyone would have access to it, and there would be no room for the subscription model to increase access further.

Second, even if the amount people can afford varies, the drug company must not be able to engage in "price discrimination" (i.e., setting different prices based on ability to pay). If the drug company can price discriminate, it could make the drug affordable to everyone by charging each a "customized price." Again, there would no room for a subscription model to increase access further.

Finally, incremental production costs must be small relative to a drug's price (as tends to be the case for small molecule drugs). With large incremental production costs, an open-ended subscription model would drive up the drug company's costs without compensating it with greater revenues. Without some sort of revenue adjustment, it would discourage the development of drugs with high incremental production costs.

Under the right conditions—varying ability to pay, no possibility for price discrimination, and low incremental production costs—the Netflix model has advantages. The fixed payments reduce uncertainty for both payers and drug

Box 10.1 Subscription (Netflix) Drug Payment Models

Appreciating how a subscription drug model increases access while preserving appropriate incentives for innovators depends on understanding how drug companies would set a per-person drug price to maximize their profits. Assuming that incremental production costs are low (as is typically the case for small molecule drugs), profits are essentially equal to revenues. Profits thus reflect the product of the drug's per-person price and the number of people who receive treatment. Consider a stylized example in which all patients can pay the same amount for the drug. In this case, the drug company will set the price equal to what everyone can afford. For example, if there are 1,000 patients and each patient can afford to pay $1,000, then the drug company will charge $1,000 for the drug and earn $1,000,000.

But suppose some patients can afford to pay more or less than $1,000 for the drug. For example, suppose that 500 patients can pay $1,500 and the other 500 can pay $500. If the drug company charges $1,500 per person treated, the first group of 500 patients will purchase the drug, and total revenues (and profits) will be $750,000. If the drug company wants all 1,000 patients to purchase the drug, it must lower the per-person price to $500. At that price, total revenue (and profits) will be $500,000. So the drug company maximizes profits by charging the higher amount of $1,500 per patient, but 500 of the 1,000 patients cannot access the treatment.

The Netflix subscription model improves the situation by capitalizing on the fact that the company cannot do better than earning $750,000 (by charging $1,500 per patient and selling drugs to half of the patients) and by setting subscription fees to supply the entire population equal to those maximum earnings. Under the model, the drug company earns the same $750,000 it would have earned had it maximized profits under a per-person-treated pricing scheme, but instead of providing drugs to only 500 patients, all 1,000 patients receive the therapy.

Understanding how the Netflix model works also sheds light on how it can fail to improve on conventional per-person pricing. Consider the following thought experiment. First, imagine everyone can afford the same price for a drug. In that case, the drug company will set the price at that level, everyone pays that price, and access to the drug is universal. The Netflix model cannot further expand access. For instance, imagine as in the previous example, that everyone places a value of $1,000 on the drug. Setting the price at $1,000 means that all 1,000 individuals will pay $1,000, yielding revenue of $1,000,000. The drug company will not accept a subscription price below $1,000,000, so the Netflix plan cannot reduce payer costs. Nor can it improve on access, which is already 100%.

Second, suppose the drug company can engage in "price discrimination"—that is, setting different prices for different individuals based on each individual's ability to pay. In this case, it will charge each person the value they place on the drug. Staying with the example, this would mean charging the first 500 people $1,500 per person and charging the other 500 people $500 each. Because total revenue will be $1,000,000, the drug company will not accept a subscription fee of less than $1,000,000. Nor can the subscription model increase access, which is already 100%.

Finally, if incremental production costs are large, then the subscription fee must cover not only the revenue the drug company would earn under the per-person pricing model, but also the added cost of production that accompanies the increased utilization accomplished under the Netflix model. This challenge is not insurmountable, but the plan needs to incorporate these added costs into the subscription fee offered in lieu of revenues they would have earned under conventional, per-person drug pricing.

companies and thus facilitate negotiated discounts. (Another way to achieve these aims is through advanced market commitments—see Box 10.2.) Like monetary prizes, however, the Netflix model does not preclude the need to measure value, even though it substitutes per-person prices with a subscription fee. Determination of the appropriate fee depends on estimating a drug's value for the population so that the total amount paid does not exceed the drug's value.

As long as pricing policies attempt to provide incentives to drug companies to innovate, drug value must be measured somehow so that resources can be appropriately channeled. But what if we could remove drug companies from the equation altogether, or at least diminish their role?

Reducing the Role of Drug Companies Altogether

Referring to the Prescription Drug Relief Act of 2018, filed by Vermont Senator Bernie Sanders and California Representative Ro Khanna, Dean Baker, senior economist at the Center for Economic and Policy Research in Washington, DC, called the bill "brilliant."[20] Baker explained that the legislation proposed by Sanders and Khanna would eliminate patent protection for drugs with prices exceeding those charged in seven large, affluent countries.[20] Because the threat of patent loss would effectively force companies to refrain

Box 10.2. Advanced Market Commitments

An advanced market commitment (AMC) commits a payer—often the government—to purchase a specified volume of a drug at a mutually agreed-upon price, before the product is available. These agreements typically tie pricing to R&D costs and build in an assumed profit margin. Governments have turned to AMCs to accelerate and reduce the risks around vaccine development, for example. During the 2009 H1N1 ("swine flu") pandemic, the US government purchased 250 million doses of a vaccine still in development, at a cost of about $2 billion.[1] More recently, the government struck several deals with vaccine developers to ensure adequate supplies of vaccines against COVID-19.[2,3] In one case, the US government arranged to purchase an initial 100 million doses of the Pfizer/BioNTech vaccine (which had just completed Phase I trials) for $1.95 billion, contingent on FDA approval or emergency use authorization.[4] The European Union announced similar agreements with other manufacturers.[5,6] AMCs are often subject to a multiple-bid process, allowing the government to select the companies willing to produce sufficient volume at the most favorable prices, and winning contracts typically include all phases of production, distribution, outreach, and delivery.[7]

The arrangements can help reduce a manufacturer's risks while ensuring widespread availability of products once approved. These agreements bring an expectation that once the volume commitment is reached, the purchase price will decrease to ensure widespread availability and affordability.[8] Subscription-based agreements, such as the one that Gilead struck with the state of Louisiana for hepatitis C treatments (see Box 6.1 in Chapter 6 of this volume and Box 10.1), are similar to advanced market commitments in many respects, but differ in two important ways. First, under a subscription-based agreement, the manufacturer typically agrees to provide an essentially *unlimited* supply of therapy for an agreed-upon price, rather than have that price change after volume commitments are met. Second, subscription-based agreements are more commonly employed for already-approved products with some certainty with regard to performance, manufacturing, and distribution.

---

[1] Bartlett, J.G. 2009. "2009 H1N1 influenza—just the facts: Vaccine essentials." *Medscape*. https://www.medscape.com/viewarticle/709468_5.

[2] Herper, M. 2020. "Sanofi and GSK land $2.1 billion deal with U.S. for Covid-19 vaccine development and 100 million doses." *STAT*. https://www.statnews.com/2020/07/31/operation-warp-speed-sanofi-gsk-covid19-vaccine/.

[3] Renauer, C. 2020, August 1. "5 Coronavirus vaccines with huge operation warp speed deals." *The Motley Fool*. https://www.fool.com/investing/2020/08/01/coronavirus-vaccines-funded-by-operation-warp-spee.aspx.

[4] Lupkin, S. 2020. "U.S. to get 100 million doses of Pfizer Coronavirus vaccine in $1.95 billion deal." *National Public Radio*. https://www.npr.org/sections/coronavirus-live-updates/2020/07/22/894184607/u-s-to-get-100-million-doses-of-pfizer-coronavirus-vaccine-in-1-95-billion-deal.

⁵ "Coronavirus: Commission concludes talks to secure future coronavirus vaccine for Europeans." 2020. *European Commission.* https://ec.europa.eu/commission/presscorner/detail/en/IP_20_1439.

⁶ "European commission reaches first agreement to buy potential COVID-19 vaccine." 2020, August 17. https://www.schengenvisainfo.com/news/european-commission-reaches-first-agreement-to-buy-potential-covid-19-vaccine/.

⁷ Bach, P.B., and Trusheim, M. 2020, March 17. "U.S. should buy coronavirus vaccines before they're invented." *Bloomberg Opinion.* https://www.bloomberg.com/opinion/articles/2020-03-17/the-u-s-should-buy-covid-19-vaccines-before-they-re-invented.

⁸ "Advanced market commitments for vaccines." 2006. *World Health Organization.* https://www.who.int/immunization/newsroom/amcs/en/.

from raising their prices above those international benchmarks, it amounted to the clever imposition of reference pricing (see Chapter 3 of this volume) that Baker estimated would reduce US brand drug prices in half.

But Baker hinted that he favored even more fundamental change. Instead of threatening the suspension of patent protection to restrain drug price increases, he suggested the removal of patent protection as a first-line strategy for all new drugs. He explained, "We should be looking to more modern and efficient mechanisms than patent monopolies for financing drug research. . . . If [the National Institutes of Health] paid for the research up front, then all new drugs could be sold at their free market price from day one."[20] That is, if the government directly funded drug development, it would obviate the need to maintain the patent protection that returned substantial profits to drug companies. Generic competition would start the day a drug received FDA approval, and prices would sink to a level just high enough to cover manufacturing costs, plus a standard profit margin. With free market competition dictating each drug's price, there would be no need for formal value assessments to determine a drug's "fair" price.

But how would innovation be funded if drug companies no longer earned considerable profits from the products they invented and developed? Baker suggested that the National Institutes of Health (NIH) could assume the role of drug developer. He observed that the pharmaceutical industry spends $70 billion annually on research, while the NIH's research budget is $40 billion. Dial up the government's spending to cover the extra $70 billion in corporate research funding and the United States could jettison drug companies altogether. (Baker estimated the plan would save around $370 billion per year—the amount drug companies spend on nonresearch activities.)

Baker's plan raises some practical concerns. First, his dismissal of all $370 billion of industry's nonresearch spending as superfluous prompts questions. Although some of the spending may be nonessential, it is hard to imagine that drug companies could successfully develop therapies if they relied only on the activities represented by research. For one thing, drug company spending on promotional activities, although often disliked and sometimes misleading, also plays an important role in educating physicians and the public about diseases and treatment options.[21-24]

Second, "research" is not a homogenous activity. One study found that the federal government had indeed funded research connected to all 210 "new molecular entities" approved by the FDA from 2010 to 2016.[25] But the same study found that over 90% of that government-funded research had addressed "basic research" topics—that is, the "general scientific knowledge" questions that can facilitate development of multiple therapies.[25] Because multiple companies can benefit from basic research findings, individual companies are typically reluctant to foot the bill for basic knowledge creation that could benefit their competitors (in economic parlance, that information is a "public good").[26pp91-96] For that reason, basic science research is well suited to government sponsorship. On the other hand, there are more limited spillovers ("positive externalities") from research supporting the development of a specific drug—the kind of work that is the focus of private, for-profit drug companies.

To be sure, the government provides some R&D funding for clinical research pertaining to drugs (i.e., not simply basic research). In 2010, 61% of pharmaceutical R&D spending came from the drug industry while about one third derived from federal sources (foundations and individual donors provided the remainder).[27] Public Citizen estimated that the federal government contributed approximately $70 million to the development of remdesivir, the first drug approved to treat COVID-19, for example.[28]

Some argue that because of these taxpayer-funded contributions to drug development, the government should retain some power over subsequent pricing to ensure that drugs remain affordable.[28] But such a policy would be inconsistent with other industries that likewise benefit from public investment. For example, the aerospace company, SpaceX, benefits from technology developed by NASA, and Google profits from algorithm work financed by the National Science Foundation, not to mention the federal government's early work on the development of the Internet.[29,30] The US Defense Advanced Research Project Agency spearheaded the early work on the Internet,[31,32] which now benefits companies like Amazon and Uber. Indeed, for decades, federal policy has promoted the privatization of discoveries and inventions based on publicly funded research. The Bayh–Dole Act of 1980 encourages institutions receiving federal funding to pursue technology patents, rather than requiring inventors to assign inventions to the government.[33]

Extending government pricing power based on the magnitude of its funding toward a drug's development also triggers many practical questions.

For one, it is difficult to trace the precise path between public spending and the ultimate marketed product.[34pp1-4] For another, tying the government's control over pricing to its contribution to the underlying R&D would give drug companies an incentive to increase that R&D spending, even if it is inefficiently deployed. Nor is it necessary to "recapture" the government's R&D investment on a product-by-product basis. Companies already compensate the government (at least in part) by paying taxes. Other possible remedies include giving the government an equity stake in companies that piggyback on federal research and then using the revenues for a "public innovation fund" that could subsidize more basic research.[30]

Importantly, even setting aside these concerns and adopting Baker's plan to substitute government resources for private funding of drug development, someone must still assess value because research must be prioritized. Given its finite budget, NIH must select which compounds should receive support, and those decisions should reflect both the anticipated value of each drug's benefits and some notion of the development costs.

Aligning Price With Value: What Payers Can Do

None of the previously described options avoids the need to assess drug value. Cost recovery models may reduce prices but ignore questions about whether reimbursement is associated with a product's health benefits. Prizes and subscription fees may increase access, but determining an appropriate prize or subscription fee depends on understanding a drug's value. Removing for-profit companies from the drug development process creates logistical challenges and puts the government rather than the private sector in the position of choosing winners and losers. More fundamentally, it also depends on estimating drug value so that finite public resources can be efficiently invested in research. In short, if efficiency is important, some sort of alignment of drug prices and value is unavoidable.

How to proceed? One option is for drug companies on their own to set prices to reflect value. That prospect is unlikely, however, in the complicated US pharmaceutical market with its myriad players, byzantine rules, and often perverse incentives for such alignment (Box 10.3). Nor is there a central US authority to set drug prices. Instead, pricing reflects untold deals between multiple drug companies and multiple public and private healthcare payers.

Some might wonder why the FDA does not incorporate value considerations into its drug approval process. For example, the FDA could make approval contingent on a "fair" price in the marketplace. But the FDA's statutory

Box 10.3. How Pharmaceutical Companies Actually Set Drug Prices

A common impression is that drug prices reflect "what the market will bear." And as we have seen, any particular drug may have multiple prices that vary across customers and change over time in seemingly mysterious ways (see Chapter 2 of this volume).

In fact, drug companies tend to say little about how they really set prices for their products. A Google search yields many advertisements from consultancies that promise to help companies strategically price their products, but not much detail on the methods. The models they use forecast product demand—which depends on both price and other attributes. Drug companies use this information so that they can predict revenue (the product of demand and per-person price) and profit (revenue minus cost).

There are a number of demand forecasting models used by marketing departments within drug companies and sometimes they are divided into two main categories: aggregate- and disaggregate-level models.[1] Aggregate-level models estimate market share based on "diffusion" (i.e., number of payers or physician groups that may extend the drug's preferred status) or projected unit sales across physicians, pharmacies, and hospitals. Disaggregate-level models rely on individual prescriber behavior. Prescription count and learning models, for example, use the prior prescribing patterns and preferences of individual physicians with similar drugs or drugs in the same disease area to forecast utilization of a new product.

Importantly, other models, such as choice models and conjoint analysis, model demand as a function of price and drug attributes, such as dosing frequency, mode of administration, magnitude of benefit (e.g., "high," "medium," "low"), and risks for serious side effects. Because the models predict demand based on both price and other attributes, they can be used to estimate the value of each attribute. For example, if a model predicts that demand will be unchanged for a drug with milder side effects even if the price increases by $100, then the mitigation of side effects must be worth $100.

But this kind of modeling does not necessarily result in value-based pricing. First, as described in Chapter 2 of this volume, a variety of factors that have little to do with perceived consumer (patient) value influence demand for drugs. A major factor is the role played by prescribing clinicians, whose incentives are often not perfectly aligned with the interests of their patients. Second, drug companies are motivated to maximize profits, rather than to align prices with value. Third, a strong factor seems to be the price of existing products, whether or not those drug prices are aligned with value.

It is one thing to use these modeling approaches to anticipate market share, but quite another to translate estimates from models into appropriate prices. Again, there is very little documentation on how drug companies ultimately set prices other than what those consultancies who serve the industry promise (the familiar "highest price the market will bear"). In the late 1990s, Lu and Comanor studied factors associated with US launch price levels and found that drugs conferring greater clinical benefit were generally priced higher, and those facing greater competition (i.e., those with several alternatives already available) were priced lower.[2] The situation seemed to resemble a traditional consumer market, but there are many exceptions to this behavior. For example, drugs introduced for more severe conditions command high prices regardless of the degree of competition.[3] Manufacturers may also employ a variety of "migration" strategies by temporarily lowering the prices of new agents to attract market share, only to raise prices later.[4] Another observed phenomenon is "sticky pricing," in which new competitors enter a crowded market at a premium price relative to its alternatives, after which all competitors raise their prices to meet the new entrant.[5,6] These pricing strategies may not only reflect relatively inelastic demand for certain products (e.g., cancer therapies) but also reveal the many vagaries and perverse incentives in the marketplace.

[1] Landsman, V., Verniers, I., and Stremersch, S. 2014. "The successful launch and diffusion of new therapies." In *Innovation and marketing in the pharmaceutical industry: Emerging practices, research, and policies*, edited by M. Ding, J. Eliashberg, and S. Stremersch, 189–224. New York: Springer Science and Business Media.

[2] Lu, Z.J., and Comanor, W.S. 1998. "Strategic pricing of new pharmaceuticals." *Review of Economics and Statistics* 80 (1): 108–118.

[3] Ekelund, M., and Persson, B. 2003. "Pharmaceutical pricing in a regulated market." *Review of Economics and Statistics* 85 (2): 298–306. https://doi.org/10.1162/003465303765299828.

[4] Tironi, P. 2010. "Pharmaceutical pricing: A review of proposals to improve access and affordability of prescription drugs." *Annals of Health Law* 19 (2). https://lawecommons.luc.edu/annals/vol19/iss2/4/.

[5] Hartung, D.M., Bourdette, D.N., Ahmed, S.M., and Whitham, R.H. 2015. "The cost of multiple sclerosis drugs in the US and the pharmaceutical industry: Too big to fail?" *Neurology* 84 (21): 2185–2192. https://doi.org/10.1212/WNL.0000000000001608.

[6] Rosenthal, E. 2018, June 21. "Why competition won't bring down drug prices." *New York Times*. https://www.nytimes.com/2018/06/21/opinion/competition-drug-prices.html.

authority does not extend to such matters. In theory, Congress could broaden the FDA's mandate, allowing it to consider potential drug prices and value in addition to overseeing a product's clinical profile. Such a change would be ill-advised, however. Determining whether a drug is safe and effective already taxes the FDA's resources. Moreover, diverting the FDA's attention away from clinical matters toward economic concerns risks eroding its considerable public support.

To be sure, the FDA can do more to encourage the collection of information that promotes competitive and efficient pricing. Activities include advancing more efficient trial designs (e.g., adaptive trials that revise their subject recruitment strategy based on preliminary results), ensuring that clinical trials include active comparators, making clinical trial recruitment more inclusive to reflect the ultimate target population for the drug, and requiring and enforcing the conduct of follow-on studies after a drug receives approval.[35,36] The FDA can also help reduce barriers to generic development and entry (e.g., by streamlining regulatory requirements and reducing review times).[37]

Judgments about value and reimbursement are better left to public and private payers because they are best positioned to consider their budget constraints and their enrollees' preferences. Next, we consider what steps Medicare, Medicaid, and commercial payers might take to promote value-based drug pricing.

Medicare

The federal Medicare program, responsible for 30% of retail prescription drug spending (roughly $100 billion annually), seems an ideal place for establishing value-based drug prices.[38] In addition to the leverage its large footprint affords, the program faces fiscal challenges: for example, in 2019, the US government projected that under current law, Medicare's hospital insurance fund would run out of money in 2026.[39] In fact, CMS has advanced a range of value-based payment initiatives, including accountable care organizations and bundled-payment models that place providers (e.g., hospitals and physicians) at risk for total patient costs and tie reimbursement to the quality of care those providers deliver.[40,41] Under the arrangements, hospitals and physicians have strong incentives to be cost-conscious purchasers for all services, although it still leaves open the question of how to value and price new drugs (see Box 10.4).

For Part B drugs (medications administered in a doctor's office, outpatient clinic, or similar setting), Medicare has encountered legal and political resistance to the use of cost-effectiveness analysis to inform decisions about which drugs are worthwhile (see Chapter 5 of this volume). While competing private Part D plans (for self-administered drugs) exert pressure on drug companies to reduce prices, the requirement that they cover protected drug classes undercuts their leverage, as does the program's fragmented nature (in 2020,

Box 10.4 Paying for Cost-Effective Drugs Under Medicare: CAR-T Revisited

In 2019, Medicare determined that it would pay for chimeric antigen receptor T-cell therapy (CAR-T) for advanced blood cancers for FDA-approved indications—and also for off-label uses recommended in CMS-approved compendia.[1] At around the same time, ICER concluded that the therapies were cost-effective for treatment of pediatric B-cell leukemias and for adult B-cell lymphomas that had proven resistant to most other treatments.[2] ICER's findings primarily reflected the substantial projected survival improvements that CAR-T conferred compared to either "salvage" (last-resort) chemotherapy or palliative care (no active treatment).

CAR-T therapies are expensive. The drugs themselves are priced at $373,000 to $475,000, and there are additional costs for their administration.[3] However, rather than reimbursing hospitals based on the drug's cost, Medicare reimbursed them based on its categorization of the treated patients into diagnostic-related groups (DRGs; i.e., groups that include clinically similar patients). Because hospitals receive a fixed payment for each patient in a DRG (corresponding to the average cost to treat patients in that group), they have an incentive to contain costs. As of mid-2020, hospitals received about $37,000 for each infusion episode for patients undergoing CAR-T. That reimbursement reflected their DRG classification as patients undergoing autologous cell infusion and the average cost of that procedure for patients in this DRG group over the preceding two years.

To address the mismatch between the reimbursement rate and the actual cost of treating patients with CAR-T, CMS implemented temporary "add-on payments" of up to 65% of the therapy's cost, and hospitals could further recoup some of the shortfall by seeking payment for costly "outlier" cases. But even with these adjustments, hospitals administering CAR-T stood to lose as much as hundreds of thousands of dollars for each patient.[4]

An alternative work-around for hospitals was to provide CAR-T in an outpatient setting (e.g., in an outpatient clinic). When the hospital changed the delivery setting in that way, Medicare treated CAR-T as a Part B product, a reclassification that made it eligible for reimbursement at its average sales price plus a markup (currently 4.3%). Although administration in an outpatient setting could ameliorate the reimbursement problem, most patients receive CAR-T as inpatients because of its complication risks. Moreover, even if patients received CAR-T as outpatients, a subsequent hospitalization within three days of the outpatient administration would reclassify the treatment as an inpatient procedure, eliminating the favorable outpatient reimbursement.[4]

Some observers proposed that Medicare provide supplemental payments to cover the full cost of the CAR-T therapy, based on the average sales price of competing CAR-T products, even though such a scheme would diminish incentives for drug companies to reduce their prices and for hospitals and physicians to be judicious stewards of resources. An alternative option was for Medicare to create a new CAR-T-specific DRG with a higher reimbursement rate, although that, too, would increase costs.[4] CMS pilot-tested an outcomes-based payment mechanism for CAR-T that would establish payment rates based on the type of cancer being treated (i.e., "indication-based" pricing), but Medicare ended the project after it drew objections.[5]

In 2020, CMS proposed the creation of a new DRG for CAR-T therapies to remedy the situation.[6] But similar dilemmas posed by other new and expensive therapies are on the horizon. Indeed, even use of CAR-T is expected to expand to other indications with larger populations, such as multiple myeloma. The experience illustrates the challenges of getting the incentives right in developing payment policy. It also underscores that even with improved incentives, there is still a need to measure value in the first place.

[1] "Trump administration makes CAR T-Cell cancer therapy available to Medicare beneficiaries nationwide." 2019. *Centers for Medicare & Medicaid Services.* https://www.cms.gov/newsroom/press-releases/trump-administration-makes-car-t-cell-cancer-therapy-available-medicare-beneficiaries-nationwide.

[2] "Chimeric antigen receptor T-Cell therapy for B-Cell cancers: Effectiveness and value." 2018. *Institute for Clinical and Economic Review.* https://icer.org/wp-content/uploads/2020/10/ICER_CAR_T_Final_Evidence_Report_032318.pdf.

[3] Nelson, R. 2019. "CAR T-cell therapy causes heavy financial losses for hospitals." *Medscape.* https://www.medscape.com/viewarticle/921315.

[4] Manz, C.R., Porter, D.L., and Bekelman, J.E. 2019. "Innovation and access at the mercy of payment policy: The future of chimeric antigen receptor therapies." *Journal of Clinical Oncology* 38 (5): 384–387. https://doi.org/10.1200/JCO.19.01691.

[5] Sagonowsky, E. 2018. "CMS quietly cancels plan for indication-based pricing on Novartis' Kymriah." *Fierce Pharma.* https://www.fiercepharma.com/pharma/cms-cancels-value-based-pricing-plan-novartis-kymriah-report.

[6] "CMS builds on commitment to transform healthcare through competition and innovation." 2020. *Centers for Medicare & Medicaid Services.* Last modified May, 11. https://www.cms.gov/newsroom/press-releases/cms-builds-commitment-transform-healthcare-through-competition-and-innovation.

each state or CMS region typically had 40 to 50 Medicare Part D drug plans, amounting to more than 1,400 plans countrywide).[42]

How then to change Medicare so the program can better influence drug prices? A variety of options are possible, each with challenges. One option would change the law to permit Medicare Part B drug coverage decisions to consider cost-effectiveness. Current law prohibits Medicare from paying "for any expenses incurred for items or services, which . . . are not reasonable and necessary for the diagnosis or treatment of illness or injury." Amending the statute so that it prohibits payment "for any *expenses which are unreasonable and which are incurred for items and services*" would allow CMS to consider costs and value openly (because *reasonable* would then modify the term "expenses" rather than "items and services").[43] Alternatively, Congress could revise the "reasonable and necessary" clause, possibly using language from the 2008 Medicare Improvements for Patients and Providers Act. That statute allows CMS to account for "the relation between predicted outcomes and expenditures" and thus to consider costs when making coverage decisions pertaining to *preventive* services.[44]

For Part D drugs, Congress could grant Medicare direct authority to conduct central negotiations over drug prices based on their value, thus eliminating the challenges posed by having dozens of separate plans in each state with limited market power trying to bargain. But for Medicare to negotiate from a position of strength, Congress would also have to allow the program to refuse coverage if pricing did not satisfy its value requirements. That threat, however, would undoubtedly provoke vocal objections from constituencies dependent on the drugs in question.

Another alternative would essentially grant Medicare power to impose price controls on Part B and Part D drugs. For example, some have proposed Medicare negotiations using arbitration techniques for selected high-priced drugs that have little or no competition.[45] Under the proposal, Medicare could impose substantial penalties unless a reasonable price were achieved—and here, "reasonable" could be defined to mean "value-based" (i.e., prices in line with conventional cost-effectiveness benchmarks).[45,46]

For Part B drugs with uncertain benefits, Medicare could expand use of its "coverage with evidence development" (CED) policy, which conditionally covers medical technology while it collects additional safety and efficacy evidence. As discussed in Chapter 9, CMS could use this policy to better align how much it pays for drugs based on data collected after the drug receives approval. CMS has used the CED policy for various medical devices, diagnostics, and procedures, although rarely for drugs.[47] The CED policy has proven challenging to implement, however, and is used sparingly, in part because data collection to support this designation is complex and costly.[47]

CMS adoption of value-based pricing would no doubt be difficult. To allow challenges to be addressed gradually and to facilitate implementation, the program could turn to its Center for Medicare and Medicaid Innovation, also known as the CMS Innovation Center, to test value-based payment models for drugs, as it has tested models for hospital and physician payment reforms. For example, although they encountered resistance from industry and medical groups and ultimately had to withdraw their proposal,[48] the Obama administration in 2016 proposed using the Center for Medicare and Medicaid Innovation to explore strategies to link drug payments to patient outcomes achieved.[49]

Medicaid

At first glance, Medicaid, the federal–state program that provides healthcare to some 75 million lower-income individuals, seems to represent another ideal opportunity for the government to establish value-based pricing for drugs used by a substantial portion of the US population. But Medicaid has already entered into a pricing agreement with some 600 drug manufacturers. That agreement states that in exchange for Medicaid's coverage of all products marketed by a drug company, the company agrees to provide their drugs at a discount to Medicaid. For most drugs, that discount amounts to either approximately 23% on the average manufacturer's price for that drug or the best price offered to any other insurer, whichever is lower.[50]

In some cases, the Medicaid discounts are still insufficient to align prices with value. Several states have sought waivers to the Medicaid program requirements so they could pursue steeper price reductions and more restrictive formularies in an effort to achieve value-based pricing. Some states also pursue their own legal channels. Notably, New York State enacted a law in 2017 allowing it to push for value-based drug prices below the discounted price required by the federal government whenever New York's Medicaid spending on drugs exceeds a certain benchmark. Using that law, New York negotiated supplemental price reductions for 30 drugs in 2018, saving the state a further $60 million beyond what it would have paid based on the basic discount mandated in the federal Medicaid law.

But one manufacturer—Vertex—refused to accept New York's terms. New York State had concluded that based on the drug Orkambi's health benefits for cystic fibrosis patients, Vertex should have discounted its $272,000 per year price by 70%. (New York's conclusion in large part reflected an analysis conducted by ICER, which had concluded that Orkambi's price should be reduced by 77%.)[51] New York could not impose value-based pricing, however, because without a federal waiver, CMS required it to cover Orkambi as long as Vertex offered the smaller discount specified by the federal government.[52] As of this writing, there has been no resolution of the disagreement between Vertex and New York State.

Other states are following New York's lead. For example, Massachusetts has sought to restrict coverage by its Medicaid program of drugs that do not satisfy its value criteria.[53] However, the federal government blocked this initiative. In this case, the problem was that Massachusetts had sought to receive the standard discount from each manufacturer (23% on the average manufacturer price or the best price offered to other insurers) while not itself adhering to the other half of the bargain (i.e., guaranteeing coverage for all drugs produced by each manufacturer). CMS offered Massachusetts its requested waiver (for outpatient drugs only) if the state agreed to forego the standard Medicaid discount.[54] As of 2020, that has not happened. However, in 2019, Massachusetts enacted its own law to evaluate prices that drug companies charged its state Medicaid program.[55] The law calls for Massachusetts to negotiate directly with manufacturers for supplemental rebates when the state finds those prices to be excessive or unreasonable, which is permissible without a waiver. How effective this approach will be remains an open question.

In short, although state Medicaid programs are large enough to use their leverage to establish value-based pricing, they must be able to exclude drugs from coverage so that they can compel drug companies to negotiate. But if states deny coverage to some drugs, CMS might declare those states no longer eligible for the standard 23% (or better) across-the-board discount that drug companies have agreed to in return for broad-based coverage. Even if the federal government were to refrain from insisting that states cover all drugs from companies that have agreed to offer discounts, companies might not continue to make the standard discounts available. What, after all, would they receive in return for those discounts? Perhaps the Medicaid populations are sufficiently large to keep the drug companies interested, but there is no guarantee. At some point, the states must decide if they want standard discounts on all drugs, or if they want to pursue discounting that tailors the price of each drug to that drug's value.

Commercial Insurers

Although the Medicare and Medicaid programs are large, the commercial payer sector is even larger, covering roughly two thirds of all individuals in the United States who have any sort of health insurance.[56] It is difficult to know the precise role that value-based pricing plays in the deals reached between private insurers and drug companies because neither side publicly reveals its concessions. At the very least, few insurers openly promote the use of formal value assessments to align drug prices with value.

There are exceptions. As Chapter 5 of this book noted, in 2010 Premera Blue Cross, a large regional health plan that covers parts of Washington State and

Alaska, implemented a value-based formulary benefit for its employees that assigned drugs to copayment tiers based on a drug's cost-effectiveness.[57] When using higher value drugs (i.e., those with more favorable cost-effectiveness ratios), plan enrollees pay lower copayments. For example, drugs found to be cost-saving or to have cost-effectiveness ratios less than $50,000 per QALY require a $20 copayment, while lower value drugs (with cost-effectiveness ratios exceeding $150,000 per QALY or with insufficient evidence to determine cost-effectiveness) have a $100 copayment. "Preventive drugs" have no copayment. Premera's value-based formulary has yielded encouraging results. According to evaluations, it has shifted members toward higher-value drugs and reduced health plan and total drug spending with no adverse impacts on hospitalization rates or adherence.[57,58]

Another exception is CVS Caremark, by some measures the nation's largest pharmacy benefit manager (a company that negotiates with drug manufacturers to buy medications on behalf of health insurers and employer-sponsored health plans; see Chapter 2).[59] In 2018, CVS Caremark announced to some fanfare that it would allow its client health plans to exclude coverage of high cost, "me-too" drugs (drugs that mimic the action of earlier, innovative medications) if those drugs had cost-effectiveness ratios exceeding $100,000 per QALY, as projected by ICER.[60] CVS exempted from the process drugs the FDA had designated as breakthrough therapies.

The Premera and CVS initiatives have attracted attention as vanguards of a value-based pricing movement for drugs. Notably, however, no other American health plan seems to have adopted the Premera model. Nor has the CVS plan gained much traction with customers.[61] Industry and patient advocacy groups have strongly criticized it, and CVS itself says that although it has enrolled its own employees and the employees of a few large clients, it has not widely promoted the plan.[61]

These experiences suggest that even as they report using ICER's value estimates in their drug pricing and management decisions, health plans are disinclined to adopt publicly strategies that deny or manage drugs based explicitly on cost-effectiveness considerations. Rather, they are inclined to keep value assessments at arm's length.

Achieving Both Access and Value Pricing

We have argued throughout this book that aligning prices with value sends pharmaceutical companies signals that can best assure they allocate resources to developing products that deliver the greatest benefit to the population.

But value-based pricing does not address the problem largely driving the national debate over drug pricing—namely, assuring that people can afford the drugs they need. The affordability or "access" problem is fundamental. A 2020 survey found that over the prior year, 10% of even wealthy Americans—those with incomes of at least $500,000 per year (i.e., the top 1%)—had not filled a prescription, or had curtailed a prescribed dosage because of drug costs.[62] Among lower-income individuals—those with annual incomes under $35,000—the proportion was 30%. In many cases, the medications were essential to the patient's health.[62]

The remedy to the access problem seems straightforward: reduce drug prices. But that imperative may conflict with the desire to align prices with value. Recall examples we have reviewed: sovosbuvir (Sovaldi®), which cures hepatitis C but initially cost nearly $100,000; CAR-T therapy, which can cure otherwise fatal childhood cancer but costs $400,000 or more; remdesivir, which reduces the risk of death among severely ill COVID-19 patients but with a price tag of more than $3,000; and a new therapy for hemophilia that costs $450,000 per year. All of these drugs are highly cost-effective, improving health at a cost of less than $50,000 per QALY gained (the therapy for hemophilia A even saves money compared to the existing prophylactic treatments).[63] Most people simply cannot afford to pay the full price of these medications, however.

Insurance, which protects against small probabilities of incurring large expenses, is supposed to address this contradiction. Policyholders (or their employers or the government) pay an "affordable" monthly premium and insurance pays (much of) the cost for pricey medications. By spreading this cost across a large group of people, insurance makes it possible for value-aligned drug prices (even if high) to coexist with affordability.

Except that it often doesn't. Even among Americans with insurance, many report being denied coverage for medications or foregoing prescriptions. For individuals earning $500,000 or more annually, 18% say they encounter this problem. For individuals earning under $35,000, the proportion climbs to 51%.[62]

Part of the problem is that even if an insurance policy covers a drug, it may impose high cost-sharing requirements on patients. As Chapter 1 of this volume described, rising out-of-pocket spending for drug copayments and coinsurance creates financial difficulties for many individuals and their families, particularly among the sickest patients. Of the $344 billion spent on retail drugs in 2018, patients were responsible for paying $61 billion.[64] The problem is particularly acute for Medicare beneficiaries. In 2016, out-of-pocket drug expenses exceeded $1,000 for 1 out of every 10 people in a Medicare Part D program.[38] Median and mean annual out-of-pocket costs in 2019 for many orally administered specialty drugs exceed $10,000 per year.[65,66]

Health plans also limit access to medications in other ways. While they generally cover FDA-approved products, they frequently restrict who can receive them by imposing patient subgroup requirements (based on a patient's age or level of disease severity) or step-therapy protocols (requirements that patients try and "fail" other medications before gaining coverage for a desired treatment). For specialty drugs ("high-cost, complex medications that require special administration, monitoring, and handling"[67p1042]) that treat orphan conditions (i.e., affecting no more than 200,000 people in the United States), some level of coverage is nearly assured (99% probability).[68] But plans impose restrictions with 29% probability. For drugs treating common conditions (i.e., affecting at least 200,000 people in the United States), restrictions are even more common. While plans provide some level of coverage with 94% probability, the chance that they impose restrictions is 41%.[68]

In theory, high co-payments and other requirements may discourage use of low-value or unnecessary therapies. Cost-sharing may encourage responsible behavior (in economic terms, to protect against "moral hazard"—the idea that insured individuals will "overutilize" care because they know insurers will pay the costs). The idea is that cost-sharing provisions give patients "skin in the game"[12p55] so that they shy away expensive brand name drugs when cheaper generic copies are available and avoid other costly drugs with limited benefits.

But there is little evidence that insurance companies design copayments to move patients toward drug therapies based on the therapy's value. For example, it makes little sense to impose financial obstacles on a patient with diabetes or cancer who requires essential medications that will protect their health or extend their life. As former FDA Commissioner Scott Gottlieb has observed, "after all, what's the point of a big copay on a costly cancer drug? Is a patient really in a position to make an economically-based decision? Is the copay going to discourage over-utilization? Is someone in this situation voluntarily seeking chemo?"[69] Rather than promoting higher value care, copayments tend to be uniform for medications within a particular pharmacy tier despite substantial differences in the drugs' clinical benefits.[70] Research suggests indiscriminate cost sharing, regardless of whether a product is high or low value.[70,71]

Nor do patient subgroup requirements or step-therapy protocols seem to promote high value healthcare. If insurers had designed these restrictions for that purpose, we would expect consistency across plans. Instead, restrictions vary substantially. For example, for specialty drugs, one large plan restricts coverage (compared to the use approved by FDA) in only 7% of cases, while another restricts coverage in 57% of cases.[67] Although plans reveal little about how they incorporate value considerations into decisions, it seems likely that they deny access to both high- and low-value products.

A better approach would design policies to encourage high-value care and discourage low-value care. Value-based insurance can align patient out-of-pocket costs with each medication's value (e.g., waiving all cost-sharing for high-value drugs).[72] Similarly, health plan restrictions on coverage should align with the value of the medications.

Ensuring low out-of-pocket costs for high value medications could mean higher premiums for commercial insurance plans, or higher taxes to support public plans like Medicare and Medicaid. Approaching half a trillion dollars a year (see Box 1.1 in Chapter 1 of this volume), spending on prescription drugs is already in the neighborhood of what the United States spends on the Department of Defense. Moreover, as we noted early in this book, drug spending is rising rapidly, making it the fastest-growing healthcare expenditure category in some recent years. Expanding coverage for insured individuals (and expanding health insurance to all Americans for that matter) would make this slice of the pie grow faster. Still, at 15% or so of total healthcare spending, it seems the system could afford to pay to ensure people have access to those drugs that deliver good value.

References

1. Roland, D. 2019, November 4. "Obscure model puts a price on good health—and drives down drug costs." *The Wall Street Journal*. https://www.wsj.com/articles/obscure-model-puts-a-price-on-good-healthand-drives-down-drug-costs-11572885123.
2. Davio, K. 2017, November 2. "ICER receives $13.9 million grant, plans to assess all new drugs." *AJMC*. https://www.ajmc.com/view/icer-receives-139-million-grant-plans-to-assess-all-new-drugs.
3. Emond, S.K., and Pearson, S.D. 2020. "Alternative policies for pricing novel vaccines and drug therapies for COVID-19." *Institute for Clinical and Economic Review*. https://icer.org/wp-content/uploads/2020/11/Alternative-Policies-for-Pricing-Novel-Vaccines-and-Drug-Therapies-for-COVID-19-_-ICER-White-Paper.pdf.
4. Neumann, P.J., Cohen, J.T., Kim, D.D., and Ollendorf, D.O. 2021. "Consideration of value-based pricing for treatments and vaccines is important, even in the COVID-19 pandemic." *Health Affairs* 40(1): 53–61 https://www.healthaffairs.org/doi/10.1377/hlthaff.2020.01548
5. Cohen, J.T., Neumann, P.J., and Ollendorf, D.A. 2020, May 20. "Valuing and pricing remdesivir: Should drug makers get paid for helping us get back to work?" *Health Affairs*. https://www.healthaffairs.org/do/10.1377/hblog20200518.966027/full/.
6. Federal Acquisition Regulation. 2019. General Services Administration, Department of Defense, National Aeronautics and Space Administration. United States Government.

https://www.acquisition.gov/sites/default/files/current/far/pdf/FAR.pdf.   Accessed January 21, 2021. Section 52.245-1 (e) (3). Page 52.2-421.

7. Siripurapu, A. 2020. "What is the Defense Production Act?." *Council on Foreign Relations.* https://www.cfr.org/in-brief/what-defense-production-act.

8. Thuray, H., Samai, O., Fofana, P., and Sengeh, P. 1997. "Establishing a cost recovery system for drugs, Bo, Sierra Leone." *International Journal of Gynecology & Obstetrics* 59 (Suppl 2): S141–S147.

9. "SOPP 8203: Evaluation of cost recovery requests for investigational new drugs and investigational device exemptions." 2019. *Center for Biologics Evaluation and Research* 2. https://www.fda.gov/media/116928/download.

10. Karst, K., R. 2009. "The rarely used 'cost recovery' path to orphan drug designation and approval." *Hyman, Phelps & McNamara: FDA Law Blog.* http://www.fdalawblog.net/2009/02/the-rarely-used-cost-recovery-path-to-orphan-drug-designation-and-approval/.

11. Quinn, K. 2014. "After the revolution: DRGs at age 30." *Annals of Internal Medicine* 160 (6): 426–429. https://doi.org/10.7326/M13-2115.

12. Kolchinsky, P. 2019. *The great American drug deal.* Boston: Evelexa Press.

13. Grootendorst, P., Hollis, A., Levine, D.K., Pogge, T., and Edwards, A.M. 2011. "New approaches to rewarding pharmaceutical innovation." *Canadian Medical Association Journal* 183 (6): 681–685. https://doi.org/10.1503/cmaj.100375.

14. Ridley, D.B. 2017. "Priorities for the priority review voucher." *The American Society of Tropical Medicine and Hygiene* 96 (1): 14–15. https://doi.org/10.4269/ajtmh.16-0600.

15. Stevens, P., and Ezell, S. 2020. "Delinkage debunked: Why replacing patents with prizes for drug development won't work." *Information Technology & Innovation Foundation.* https://itif.org/publications/2020/02/03/delinkage-debunked-why-replacing-patents-prizes-drug-development-wont-work.

16. Abramowicz, M.B. 2019. "Prize and reward alternatives to intellectual property." In *Research handbook on the economics of intellectual property law.* GWU Law School Public Law Research Paper No. 2019-13; GWU Legal Studies Research Paper No. 2019-13. https://scholarship.law.gwu.edu/cgi/viewcontent.cgi?article=2672&context=faculty_publications.

17. "Prizes as an alternative to patents." *Wikipedia.* Last modified April 19, 2020. Accessed August 6, 2020. https://en.wikipedia.org/wiki/Prizes_as_an_alternative_to_patents#cite_note-globalipcenter-9.

18. Trusheim, M.R., Cassidy, W.M., and Bach, P.B. 2018. "Alternative state-level financing for Hepatitis C treatment—the 'Netflix model.'" *JAMA* 320 (19): 1977–1978. https://doi.org/10.1001/jama.2018.15782.

19. Goldman, D. 2013. "What healthcare can learn from Netflix." *USC Schaeffer: Leonard D. Schaeffer Center for Health Policy & Economics.* https://healthpolicy.usc.edu/article/what-health-care-can-learn-from-netflix/.

20. Baker, D. 2018. "Sanders-Khanna bill would stop monopoly drug pricing in the US." *Truthout.* https://truthout.org/articles/sanders-khanna-bill-would-stop-propping-up-drug-prices/.

21. Packer, M. 2018. "Does anyone read medical journals anymore?" *Medpage Today.* https://www.medpagetoday.com/blogs/revolutionandrevelation/72029.

22. Ruiz, R. 2010, February 2. "Ten misleading drug ads." *Forbes.* https://www.forbes.com/2010/02/02/drug-advertising-lipitor-lifestyle-health-pharmaceuticals-safety_slide.html#134082fd2398.

23. Sinkinson, M., and Starc, A. 2016. "The hidden benefits of TV drug ads." *KelloggInsight: Kellogg School of Management at Northwestern University.* https://insight.kellogg.northwestern.edu/article/the-hidden-benefits-of-tv-drug-ads1.

24. "The impact of direct-to-consumer advertising." US Food & Drug Administration. Last modified October 23, 2015. https://www.fda.gov/drugs/drug-information-consumers/impact-direct-consumer-advertising.
25. Galkina Cleary, E., Beierlein, J.M., Khanuja, N.S., McNamee, L.M., and Ledley, F.D. 2018. "Contribution of NIH funding to new drug approvals 2010–2016." *Proceedings of the National Academy of Sciences* 115 (10): 2329. https://doi.org/10.1073/pnas.1715368115.
26. Gruber, J., and Johnson, S. 2019. *Jump-starting America: How breakthrough science can revive economic growth and the American dream*. New York: Hachette.
27. Stone, K. 2019. "Who funds biomedical research?" *The Balance*. https://www.thebalance.com/who-funds-biomedical-research-2663193.
28. Silverman, E. 2020, May 8. "The U.S. government contributed research to a Gilead remdesivir patent—but didn't get credit." *STAT*. https://www.statnews.com/pharmalot/2020/05/08/gilead-remdesivir-covid19-coronavirus-patents/.
29. Mazzucato, M. 2013. *The entrepreneurial state: Debunking public vs. private sector myths*. London: Anthem Press.
30. Porter, E. 2015, May 27. "Government R&D, private profits and the American taxpayer." *The New York Times*. https://www.nytimes.com/2015/05/27/business/giving-taxpayers-a-cut-when-government-rd-pays-off-for-industry.html.
31. Fritzinger, S. 2012. "How government sort of created the internet." *Foundation for Economic Education*. https://fee.org/articles/how-government-sort-of-created-the-internet/.
32. Cerf, V. "A brief history of the internet & related networks." *Internet Society*. https://www.internetsociety.org/internet/history-internet/brief-history-internet-related-networks.
33. Public Law 96-517. 96th Congr. (1980).
34. Mowery, D.C., and Rosenberg, N. 1998. *Paths of innovation: Technological change in 20th-century America*. Cambridge, UK: Cambridge University Press.
35. "Adaptive design clinical trials for drugs and biologics guidance for industry." 2019. *US Food & Drug Administration: Center for Biologics Evaluation and Research. Center for Drug Evaluation and Research*. https://www.fda.gov/regulatory-information/search-fda-guidance-documents/adaptive-design-clinical-trials-drugs-and-biologics-guidance-industry.
36. Skydel, J.J., Luxkaranayagam, A.T., Dhruva, S.S., Ross, J.S., and Wallach, J.D. 2019. "Analysis of postapproval clinical trials of therapeutics approved by the US Food and Drug Administration without clinical postmarketing requirements or commitments." *JAMA Network Open* 2 (5): e193410–e193410. https://doi.org/10.1001/jamanetworkopen.2019.3410.
37. "Statement from FDA Commissioner Scott Gottlieb, M.D., on new policy to improve access and foster price competition for drugs that face inadequate generic competition." 2019. US Food & Drug Administration. https://www.fda.gov/news-events/press-announcements/statement-fda-commissioner-scott-gottlieb-md-new-policy-improve-access-and-foster-price-competition.
38. Cubanski, J., Rae, M., Young, K., and Damico, A. 2019. "How does prescription drug spending and use compare across large employer plans, Medicare Part D, and Medicaid?" *Kaiser Family Foundation*. https://www.kff.org/medicare/issue-brief/how-does-prescription-drug-spending-and-use-compare-across-large-employer-plans-medicare-part-d-and-medicaid/.
39. "2019 annual report of the boards of trustees of the federal hospital insurance and federal supplementary medical insurance trust funds." *Centers for Medicare & Medicaid Services*. https://www.cms.gov/Research-Statistics-Data-and-Systems/Statistics-Trends-and-Reports/ReportsTrustFunds/Downloads/TR2019.pdf.
40. "What are the value-based programs?" *Centers for Medicare & Medicaid Services*. Accessed September 8, 2020. https://www.cms.gov/Medicare/Quality-Initiatives-Patient-Assessment-Instruments/Value-Based-Programs/Value-Based-Programs.

41. "Innovation models." *Centers for Medicare & Medicaid Services.* Accessed September 8, 2020. https://innovation.cms.gov/innovation-models#views=models.
42. "The background and basics of Medicare Part D prescription drug plans." *Q1Group LLC.* Accessed September 8, 2020. https://q1medicare.com/PartD-History-MedicarePartD-ProgramPDP.php.
43. Fox, J. 2011. "The hidden role of cost: Medicare decisions, transparency and public trust." *University of Cincinnati Law Review* 79 (1). http://scholarship.law.uc.edu/uclr/vol79/iss1/1.
44. Neumann, P.J., and Chambers, J.D. 2012. "Medicare's enduring struggle to define "reasonable and necessary" care." *New England Journal of Medicine* 367 (19): 1775–1777. https://doi.org/10.1056/NEJMp1208386.
45. Frank, R.G., and Nichols, L.M. 2019. "Medicare drug-price negotiation—why now . . . and how." *New England Journal of Medicine* 381 (15): 1404–1406. https://doi.org/10.1056/NEJMp1909798.
46. Frank, R.G., and Zeckhauser, R.J. 2017. "A framework for negotiation in Part D of Medicare." Hutchins Center Working Paper No. 28. https://pdfs.semanticscholar.org/db48/4e8f900b2083c4108ae74ea261392716813b.pdf.
47. Chambers, J.D., Chenoweth, M.D., Pyo, J., Cangelosi, M.J., and Neumann, P.J. 2015. "Changing face of Medicare's national coverage determinations for technology." *International Journal of Technology Assessment in Health Care* 31 (5): 347–354. https://doi.org/10.1017/S0266462315000525.
48. Sullivan, T. 2018. "CMS announces the end of part B demonstration." *Policy & Medicine.* Accessed September 9, 2020. https://www.policymed.com/2017/10/cms-announces-the-end-of-part-b-demonstration.html.
49. Appleby, J. 2016. "Medicare to experiment with tying drug costs to effectiveness." *KCUR 89.3.* https://www.kcur.org/2016-03-17/medicare-to-experiment-with-tying-drug-costs-to-effectiveness.
50. "Medicaid drug rebate program." *US Department of Health and Human Services.* Last modified November 13, 2018. Accessed July 24, 2020. https://www.medicaid.gov/medicaid/prescription-drugs/medicaid-drug-rebate-program/index.html.
51. Thomas, K. 2018, June 24. "A drug costs $272,000 a year: Not so fast, says New York State." *The New York Times.* https://www.nytimes.com/2018/06/24/health/drug-prices-orkambi-new-york.html.
52. Sachs, R. 2019, January 3. "Prescription drug policy: The year in review, and the year ahead." *Health Affairs.* https://www.healthaffairs.org/do/10.1377/hblog20190103.183538/full/
53. McCluskey, P.D. 2019, August 27. "Reining in the spending on drugs: What Mass. can learn from other states." *The Boston Globe.* https://www.bostonglobe.com/business/2019/08/27/reining-spending-drugs-what-mass-can-learn-from-other-states/cEfQNNKOW66xbqKwA861BM/story.html.
54. Cohen, J. 2018, September 4. "Medicaid to introduce value-based drug pricing." *Forbes.* https://www.forbes.com/sites/joshuacohen/2018/09/04/medicaid-to-introduce-value-based-drug-pricing/#12137af13234.
55. Drug pricing review. 2020. Massachusetts Health Policy Commission. https://www.mass.gov/service-details/drug-pricing-review.
56. Berchick, E.R., Barnett, J.C., and Upton, R.D. 2019. "Health insurance coverage in the United States: 2018." *US Census Bureau.* https://www.census.gov/library/publications/2019/demo/p60-267.html.
57. Sullivan, S.D., Yeung, K., Vogeler, C., Ramsey, S.D., Wong, E., Murphy, C.O., Danielson, D., Veenstra, D.L., Garrison, L.P., Burke, W., and Watkins, J.B. 2015. "Design, implementation,

and first-year outcomes of a value-based drug formulary." *Journal of Managed Care & Specialty Pharmacy* 21 (4): 269–275. https://doi.org/10.18553/jmcp.2015.21.4.269.

58. Yeung, K., Basu, A., Hansen, R.N., Watkins, J.B., and Sullivan, S.D. 2017. "Impact of a value-based formulary on medication utilization, health services utilization, and expenditures." *Medical Care* 55 (2): 191–198. https://doi.org/10.1097/MLR.0000000000000630.

59. Paavola, A. 2019. "Top PBMs by market share." *Becker Hospital Review*. https://www.beckershospitalreview.com/pharmacy/top-pbms-by-market-share.html.

60. Gopalan, A. 2018. "CVS announcement of cost-effective benchmarks puts ICER in the spotlight." *STAT*. https://www.statnews.com/2018/08/22/cvs-cost-effectiveness-benchmarks-puts-icer/.

61. Humer, C. 2019. "CVS drug coverage plan based on outside pricing review is off to a slow start." *Reuters*. https://www.reuters.com/article/us-cvs-health-drugpricing-focus-idUSKBN1WI2IO.

62. "Life experiences and income inequality in the United States." 2020. *Robert Wood Johnson Foundation*. https://www.rwjf.org/en/library/research/2019/12/life-experiences-and-income-inequality-in-the-united-states.html.

63. "Emicizumab for hemophilia A with inhibitors: Effectiveness and value final evidence report." 2018, April 16. *Institute for Clinical and Economic Review*. https://icer.org/wp-content/uploads/2020/10/ICER_Hemophilia_Final_Evidence_Report_041618.pdf.

64. Aitken, M., and Kleinrock, M. 2019. "Medicine use and spending in the U.S.: A review of 2018 and outlook to 2023." *IQVIA Institute for Human Data Science*. https://www.iqvia.com/-/media/iqvia/pdfs/institute-reports/medicine-use-and-spending-in-the-us---a-review-of-2018-outlook-to-2023.pdf?&_=1599158924142.

65. Cubanski, J., Koma, W., and Neuman, T. 2019. "The out-of-pocket cost burden for specialty drugs in Medicare Part D in 2019." *Kaiser Family Foundation*. https://www.kff.org/medicare/issue-brief/the-out-of-pocket-cost-burden-for-specialty-drugs-in-medicare-part-d-in-2019/.

66. Dusetzina, S.B., Huskamp, H.A., and Keating, N.L. 2019. "Specialty drug pricing and out-of-pocket spending on orally administered anticancer drugs in Medicare Part D, 2010 to 2019." *JAMA* 321 (20): 2025–2028. https://doi.org/10.1001/jama.2019.4492.

67. Chambers, J.D., Kim, D.D., Pope, E.F., Graff, J.S., Wilkinson, C.L., and Neumann, P.J. 2018. "Specialty drug coverage varies across commercial health plans in the US." *Health Affairs (Millwood)* 37 (7): 1041–1047. https://doi.org/10.1377/hlthaff.2017.1553.

68. Chambers, J.D., Panzer, A.D., Kim, D.D., Margaretos, N.M., and Neumann, P.J. 2019. "Variation in US private health plans' coverage of orphan drugs." *American Journal of Managed Care* 25 (10): 508–512. https://pubmed.ncbi.nlm.nih.gov/31622066/.

69. Gottlieb, S. 2018. "Capturing the benefits of competition for patients." *US Food & Drug Administration*. https://www.fda.gov/news-events/speeches/fda-officials/capturing-benefits-competition-patients-03072018.

70. Chernew, M.E., Rosen, A.B., and Fendrick, A.M. 2007. "Value-based insurance design." *Health Affairs* 26 (Suppl 2): w195–w203. https://doi.org/10.1377/hlthaff.26.2.w195.

71. Neumann, P.J., Lin, P.-J., Greenberg, D., Berger, M.L., Teutsch, S.M., Mansley, E., Weinstein, M.C., and Rosen, A.B. 2006. "Do drug formulary policies reflect evidence of value." *American Journal of Managed Care*. https://www.ajmc.com/view/jan06-2245p30-36.

72. "What is value-based insurance design?" n.d. *University of Michigan Center for Value-Based Insurance*. https://vbidcenter.org/about-v-bid/.

11
The Path Forward

The urgency to address prescription drug pricing stems from the fact that the United States spends so much on drugs and because drugs play such a large role in improving and sustaining people's health. As Chapter 2 of this volume explained, the importance to act also reflects the unusual characteristics of pharmaceutical markets that interfere with mechanisms that typically keep prices in check. Consumers have little agency because they must rely on clinicians to tell them which drugs to use and even for permission to use those drugs. Health insurance shields consumers from the costs and insurers often restrict access to products. When drug companies introduce new products, patent and exclusivity protections provided by the government remove price competition.

As Chapter 3 of this volume described, the urgency has led to various proposals to restrain drug prices. Among many observers, the presumption is that most drug company revenue is superfluous, fueling excessive profits, inflated executive compensation, and wasteful spending on marketing and advertising. The implication is that drug companies' revenues could be lower without affecting vital innovation. But attempting to discern how much revenue the drug industry "needs" for important innovation is an endless conundrum. It is most realistic to view revenue as a potent if imperfect signal to stimulate worthy technological advances. Prices and innovation are inextricably linked: higher prices and profits attract more investment, which in turn gives rise to more rapid innovation and more therapies.

The critical question is not how we can keep drug prices down. Constraining drug prices is easy, as the government could readily impose price controls and other measures, as described in Chapter 3 of this volume. The important question is, What is a *reasonable* price for each drug? We have argued that prices should correspond to value because this incentivizes companies to spend more on highly beneficial drugs and less on drugs that deliver fewer benefits. It also means that society should pay no more for drugs than they are

The Right Price. Peter J. Neumann, Joshua T. Cohen, and Daniel A. Ollendorf, Oxford University Press (2021).
© Peter J. Neumann, Joshua T. Cohen, and Daniel A. Ollendorf. DOI: 10.1093/oso/9780197512883.003.0011

worth. For this approach to work, value must be measured appropriately, and payers must pursue value-based pricing. Our recommendations follow.

Measuring Value

Measuring value credibly means accounting for the impacts people care about. Although people debate the appropriate components, length of life and quality of life (including ability to function and freedom from pain) represent fundamental outcomes upon which virtually everyone agrees. That makes the quality-adjusted life-year (QALY) a good starting point as a measure of health benefits. Augmenting QALYs to account for other outcomes would help, but as the core set of benefits it represents expands, dollar-per-QALY benchmarks must be appropriately adjusted downward (made more stringent) to align the same (hypothetical) healthcare budget with a now greater supply of QALYs. Criticism regarding the fairness of the QALY will persist, but researchers have struggled to develop an alternative that shares its advantages, including its broad applicability to a wide range of diseases and therapies and its relatively intuitive incorporation of both longevity and quality of life. While other representations of value are worthy of consideration, the cost-per-QALY measure serves as a useful standard and measure of efficiency and can play a key role in informing drug pricing decisions alongside other considerations.

Cost represents the other side of the value equation. Methods for proper cost measurement span domains transcending drugs and even healthcare. And yet a fundamental aspect of drug cost has received relatively little attention in value measurement—namely, a recognition that prices for prescription drugs tend to decline when they lose market exclusivity (and yes, prices can and do sometimes increase both before and after exclusivity ends). A distinguishing feature is that a drug's lifetime costs tend to be "front-loaded," rather than spread more evenly over time, as with many other products and services. When considering drug costs, what matters is the total payments made over a drug's life cycle (properly discounted)—and how that amount compares to the drug's total benefits. Failing to recognize the front-loading that results from government-protected market exclusivity can erroneously inflate drug cost estimates, distorting resource allocation decisions. On the other hand, if value assessments must properly project drug costs and account for future market exclusivity loss, analyses need better information about the likely trajectory of drug prices over a therapy's life cycle and how these patterns depend on factors such as the nature of the drug (whether small molecule vs. biologic) and market size. Opportunities for drug companies to delay exclusivity protection must be controlled as well. Otherwise, value assessments must assume that elevated, monopolistic pricing power will persist for longer than government regulations suggest, thus reducing value-aligned prices for drugs at launch.

Because value assessment should reflect all impacts that matter to people, evaluations should consider a societal perspective—that is, consequences extending beyond the healthcare system and benefits to the primary patient population and health condition. For some drugs, expanding the perspective beyond the healthcare sector may have relatively little effect on value assessment. In many cases, however, such as treatments for Alzheimer's disease, the difference can be substantial. (The COVID-19 pandemic serves as a reminder that societal costs associated with a disease can dwarf costs to the healthcare system.) Importantly, measuring a drug's value from a societal perspective does not mean that all of the societal consequences (e.g., cost offsets) should be reflected in a therapy's price. Indeed, this may be impractical in many cases, because the resultant value-based price will be extravagantly large. But societal value should be calculated and reported. The analysis can serve as an important input into pricing discussions, helping policymakers to consider each drug's full costs and benefits and the wider implications of their actions. Decisions about how much of that value is reflected in the price should consider the signals that are sent to the drug industry in terms of how innovation to prevent or address future health crises will be valued.

There is also the important question of whether drug prices should reflect contributions the government makes to their development.[1] For example, the National Institutes of Health supports broadly applicable basic research.[2] But virtually all other industries also benefit from basic government research and "infrastructure" investments (e.g., Google benefits from the government's development of the early Internet).[3] Government invests in "risky" basic research because it is a public good, and the private sector left to its own devices would underinvest from a society's perspective, because companies cannot easily capture the full benefits of their investments (i.e., other companies "free ride"). Businesses "pay" for these contributions through taxes, rather than by lowering their prices. It would be difficult in any case to trace the links between the government's basic research investment and ultimately marketed products and then to adjust prices.

The matter is different when the government invests in later stage clinical research. In that case, the argument for adjusting product prices is stronger: returning all of a compound's revenue to a private company even when it pays only a portion of the development costs will lead to inappropriately high returns and subsequently to overinvestment in future products; that is, the pricing signals would be too strong. For example, the US government contributed $483 million to the development of Moderna's COVID-19 vaccine.[4] Perhaps Moderna's revenue should be split with the government according to the percentage of development costs the government funded; in other words, if that $483 million represented 30% of total development costs, 30% of the revenue should go to the government.

Value assessment must also recognize uncertainty. In some cases, assessments can help determine that a drug represents good value or poor value—even if it is not possible to determine exactly how good or poor. In other cases, uncertainty analysis will identify the factors for which more information will best reduce the ambiguity. In many cases, only more evidence will adequately address uncertainty. In those cases, outcomes-based risk sharing agreements should be considered.

Finally, there is the question of *who* should measure value. In many countries, the government assumes this task, providing this "public good" that its own, typically publicly funded health insurance programs depend on. That approach has worked well in many nations. In the United States, however, public generation of value assessments has proven unpopular. As a result, the United States has, to its detriment, gone without public value assessment for decision-making purposes for decades. The emergence and influence of the Institute for Clinical and Economic Review (ICER) point to the feasibility and sustainability of a private sector solution. Still, as a private organization lacking public accountability, the question of the legitimacy of ICER's role remains.

Some have proposed enhancements to ICER's process to increase the role that other stakeholders might play. We make two recommendations. First, ICER's analyses should be as transparent as possible so others can readily explore the extent to which alternative assumptions influence its findings. That means that the source code for the computer simulation models that underlie its projections must be made public. Second, ICER should provide value price estimates corresponding to a wide range of cost-per-QALY benchmarks. Rather than favoring a single value benchmark, it should defer to the payers, who represent enrollees, subscribers, and taxpayers, to determine what health resource trade-offs are appropriate.

Toward Value-Based Pricing

Although other actors could align drug prices and value in the United States, it makes sense for the parties paying the bills for those drugs—primarily

Medicare, Medicaid, and commercial payers—to assume the lead. They are best positioned to understand the priorities of the people they serve and the entities who provide their funding. They also have the closest proximity to the healthcare system's purse strings, thus positioning them to exert leverage. Indeed, payers have the means to establish value-based pricing—but doing so can involve trade-offs.

The Massachusetts Medicaid program's experience with value-based pricing highlights the dilemma. Federal law has forced Massachusetts to choose between value-based pricing and a (near) uniform discount on all drugs (approximately 23% on the drug's average manufacturer's price or the "best price" offered by the manufacturer to any other insurer). A seemingly straightforward solution would allow Massachusetts to pay either the value-based price or the standard discount and to select which pricing scheme it will use for each drug separately. Presumably, however, the drug industry would not have agreed to a standard 23% discount had it not been accompanied by guaranteed coverage of all of its products approved by the US Food and Drug Administration.

More fundamentally, providing state Medicaid programs the option to select either the value-based price or the standard discount misses the point. In practice, state programs would opt for the lesser of the two prices. Whenever the standard discount is the lesser of the two prices, its selection would mean a deviation away from value-based pricing; it would mean that the state is paying less than it should and sending a signal that inappropriately discourages development of similar, future therapies.

The trade-offs discouraging commercial plans from embracing value-based pricing are less obvious. Perhaps private payers are reluctant to commit to a value-based price because it means foregoing latitude to negotiate either lower prices (that save money) or higher prices (in exchange for other concessions—perhaps related to other therapies). Private health plans also wish to avoid being tagged as the party that exits the negotiating table when it comes to covering important therapies.

For too long, health insurers and drug companies have viewed value-based pricing as simply a means to reduce drug prices. This is why some have celebrated and others reviled bodies like the National Institute for Health and Care Excellence in the United Kingdom and ICER in the United States. But the purpose of value-based pricing is not to reduce drug prices as much as possible. Instead, the main goal should be getting to the "right" price. Paying too high a price diverts resources from better uses elsewhere. Paying too little fails to send industry suitable signals to incentivize the development of new drugs.

That view of value assessment still does not address the goal of promoting widespread access to crucial medications. Here, health insurers must play a crucial role by committing to make drugs that confer benefits at a reasonable value available to those who need them. This may mean society pays higher premiums, and if this raises questions of affordability, it suggests a need to examine the value conferred by other healthcare spending as well as the value conferred by spending on nonhealth priorities.

We are living in a time of remarkable scientific breakthroughs, but these advances come at a cost. As drug prices have steadily risen, payers, clinicians and patients have lacked reliable information to allow comparisons of the benefits with the costs. In the end, paying value-based prices, even as we strive to encourage innovation, makes sense because it helps ensure that drug companies produce more of what people want—products that improve people's health—while considering society's other pressing priorities.

References

1. Neumann, P.J., Cohen, J., Ollendorf, D.A., and Kim, D. 2021. "Consideration of value-based pricing for treatments and vaccines is important, even in the COVID-19 pandemic." *Health Affairs*. https://www.healthaffairs.org/doi/10.1377/hlthaff.2020.01548
2. Galkina Cleary, E., Beierlein, J.M., Khanuja, N.S., McNamee, L.M., and Ledley, F.D. 2018. "Contribution of NIH funding to new drug approvals 2010-2016." *Proceedings of the National Academy of Sciences of the United States of America*.115 (10): 2329–2334. https://doi.org/10.1073/pnas.1715368115.
3. Porter, E. 2015, May 27. "Government R&D, Private Profits and the American Taxpayer." *The New York Times.* https://www.nytimes.com/2015/05/27/business/giving-taxpayers-a-cut-when-government-rd-pays-off-for-industry.html.
4. Balfour, H. 2020, April 21. "BARDA to give Moderna up to $483 million for COVID-19 vaccine development." *European Pharmaceutical Review*. https://www.europeanpharmaceuticalreview.com/news/117327/barda-to-give-moderna-up-to-483-million-for-covid-19-vaccine-development.

That view of value assessment still does not address the goal of promoting widespread access to crucial medications. Here, health insurers must play a crucial role by committing to make drugs that confer benefits at a reasonable value available to those who need them. This may mean society pays higher premiums, and if this raises questions of affordability, it suggests a need to examine the value conferred by other healthcare spending as well as the value conferred by spending on nonhealth priorities.

We are living in a time of remarkable scientific breakthroughs, but these advances come at a cost. As drug prices have steadily risen, payers, clinicians and patients have lacked reliable information to allow comparisons of the benefits with the costs. In the end, paying value-based prices, even as we strive to encourage innovation, makes sense because it helps ensure that drug companies produce more of what people want—products that improve people's health—while considering society's other pressing priorities.

References

1. Neumann, P.J., Cohen, J.T., Ollendorf, D.A., and Kim, D.D. 2020. [illegible] pricing for treatments and vaccines is important, even in the COVID-19 [illegible]. Health Affairs. https://www.healthaffairs.org/do/10.1377/hblog20200518 [illegible]
2. Galkina Cleary, E., Beierlein, J.M., Khanuja, N.S., McNamee, L.M., and Ledley, F.D. 2018. "Contribution of NIH funding to new drug approvals 2010–2016." Proceedings of the National Academy of Sciences of the United States of America 115 (10): 2329–2334. https://doi.org/10.1073/pnas.1715368115.
3. [illegible] E. 2020, May 27. "Government [illegible], Private Profit and the American Taxpayer." The New York Times. https://www.nytimes.com/2020/05/27/business/giving-taxpayers-a- [illegible]
4. [illegible] H. 2020, April [illegible]. "[illegible] COVID-19 vaccine development." European Pharmaceutical Review. [illegible] -covid-19-vaccine-development.

Index

For the benefit of digital users, indexed terms that span two pages (e.g., 52–53) may, on occasion, appear on only one of those pages.

Tables, figures and boxes are indicated by *t*, *f* and *b* following the page number

Printed in the USA/Agawam, MA
May 6, 2021

774219.005